ADVANCED PAEDIATRIC LIFE SUPPORT

Third edition

ADVANCED PAEDIATRIC LIFE SUPPORT

The Practical Approach

Third edition

Advanced Life Support Group

Edited by
Kevin Mackway-Jones
Elizabeth Molyneux
Barbara Phillips
Susan Wieteska

BMJ Books is an imprint of the BMJ Publishing Group,
BMA House, Tavistock Square, London WC1H 9JR
www.bmjbooks.com

First published in 1993 by the BMJ Publishing Group
Reprinted 1994
Reprinted 1995
Reprinted 1996

Second edition 1997
Reprinted 1998
Reprinted with revisions 1998
Reprinted 1999
Reprinted 2000

Third edition 2001

British Library Cataloguing in Publication Data

A catalogue record for this book is available from the British Library

ISBN 0-7279-1554-1

Typeset in Great Britain by FiSH Books, London
Printed and bound by Selwood Printing Ltd, Burgess Hill, West Sussex

CONTENTS

WORKING GROUP

A. Argent	Paediatric ICU, Cape Town
A. Charters	Emergency Nursing, Sheffield
M. Felix	Paediatrics, Coimbra
J. Fothergill	Emergency Medicine, London
G. Hughes	Emergency Medicine, Wellington
F. Jewkes	Paediatric Nephrology, Cardiff
J. Leigh	Anaesthesia, Bristol
K. Mackway-Jones	Emergency Medicine, Manchester
E. Molyneux	Paediatric Emergency Medicine, Malawi
P. Oakley	Anaesthesia/Trauma, Stoke on Trent
B. Phillips	Paediatric Emergency Medicine, Liverpool and Manchester
C. Tozer	Emergency Nursing, Abergavenny
N. Turner	Anaesthesia, Amsterdam
J. Walker	Paediatric Surgery, Sheffield
S. Wieteska	Course Co-ordinator, Manchester
K. Williams	Paediatric Emergency Nursing, Liverpool
S. Young	Paediatric Emergency Medicine, Melbourne
D. Zideman	Paediatric Anaesthesia, London

CONTRIBUTORS

R. Appleton	Paediatric Neurology, Liverpool
P. Baines	Paediatric Intensive Care, Liverpool
I. Barker	Paediatric Anaesthesia, Sheffield
D. Bickerstaff	Paediatric Orthopaedics, Sheffield
R. Bingham	Paediatric Anaesthesia, London
P. Brennan	Paediatric Emergency Medicine, Sheffield
J. Britto	Paediatric Intensive Care, London
C. Cahill	Emergency Medicine, Portsmouth
H. Carty	Paediatric Radiology, Liverpool
M. Clarke	Paediatric Neurology, Manchester
J. Couriel	Paediatric Respiratory Medicine, Liverpool
P. Driscoll	Emergency Medicine, Manchester
J. Fothergill	Emergency Medicine, London
P. Habibi	Paediatric Intensive Care, London
D. Heaf	Paediatric Respiratory Medicine, Liverpool
F. Jewkes	Paediatric Nephrology, Cardiff
E. Ladusans	Paediatric Cardiology, Manchester
J. Leggatte	Paediatric Neurosurgery, Manchester
J. Leigh	Anaesthesia, Bristol

CONTRIBUTORS

S. Levene   Child Accident Prevention Trust, London

M. Lewis   Paediatric Nephrology, Manchester

K. Mackway-Jones   Emergency Medicine, Manchester

J. Madar   Neonatology, Plymouth

T. Martland   Paediatric Neurologist, Manchester

E. Molyneux   Paediatric Emergency Medicine, Malawi

D. Nicholson   Radiology, Manchester

A. Nunn   Pharmacy, Liverpool

P. Oakley   Anaesthesia, Stoke on Trent

B. Phillips   Paediatric Emergency Medicine, Manchester and Liverpool

J. Robson   Paediatric Emergency Medicine, Liverpool

D. Sims   Neonatology, Manchester

A. Sprigg   Paediatric Radiology, Sheffield

J. Stuart   Emergency Medicine, Manchester

J. Tibballs   Paediatric Intensive Care, Melbourne

J. Walker   Paediatric Surgery, Sheffield

W. Whitehouse   Paediatric Neurologist, Birmingham

S. Wieteska   Course Co-ordinator, Manchester

M. Williams   Emergency Medicine, York

B. Wilson   Paediatric Radiology, Manchester

J. Wyllie   Neonatology, Middlesbrough

S. Young   Paediatric Emergency Medicine, Melbourne

D. Zideman   Anaesthesia, London

PREFACE TO THIRD EDITION

Since this book was first published in 1993, the Advanced Paediatric Life Support (APLS) concept and courses have gone a great way towards their aim of bringing simple guidelines for the management of ill and injured children to front-line doctors and nurses.

Over the years an increasing number of experts have contributed to the work and we extend our thanks both to them and also to our instructors who unceasingly provide helpful feedback. The Advanced Paediatric Life Support Course is now well established in several countries outside the United Kingdom. These include Australia, New Zealand, the Netherlands, Portugal and South Africa. APLS is also the recommended paediatric course for the European Resuscitation Council. Furthermore, material from APLS is being successfully used in countries with under-resourced health care systems such as Bosnia-Herzegovina, Malawi and Uganda.

A small "family" of courses have developed from APLS in response to different training needs. One is the Paediatric Life Support (PLS) course, a one-day locally delivered course designed for doctors and nurses who have only subsidiary responsibility for seriously ill or injured children (see note, page xvi). Another is Pre-Hospital Paediatric Life Support (PHPLS), which has its own textbook and is for the pre-hospital provider.

Readers will find significant changes in the third edition. The chapters on resuscitation and the management of arrhythmias have been informed by the new International Guidelines, produced by an evidence-based process from the collaboration of many international experts under the umbrella of the International Liaison Committee on Resuscitation (ILCOR). The chapters on serious illness have been rewritten both to include new knowledge and practice and also to reflect the problem-based approach used in teaching. In addition there are some new chapters.

In the past the editors have been criticised for the decision not to include in the text the many references which support its assertions. We have not changed this now – but have harnessed the power of the World Wide Web to allow us (and you the reader, the candidate and the instructor) to keep the evidence available and up to date. Log on to *www.bestbets.org* to see how far we have got and how you can help.

KMJ
EM
BP
SW

Manchester 2001

PREFACE TO THE FIRST EDITION

Advanced Paediatric Life Support: The Practical Approach was written to improve the emergency care of children, and has been developed by a number of paediatricians, paediatric surgeons, emergency physicians, and anaesthetists from several UK centres. It is the core text for the APLS (UK) course, and will also be of value to medical and allied personnel unable to attend the course. It is designed to include all the common emergencies, and also covers a number of less common diagnoses that are amenable to good initial treatment. The remit is the first hour of care, because it is during this time that the subsequent course of the child is set.

The book is divided into six parts. Part I introduces the subject by discussing the causes of childhood emergencies, the reasons why children need to be treated differently, and the ways in which a seriously ill child can be recognised quickly. Part II deals with the techniques of life support. Both basic and advanced techniques are covered, and there is a separate section on resuscitation of the newborn. Part III deals with children who present with serious illness. Shock is dealt with in detail, because recognition and treatment can be particularly difficult. Cardiac and respiratory emergencies, and coma and convulsions, are also discussed. Part IV concentrates on the child who has been seriously injured. Injury is the most common cause of death in the 1–14 year age group and the importance of this topic cannot be overemphasised. Part V gives practical guidance on performing the procedures mentioned elsewhere in the text. Finally, Part VI (the Appendices) deals with other areas of importance.

Emergencies in children generate a great deal of anxiety – in the child, the parents, and in the medical and nursing staff who have to deal with them. We hope that this book will shed some light on the subject of paediatric emergency care, and that it will raise the standard of paediatric life support. An understanding of the contents will allow doctors, nurses, and paramedics dealing with seriously ill and injured children to approach their care with confidence.

Kevin Mackway-Jones
Elizabeth Molyneux
Barbara Phillips
Susan Wieteska
(*Editorial Board*)

1993

ACKNOWLEDGEMENTS

A great many people have put a lot of hard work into the production of this book, and the accompanying advanced life support course. The editors would like to thank all the contributors for their efforts and all the APLS instructors who took the time to send their comments on the first and second editions to us.

We are greatly indebted to Helen Carruthers MMAA and Mary Harrison MMAA for producing the excellent line drawings that illustrate the text. Thanks to the British Paediatric Neurology Group for the status epilecticus protocol and the Child's Glasgow Coma Scale.

Finally, we would like to thank, in advance, those of you who will attend the Advanced Paediatric Life Support course and other courses using this text; no doubt, you will have much constructive criticism to offer.

CONTACT DETAILS AND WEBSITE INFORMATION

ALSG: www.aslg.org
Best bets: www.bestbets.org

For details on ALSG courses visit the website or contact:

Advanced Life Support Group
Second Floor, The Dock Office
Trafford Road
Salford Quays
Manchester, M5 2XB
UK

Tel: +44 (0)161 877 1999
Fax: +44 (0)161 877 1666
Email:@alsg.org

Clinicians practising in tropical and under-resourced health care systems are advised to read *A Manual for International Child Health Care* (0 7279 1476 6) published by BMJ Books which gives details of additional relevant illnesses not included in this text.

NOTE

Sections with the grey marginal tint are relevant for the Paediatric Life Support (PLS) Course.

INTRODUCTION

CHAPTER

1

Introduction

CAUSES OF DEATH IN CHILDHOOD

As can be seen from Table 1.1, the greatest mortality during childhood occurs in the first year of life with the highest death rate of all happening in the first month.

Table 1.1. Number of deaths by age group

Age group	Number of deaths (rate)		
	1991 (E&W)	1998 (E&W)	1998 (Australia)
0–28 days	3052 (4·4)	24189 (3·8)	842 (5·02)
4–52 weeks	2106 (3·0)	1207 (1·9)	410
1–4 years	993 (36)	722 (28)	347
5–14 years	1165 (19)	897 (13)	376
1–14 years	2158 (24)	1619 (17)	723 (19·7)

The rate for under ones is per 1 000 population and for over ones per 100 000 population
England and Wales, 1991 and 1998 Office of National Statistics (ONS) Australia 1998

The causes of death vary with age as shown in Table 1.2. In the newborn period the most common causes are congenital abnormalities and factors associated with prematurity, such as respiratory immaturity, cerebral haemorrhage, and infection due to immaturity of the immune response.

From 1 month to 1 year of age the condition known as "cot death" is the most common cause of death. Some victims of this condition have previously unrecognised respiratory or metabolic disease, but some have no specific cause of death found at detailed postmortem examination. This latter group is described as suffering from the sudden infant death syndrome. There has been a striking reduction in the incidence of the sudden infant death syndrome over the last few years in the UK, Holland, Australia and New Zealand. In England and Wales the decrease has been from 1597 in 1988 to 454 in 1994 and to 239 in 1998. The reduction has followed national campaigns to inform parents of known risk factors such as the prone sleeping position in the infant and parental smoking. The next most common causes in this age group are congenital abnormalities and infections (Table 1.2).

3

Table 1.2 Common causes of death by age group

Cause	Number of deaths* at		
	4–52 weeks	1–4 years	5–14 years
Cot death	239 (20)	0 (0)	0 (0)
Congenital abnormality	285 (24)	102 (14)	66 (7)
Infection	228 (19)	69 (10)	35 (4)
Trauma	53 (4)	143 (20)	219 (25)
Neoplasms	22 (2)	94 (13)	232 (25)

England and Wales, 1998, ONS.
*Numbers in parentheses are the percentage.

After 1 year of age trauma is the most frequent cause of death, and remains so until well into adult life. Deaths from trauma have been described as falling into three groups. In the first group there is overwhelming damage at the time of trauma, and the injury caused is incompatible with life; children with such massive injuries will die within minutes whatever is done. Those in the second group die because of progressive respiratory failure, circulatory insufficiency, or raised intracranial pressure secondary to the effects of injury; death occurs within a few hours if no treatment is administered, but may be avoided if treatment is prompt and effective. The final group consists of late deaths due to raised intracranial pressure, infection or multiple organ failure. Appropriate management in the first few hours will decrease mortality in this group also. The trimodal distribution of trauma deaths is illustrated in Figure 1.1.

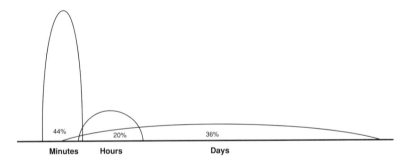

Figure 1.1. Trimodal distribution of deaths from trauma

Only a minority of childhood deaths, such as those due to unresponsive end-stage neoplastic disease, are expected and "managed". Most children with potentially fatal diseases such as complex congenital heart disease, inborn errors of metabolism, or cystic fibrosis are treated or "cured" by operation, diet, transplant or, soon, even gene therapy. The approach to these children is to treat vigorously incidental illnesses (such as respiratory infections) to which many are especially prone. Therefore, some children presenting to hospital with serious life-threatening acute illness also have an underlying chronic disease.

PATHWAYS LEADING TO CARDIORESPIRATORY ARREST

Cardiac arrest in infancy and childhood is rarely due to primary cardiac disease. This is different from the adult situation where the primary arrest is often cardiac, and cardiorespiratory function may remain near normal until the moment of arrest. In childhood most cardiac arrests are secondary to hypoxia, underlying causes including birth asphyxia, inhalation of foreign body, bronchiolitis, asthma, and pneumothorax. Respiratory arrest also occurs secondary to neurological dysfunction such as that caused by some poisons or during convulsions. Raised intracranial pressure (ICP) due to head injury or acute encephalopathy eventually leads to respiratory arrest, but severe neuronal damage has already been sustained before the arrest occurs.

Whatever the cause, by the time of cardiac arrest the child has had a period of respiratory insufficiency which will have caused hypoxia and respiratory acidosis. The combination of hypoxia and acidosis causes cell damage and death (particularly in more sensitive organs such as the brain, liver, and kidney), before myocardial damage is severe enough to cause cardiac arrest.

Most other cardiac arrests are secondary to circulatory failure (shock). This will have resulted often from fluid or blood loss, or from fluid maldistribution within the circulatory system. The former may be due to gastroenteritis, burns, or trauma whilst the latter is often caused by sepsis or anaphylaxis. As all organs are deprived of essential nutrients and oxygen as shock progresses to cardiac arrest, circulatory failure, like respiratory failure, causes tissue hypoxia and acidosis. In fact, both pathways may occur in the same condition. The pathways leading to cardiac arrest in children are summarised in Figure 1.2.

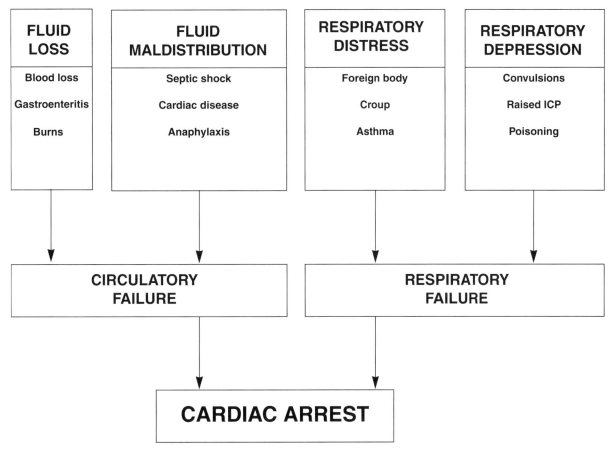

Figure 1.2. Pathways leading to cardiac arrest in childhood (with examples of underlying causes)

The worst outcome is in children who have had an out-of-hospital arrest and who arrive apnoeic and pulseless. These children have a poor chance of intact neurological survival. There has often been a prolonged period of hypoxia and ischaemia before the start of adequate cardiopulmonary resuscitation. Earlier recognition of seriously ill children and paediatric cardiopulmonary resuscitation training for the public could improve the outcome for these children.

CHAPTER
2

Why treat children differently?

INTRODUCTION

Children are not little adults. The spectrum of diseases that they suffer from is different, and their responses to disease and injury may differ both physically and psychologically. This chapter deals with some specific points that have particular relevance to emergency care.

SIZE

The most obvious reason for treating children differently is their size, and its variation with age.

Weight

The most rapid changes in size occur in the first year of life. An average birth weight of 3·5 kg has increased to 10·3 kg by the age of 1 year. After that time weight increases more slowly until the pubertal growth spurt. This is illustrated in the weight chart for boys shown in Figure 2.1.

As most therapies are given as the dose per kilogram, it is important to get some idea of a child's weight as soon as possible. In the emergency situation this is especially difficult because it is often impracticable to weigh the child. To overcome this problem a number of methods can be used to derive a weight estimate. If the age is known the formula:

$$\text{Weight (kg)} = 2 \, (\text{Age} + 4)$$

can be used if the child is aged between 1 and 10 years old. In addition various charts (such as the Oakley chart) are available which allow an approximation of weight to be derived from the age. Finally, the Broselow tape (which relates weight to height) can be used. Whatever the method, it is essential that the carer is sufficiently familiar with it to be able to use it quickly and accurately.

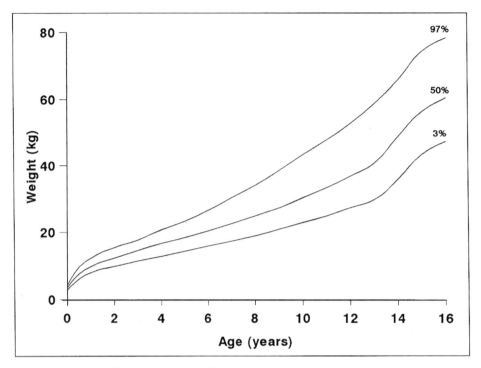

Figure 2.1 Centile chart for weight in boys

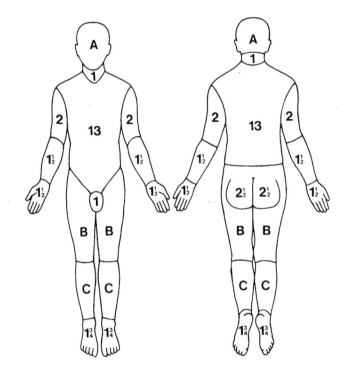

Areas indicated	Surface area at				
	0	1 year	5 years	10 years	15 years
A	9·5	8·5	6·5	5·5	4·5
B	2·75	3·25	4·0	4·5	4·5
C	2·5	2·5	2·75	3·0	3·25

Figure 2.2 Body surface area (per cent). (Reproduced courtesy of Smith & Nephew Pharmaceuticals Ltd)

Body proportions

The body proportions change with age. This is most graphically illustrated by considering the body surface area (BSA). At birth the head accounts for 19% of BSA; this falls to 9% by the age of 15 years. Figure 2.2 shows these changes.

The BSA to weight ratio decreases with age. Small children, with a high ratio, lose heat more rapidly and consequently are relatively more prone to hypothermia.

Certain specific changes in body proportions also have a bearing on emergency care. For example, the relatively large head and short neck of the infant tend to cause neck flexion and this, together with the relatively large tongue, make airway care difficult. Specific problems such as this are highlighted in the relevant chapters.

ANATOMY AND PHYSIOLOGY

Particular anatomical and physiological features, and the way they change with age, can have a bearing on emergency care. Although there are changes in most areas, the most important from this perspective are those that occur in the respiratory and cardiovascular systems. These are discussed in more detail below.

Anatomy

Airway

Anatomical features outside the airway have some relevance to its care. As mentioned above the head is large and the neck short, tending to cause neck flexion. The face and mandible are small and teeth or orthodontic appliances may be loose. The relatively large tongue not only tends to obstruct the airway in an unconscious child, but may also impede the view at laryngoscopy. Finally, the floor of the mouth is easily compressible, requiring care in the positioning of fingers when holding the jaw for airway positioning. These features are summarised in Figure 2.3.

The anatomy of the airway itself changes with age, and consequently different problems affect different age groups. Infants less than 6 months old are obligate nasal breathers. As the narrow nasal passages are easily obstructed by mucus secretions, and upper respiratory tract infections are common in this age group, these children are at particular risk of airway compromise. In 3 to 8 year olds adenotonsillar hypertrophy is a problem. This not only tends to cause obstruction, but also causes difficulty when the nasal route is used to pass pharyngeal, gastric, or tracheal tubes.

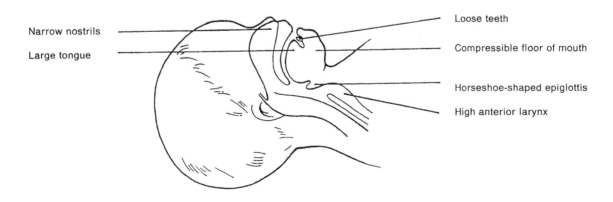

Figure 2.3 Summary of significant upper airway anatomy

In all young children the epiglottis is horseshoe-shaped, and projects posteriorly at 45° making tracheal intubation more difficult. This, together with the fact that the larynx is high and anterior (at the level of the second and third cervical vertebrae in the infant, compared with the fifth and sixth vertebrae in the adult), means that it is easier to intubate an infant using a straight-blade laryngoscope. The cricoid ring is the narrowest part of the upper airway (as opposed to the larynx in an adult). The narrow cross-sectional area at this point, together with the fact that the cricoid ring is lined by pseudostratified ciliated epithelium loosely bound to areolar tissue, makes it particularly susceptible to oedema. As tracheal tube cuffs tend to lie at this level, uncuffed tubes are preferred in pre-pubertal children.

The trachea is short and soft. Over-extension of the neck may therefore cause tracheal compression. The short trachea and the symmetry of the carinal angles mean that, not only is tube displacement more likely, but also a tube or a foreign body is just as likely to be displaced into the left as the right main-stem bronchus.

Breathing

The lungs are relatively immature at birth. The air tissue interface has a relatively small total surface area in the infant (less than 3 m^2). In addition, there is a tenfold increase in the number of small airways from birth to adulthood.

Both the upper and lower airways are relatively small, and are consequently more easily obstructed. As resistance to flow is inversely proportional to the fourth power of the airway radius (halving the radius increases the resistance sixteenfold), seemingly small obstructions can have significant effects on air entry in children.

Infants rely mainly on diaphragmatic breathing. Their muscles are more likely to fatigue, as they have fewer type I (slow twitch, highly oxidative, fatigue-resistant) fibres compared with adults. Pre-term infants' muscles have even less type I fibres. These children are consequently more prone to respiratory failure.

The ribs lie more horizontally in infants, and therefore contribute less to chest expansion. In the injured child, the compliant chest wall may allow serious parenchymal injuries to occur without necessarily incurring rib fractures. For multiple rib fractures to occur the force must be very large; the parenchymal injury that results is consequently very severe and flail chest is tolerated badly.

Circulation

At birth the two cardiac ventricles are of similar weight; by 2 months of age the RV/LV weight ratio is 0·5. These changes are reflected in the infant's ECG. During the first months of life the right ventricle (RV) dominance is apparent, but by 4–6 months of age the left ventricle (LV) is dominant. As the heart develops during childhood, the sizes of the P wave and QRS complex increase, and the P–R interval and QRS duration become longer.

The child's circulating blood volume is higher per kilogram body weight (70–80 ml/kg) than that of an adult, but the actual volume is small. This means that in infants and small children relatively small absolute amounts of blood loss can be critically important.

Physiology

Airway and breathing

The infant has a relatively greater metabolic rate and oxygen consumption. This is one reason for an increased respiratory rate. However, the tidal volume remains relatively constant in relation to body weight (5–7 ml/kg) through to adulthood. The work of breathing is also relatively unchanged at about 1% of the metabolic rate, although it is increased in the pre-term infant.

Table 2.1 Respiratory rate by age at rest

Age (years)	Respiratory rate (breaths per minute)
<1	30–40
1–2	25–35
2–5	25–30
5–12	20–25
>12	15–20

In the adult, the lung and chest wall contribute equally to the total compliance. In the newborn, most of the impedance to expansion is due to the lung, and is critically dependent on surfactant. The lung compliance increases over the first week of life as fluid is removed from the lung. The child's compliant chest wall leads to prominent sternal recession and rib space indrawing when the airway is obstructed or lung compliance decreases. It also allows the intrathoracic pressure to be less "negative". This reduces small airway patency. As a result, the lung volume at the end of expiration is similar to the closing volume (the volume at which small airway closure starts to take place).

At birth, the oxygen dissociation curve is shifted to the left and P_{50} (Po_2 at 50% oxygen saturation) is greatly reduced. This is due to the fact that 70% of the haemoglobin is in the form of HbF; this gradually declines to negligible amounts by the age of 6 months.

Circulation

The infant has a relatively small stroke volume (1·5 ml/kg at birth) but has the highest cardiac index seen at any stage of life (300 ml/min/kg). Cardiac index decreases with age and is 100 ml/min/kg in adolescence and 70–80 ml/min/kg in the adult. At the same time the stroke volume increases as the heart gets bigger. As cardiac output is the product of stroke volume and heart rate, these changes underlie the heart rate changes seen during childhood (shown in Table 2.2).

Table 2.2. Heart rate by age

Age (years)	Heart rate (beats per minute)
<1	110–160
1–2	100–150
2–5	95–140
5–12	80–120
>12	60–100

As the stroke volume is small and relatively fixed in infants, cardiac output is directly related to heart rate. The practical importance of this is that the response to volume therapy is blunted because stroke volume cannot increase greatly to improve cardiac output. By the age of 2 years myocardial function and response to fluid are similar to those of an adult.

Systemic vascular resistance rises after birth and continues to do so until adulthood is reached. This is reflected in the changes seen in blood pressure – shown in Table 2.3.

Table 2.3. Systolic blood pressure by age

Age (years)	Systolic blood pressure (mmHg)
<1	70–90
1–2	80–95
2–5	80–100
5–12	90–110
>12	100–120

PSYCHOLOGY

Children who are ill or injured present particular problems during emergency management because of difficulties in communicating with them, and because of the fear that they feel.

Communication

Infants and young children either have no language ability or are still developing their speech. This causes difficulty when symptoms such as pain need to be described. Even children who are usually fluent may remain silent. Information has to be gleaned from the limited verbal communication, and from the many non-verbal cues (such as facial expression and posture) that are available.

Fear

All emergency situations, and many other situations that adults would not classify as emergencies, engender fear in children. This causes additional distress to the child and adds to parental anxiety. Physiological parameters, such as pulse rate and respiratory rate, are altered because of it, and this in turn makes clinical assessment more difficult.

Fear is a particular problem in the pre-school child who often has a "magical" concept of illness and injury. This means that the child may think that the problem has been caused by some bad wish or thought that he or she has had. School-age children and adolescents may have fearsome concepts of what might happen to them because of ideas they have picked up from adult conversation, films, and television.

Knowledge allays fear and it is therefore important to explain things as clearly as possible to the child. Explanations must be phrased in a way that the child can understand. Play can be used to do this (e.g. applying a bandage to a teddy first), and also helps to maintain some semblance of normality in a strange and stressful situation Finally, parents must be allowed to stay with the child at all times; their absence from the bedside will only add additional fears both to the child and to the parents themselves.

Summary

- Absolute size and relative body proportions change with age
- Observations on children must be related to their age
- Therapy in children must be related to their age and weight
- The special psychological needs of children must be considered

3

Recognition of the seriously ill child

As described in Chapter 1, the outcome for children following cardiac arrest is, in general, very poor. Earlier recognition and management of potential respiratory, circulatory, or central neurological failure will reduce mortality and secondary morbidity. This chapter describes the physical signs that should be used for rapid assessment of children. These combine to make the primary assessment.

PRIMARY ASSESSMENT OF AIRWAY AND BREATHING
Recognition of potential respiratory failure

Effort of breathing

The degree of increase in the effort of breathing allows clinical assessment of the severity of respiratory disease. It is important to assess the following.

Respiratory rate
At rest tachypnoea indicates that increased ventilation is needed because of either lung or airway disease, or metabolic acidosis. Normal respiratory rates at differing ages are shown in Table 3.1.

Table 3.1. Respiratory rate by age at rest

Age (years)	Respiratory rate (beats per minute)
<1	30–40
1–2	25–35
2–5	25–30
5–12	20–25
>12	15–20

Recession

Intercostal, subcostal, or sternal recession shows increased effort of breathing. This sign is more easily seen in younger infants as they have a more compliant chest wall. Its presence in older children (i.e. over 6 or 7 years) suggests severe respiratory problems. The degree of recession gives an indication of the severity of respiratory difficulty.

Inspiratory or expiratory noises

An inspiratory noise while breathing (stridor) is a sign of laryngeal or tracheal obstruction. In severe obstruction the stridor may also occur in expiration, but the inspiratory component is usually more pronounced. Wheezing indicates lower airway narrowing and is more pronounced in expiration. A prolonged expiratory phase also indicates lower airway narrowing. The volume of the noise is not an indicator of severity.

Grunting

Grunting is produced by exhalation against a partially closed glottis. It is an attempt to generate a positive end-expiratory pressure and prevent airway collapse at the end of expiration in children with "stiff" lungs. This is a sign of severe respiratory distress and is characteristically seen in infants.

Accessory muscle use

As in adult life, the sternomastoid muscle may be used as an accessory respiratory muscle when the effort of breathing is increased. In infants this may cause the head to bob up and down with each breath, making it ineffectual.

Flare of the alae nasi

Flaring of the alae nasi is seen especially in infants with respiratory distress.

Exceptions

There may be absent or decreased evidence of increased effort of breathing in three circumstances:

1. In the infant or child who has had severe respiratory problems for some time, fatigue may occur and the signs of increased effort of breathing will decrease. *Exhaustion is a pre-terminal sign.*
2. Children with cerebral depression from raised intracranial pressure, poisoning or encephalopathy will have respiratory inadequacy without increased effort of breathing. The respiratory inadequacy in this case is caused by decreased respiratory drive.
3. Children who have neuromuscular disease (such as Werdnig–Hoffman disease or muscular dystrophy) may present in respiratory failure without increased effort of breathing.

The diagnosis of respiratory failure in such children is made by observing the efficacy of breathing, and looking for other signs of respiratory inadequacy. These are discussed in the text.

Efficacy of breathing

Auscultation of the chest will give an indication of the amount of air being inspired and expired. *A silent chest is an extremely worrying sign.* Similarly, observations of the degree of *chest expansion* (or, in infants, abdominal excursion) adds useful information.

Pulse oximetry can be used to measure the arterial oxygen saturation (SaO_2). The instruments are less accurate when SaO_2 is less than 70%, when shock is present, and in the presence of carboxyhaemoglobin. Oximetry in air gives a good indication of the efficacy of breathing. Supplemented oxygen will mask this information unless the hypoxia is severe.

Effects of respiratory inadequacy on other organs

Heart rate

Hypoxia produces tachycardia in the older infant and child. Anxiety and a fever will also contribute to tachycardia making this a non-specific sign. Severe or prolonged hypoxia leads to bradycardia. *This is a pre-terminal sign.*

Skin colour

Hypoxia (via catecholamine release) produces vasoconstriction and skin pallor. *Cyanosis is a late and pre-terminal sign of hypoxia.* By the time central cyanosis is visible in acute respiratory disease, the patient is close to respiratory arrest. In the anaemic child cyanosis may never be visible despite profound hypoxia. A few children will be cyanosed because of cyanotic heart disease. Their cyanosis will be largely unchanged by oxygen therapy.

Mental status

The hypoxic or hypercapnic child will be agitated and/or drowsy. Gradually drowsiness increases and eventually consciousness is lost. These extremely useful and important signs are often more difficult to detect in small infants. The parents may say that the infant is just "not himself". The doctor must assess the child's state of alertness by gaining eye contact, and noting the response to voice and, if necessary, to painful stimuli. A generalised muscular hypotonia also accompanies hypoxic cerebral depression.

Reassessment

Single observations on respiratory rate, etc. are useful but much more information can be gained by frequent repeated observations to detect a trend in the patient's condition.

PRIMARY ASSESSMENT OF THE CIRCULATION
Recognition of potential circulatory failure

Cardiovascular status

Heart rate

The heart rate initially increases in shock due to catecholamine release and as compensation for decreased stroke volume. The rate, particularly in small infants, may be extremely high (up to 220 per minute). Normal rates are shown in Table 3.2.

Bradycardia is a pre-terminal sign.

Table 3.2. Heart rate by age

Age (years)	Heart rate (beats per minute)
<1	110–160
1–2	100–150
2–5	95–140
5–12	80–120
>12	60–100

Pulse volume

Although blood pressure is maintained until shock is severe, an indication of perfusion can be gained by comparative palpation of both peripheral and central pulses. Absent peripheral pulses and weak central pulses are serious signs of advanced shock, and indicate that hypotension is already present.

Capillary refill

Following cutaneous pressure on a digit or, preferably, on the centre of the sternum for 5 seconds, capillary refill should occur within 2 seconds. A slower refill time than this indicates poor skin perfusion. This is a particularly useful sign in early septic shock, when the child may otherwise be apparently well with warm peripheries. The presence of fever does not affect the sensitivity of delayed capillary refill in children with hypovolaemia but a low ambient temperature reduces its specificity, so the sign should be used with caution in trauma patients who have been in a cold environment. Poor capillary refill and differential pulse volumes are neither sensitive nor specific indicators of shock in infants and children, but are useful clinical signs when used in conjunction with the other signs described. They should not be used as the only indicators of shock nor as quantitative measures of the response to treatment.

Blood pressure

Hypotension is a late and pre-terminal sign of circulatory failure. Once a child's blood pressure has fallen cardiac arrest is imminent. Expected systolic blood pressure can be estimated by the formula:

$$\text{Blood pressure} = 80 + (\text{Age in years} \times 2)$$

Normal systolic pressures are shown in Table 3.3.

Table 3.3. Systolic blood pressure by age

Age (years)	Systolic blood pressure (mmHg)
<1	70–90
1–2	80–95
2–5	80–100
5–12	90–110
>12	100–120

Use of the correct cuff size is crucial if an accurate blood pressure measurement is to be obtained. This caveat applies both to auscultatory and to oscillometric devices. The width of the cuff should be more than 80% of the length of the upper arm and the bladder more than 40% of the arm's circumference.

Effects of circulatory inadequacy on other organs

Respiratory system

A rapid respiration rate with an increased tidal volume, but without recession, is caused by the metabolic acidosis resulting from circulatory failure.

Skin

Mottled, cold, pale skin peripherally indicates poor perfusion. A line of coldness may be felt to move centrally as circulatory failure progresses.

Mental status

Agitation and then drowsiness leading to unconsciousness are characteristic of circulatory failure. These signs are caused by poor cerebral perfusion. In an infant parents may say that he is "not himself".

Urinary output

A urine output of less than 1 ml/kg/hour in children and less than 2 ml/kg/hour in infants indicates inadequate renal perfusion during shock. A history of oliguria or anuria should be sought.

PRIMARY ASSESSMENT OF DISABILITY
Recognition of potential central neurological failure

Neurological assessment should only be performed after airway (A), breathing (B), and circulation (C) have been assessed and treated. There are no neurological problems that take priority over ABC.

Both respiratory and circulatory failure will have central neurological effects. Conversely, some conditions with direct central neurological effects (such as meningitis, raised intracranial pressure from trauma, and status epilepticus) may also have respiratory and circulatory consequences.

Neurological function

Conscious level

A rapid assessment of conscious level can be made by assigning the patient to one of the categories shown in the box.

A	ALERT
V	responds to VOICE
P	responds to PAIN
U	UNRESPONSIVE

The painful central stimulus should be delivered either by sternal pressure or by pulling frontal hair. A child who is unresponsive or who only responds to pain has a significant degree of coma equivalent to 8 or less on the Glasgow Coma Scale.

Posture

Many children who are suffering from a serious illness in any system are hypotonic. Stiff posturing such as that shown by decorticate (flexed arms, extended legs) or decerebrate (extended arms, extended legs) children is a sign of serious brain dysfunction. A painful stimulus may be necessary to elicit the posturing sign.

Pupils

Many drugs and cerebral lesions have effects on pupil size and reactions. However, the most important pupillary signs to seek are dilatation, unreactivity, and inequality, which indicate possible serious brain disorders.

Respiratory effects of central neurological failure

There are several recognisable breathing pattern abnormalities with raised intracranial pressure. However, they are often changeable and may vary from hyperventilation to Cheyne–Stokes breathing to apnoea. The presence of any abnormal respiratory pattern in a patient with coma suggests mid- or hind-brain dysfunction.

Circulatory effects of central neurological failure

Systemic hypertension with sinus bradycardia (Cushing's response) indicates compression of the medulla oblongata caused by herniation of the cerebellar tonsils through the foramen magnum. *This is a late and pre-terminal sign.*

Summary: the rapid clinical assessment of an infant or child

      Airway and **B**reathing
         Effort of breathing
         Respiratory rate/rhythm
         Stridor/wheeze
         Auscultation
         Skin colour
      Circulation
         Heart rate
         Pulse volume
         Capillary refill
         Skin temperature
      Disability
         Mental status/conscious level
         Posture
         Pupils
      The whole assessment should take less than a minute

Once airway (A), breathing (B), and circulation (C) are clearly recognised as being stable or have been stabilised, then definitive management of the underlying condition can proceed. During definitive management reassessment of ABCD at frequent intervals will be necessary to assess progress and detect deterioration.

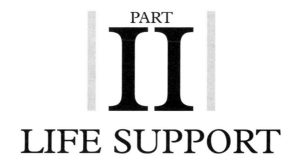

PART II

LIFE SUPPORT

CHAPTER

4

Basic life support

Paediatric basic life support (BLS) is not simply a scaled-down version of that provided for adults. Although the general principles are the same, specific techniques are required if the optimum support is to be given. The exact techniques employed need to be varied according to the size of the child. A somewhat artificial line is generally drawn between infants (less than 1 year old) and small children (less than 8 years old), and this chapter follows that approach. The preponderance of hypoxic causes of paediatric cardiorespiratory arrest means that oxygen delivery rather than defibrillation is the critical step in children. This underlines the major differences with the adult algorithm.

By applying the basic techniques described, a single rescuer can support the vital respiratory and circulatory functions of a collapsed child with no equipment.

Basic life support is the foundation on which advanced life support is built. Therefore it is essential that all advanced life support providers are proficient at basic techniques, and that they are capable of ensuring that basic support is provided continuously and well during resuscitation.

ASSESSMENT AND TREATMENT

Once the child has been approached correctly and a simple test for unresponsiveness has been carried out, assessment and treatment follow the familiar A, B, C pattern. The overall sequence of basic life support in paediatric cardiopulmonary arrest is summarised in Figure 4.1.

The SAFE approach

Additional help should be summoned rapidly. Furthermore, it is essential that the rescuer does not become a second victim, and that the child is removed from continuing danger as quickly as possible. These considerations should precede the initial airway assessment. They are summarised in Figure 4.2.

21

Are you alright?

The initial simple assessment of responsiveness consists of asking the child "Are you alright?", and *gently* shaking him or her by the shoulders. Infants and very small children who cannot talk yet, and older children who are very scared, are unlikely to reply meaningfully, but may make some sound or open their eyes to the rescuer's voice.

In case associated with trauma, the neck and spine should be immobilised during this manoeuvre. This is achieved by placing one hand firmly on the forehead, while one of the child's arms is shaken gently.

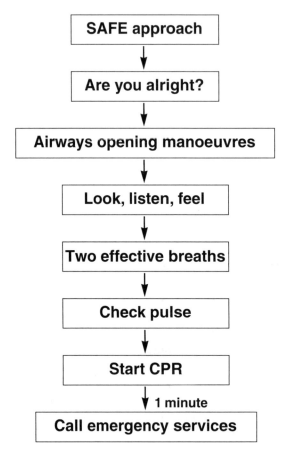

Figure 4.1. The overall sequence of basic life support in cardiopulmonary arrest (CPR = cardiopulmonary resuscitation)

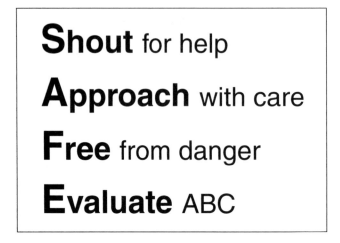

Figure 4.2. The SAFE approach

Airway (A)

An obstructed airway may be the primary problem, and correction of the obstruction can result in recovery without further intervention.

If a child is having difficulty breathing, but is conscious, then transport to hospital should be arranged as quickly as possible. A child will often find the best position to maintain his or her own airway, and should not be forced to adopt a position that may be less comfortable. Attempts to improve a partially maintained airway in an environment where immediate advanced support is not available can be dangerous, because total obstruction may occur.

If the child is not breathing it may be because the airway has been blocked by the tongue falling back to obstruct the pharynx. An attempt to open the airway should be made using the head tilt/chin lift manoeuvre. The rescuer places the hand nearest to the child's head on the forehead, and applies pressure to tilt the head back gently. The desirable degrees of tilt are: *neutral* in the infant and *sniffing* in the child.

These are shown in Figures 4.3 and 4.4.

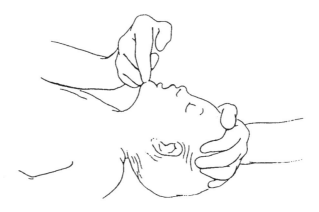

Figure 4.3.   Chin lift in infants

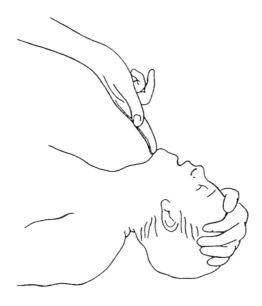

Figure 4.4.   Chin lift in children

The fingers of the other hand should then be placed under the chin and the chin should be lifted upwards. Care should be taken not to injure the soft tissue by gripping too hard. As this action can close the child's mouth, it may be necessary to use the thumb of the same hand to part the lips slightly.

The patency of the airway should then be assessed. This is done by:

LOOKing   for chest and/or abdominal movement
LISTENing   for breath sounds
FEELing   for breath

and is best achieved by the rescuer placing his or her face above the child's, with the ear over the nose, the cheek over the mouth, and the eyes looking along the line of the chest for up to 10 seconds.

If the head tilt/chin lift is not possible or is contraindicated, then the jaw thrust manoeuvre can be performed. This is achieved by placing two or three fingers under the angle of the mandible bilaterally, and lifting the jaw upwards. This technique may be easier if the rescuer's elbows are resting on the same surface as the child is lying on. A small degree of head tilt may also be applied. This is shown in Figure 4.5.

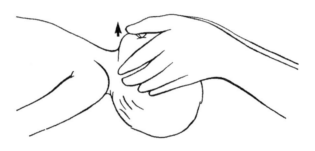

Figure 4.5.   Jaw thrust

As before the success or failure of the intervention is assessed using the

LOOK
LISTEN
FEEL

technique described above.

It should be noted that, if there is a history of trauma, then the head tilt/chin lift manoeuvre may exacerbate cervical spine injury. The safest airway intervention in these circumstances is jaw thrust without head tilt. Proper cervical spine control can only be achieved in such cases by a second rescuer maintaining in-line cervical stabilisation throughout.

The finger sweep technique often recommended in adults should not be used in children. The child's soft palate is easily damaged and bleeding from within the mouth can worsen the situation. Furthermore, foreign bodies may be forced further down the airway; they can become lodged below the vocal cords (vocal folds) and be even more difficult to remove.

If a foreign body is not obvious, inspection should be done under direct vision in hospital and, if appropriate, removal should be attempted using Magill's forceps.

Breathing (B)

If the airway opening techniques described above do not result in the resumption of adequate breathing within 10 seconds, exhaled air resuscitation should be commenced. The rescuer should distinguish between adequate and ineffective, gasping or obstructed breathing. If in doubt, attempt rescue breathing.

**Up to five initial rescue breaths should be given
to achieve two effective breaths.**

While the airway is kept open as described above, the rescuer breathes in and seals his or her mouth around the victim's mouth, or mouth and nose as shown in Figure 4.6. If the mouth alone is used then the nose should be pinched closed using the thumb and index fingers of the hand that is maintaining head tilt. Slow exhalation (1–1·5 seconds) by the rescuer should result in the victim's chest rising. The rescuer should take a breath between rescue breaths to maximise oxygenation of the victim.

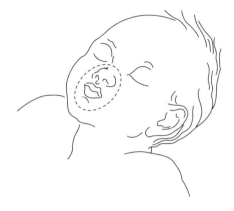

Figure 4.6. Mouth-to-mouth-and-nose in an infant

If the rescuer is unable to cover the mouth and nose in an infant he or she may attempt to seal only the infant's nose with his or her mouth.

As children vary in size only general guidance can be given regarding the volume and pressure of inflation (see the box).

General guidance for exhaled air resuscitation

- The chest should be seen to rise
- Inflation pressure may be higher because the airway is small
- Slow breaths at the lowest pressure reduce gastric distension
- Firm, gentle pressure on the cricoid cartilage may reduce gastric insufflation

---

If the chest does not rise then the airway is not clear. The usual cause is failure to apply correctly the airway opening techniques discussed above. Thus the first thing to do is to readjust the head tilt/chin lift position, and try again. If this does not work jaw thrust should be tried. It is quite possible for a single rescuer to open the airway using this technique and perform exhaled air resuscitation; however, if two rescuers are present one should maintain the airway whilst the other breathes for the child. Up to five rescue breaths may be attempted so that for the inexperienced rescuer two are effective.

Failure of both head tilt/chin and jaw thrust should lead to the suspicion that a foreign body is causing the obstruction, and the appropriate action should be taken.

Circulation (C)

Once the rescue breaths have been given as above, attention should be turned to the circulation.

Assessment

Inadequacy of the circulation is recognised by the absence of a central pulse for up to 10 seconds, by the presence of a pulse at an insufficient rate and by the absence of other signs of circulation, i.e. no breaths or cough in response to rescue breaths and no spontaneous movement. In children, as in adults, the carotid artery in the neck can be palpated.

In infants the neck is generally short and fat, and the carotid artery may be difficult to identify. Therefore the brachial artery in the medical aspect of the anecubital fossa (Figure 4.7), or the femoral artery in the groin, should be felt.

Start chest compressions if

- no pulse
- slow pulse
- no signs of circulation

"Unnecessary" chest compressions are almost never damaging.

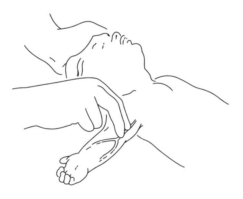

Figure 4.7. Feeling for the brachial pulse

If the pulse is absent for up to 10 seconds or inadequate (less than 60 beats/min with signs of poor perfusion) and/or there are no other signs of circulation, then cardiac compression is required. If the pulse is present and at an adequate rate, with good perfusion but apnoea persists, exhaled air resuscitation must be continued until spontaneous breathing resumes. Signs of poor perfusion include pallor, lack of responsiveness and poor muscle tone.

Cardiac compression

For the best output the child must be placed lying flat on his or her back, on a hard surface. In infants it is said that the palm of the rescuer's hand can be used for this purpose, but this may prove difficult in practice.

Children vary in size, and the exact nature of the compressions given should reflect this. In general, infants (less than 1 year) require a different technique from small children. In children over 8 years of age, the method used in adults can be applied with appropriate modifications for their size. Compressions should be approximately one third to one half of the depth of the child's or infant's chest.

Infants As the infant heart is lower with relation to external landmarks when compared to older children and adults, the area of compression is found by imagining a line between the nipples and compressing over the sternum one finger-breadth below this line. Two fingers are used to compress the chest. This is shown in Figure 4.8. There is some evidence that infant cardiac compression can be more effectively achieved using the hand-encircling technique: the infant is held with both the rescuer's hands encircling or partially encircling the chest. The thumbs are placed over the correct part of the sternum (as detailed above) and compression carried out, as shown in Figure 4.9. This method is only possible when there are two rescuers, as the time needed to re-position the airway precludes its use by a single rescuer if the recommended rates of compression and ventilation are to be achieved. The single rescuer should use the two-finger method, employing the other hand to maintain the airway position as shown in Figure 4.8.

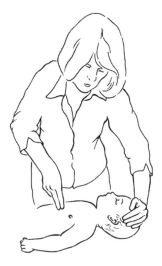

Figure 4.8. Infant chest compression: two-finger technique

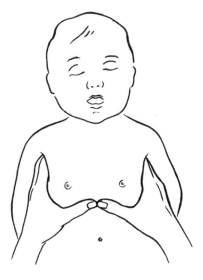

Figure 4.9. Infant chest compression: hand-encircling technique

Small children The area of compression is one finger-breadth above the xiphisternum. The heel of one hand is used to depress the sternum (Figure 4.10).

27

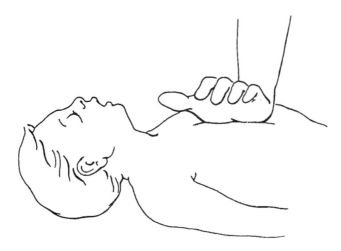

Figure 4.10. Chest compression in small children

Larger children The area of compression is two finger-breadths above the xiphisternum. The heels of both hands are used to depress the sternum (Figure 4.11).

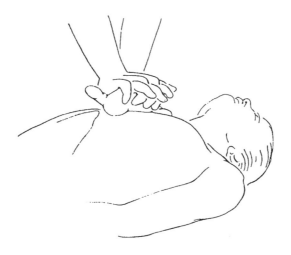

Figure 4.11. Chest compression in older children

Once the correction technique has been chosen and the area for compression identified, five compressions should be given.

Continuing cardiopulmonary resuscitation

The compression rate at all ages is 100/minute. A ratio of five compressions to one ventilation is maintained whatever the number of rescuers, except in older children who should receive a ratio of 15 compressions to 2 ventilations with any number of rescuers. If no help has arrived the emergency services must be contacted after 1 minute of cardiopulmonary resuscitation. With pauses for ventilation there will be less than 100 compressions per minute although the *rate* should be 100/min. Compressions can be recommended at the end of inspiration and may augment exhalation. *Apart from this interruption to summon help, basic life support must not be interrupted unless the child moves or takes a breath.*

Any time spent readjusting the airway or re-establishing the correct position for compressions will seriously decrease the number of cycles given per minute. This can be a very real problem for the solo rescuer and there is no easy solution. In the infant and small child, the free hand can maintain the head position. The correct position for compressions should not be re-measured after each ventilation.

The cardiopulmonary resuscitation manoeuvres recommended for infants and children are summarised in Table 4.1.

Table 4.1. Summary of basic life support techniques in infants and children

	Infant	Small child	Larger child
Airway			
Head-tilt position	Neutral	Sniffing	Sniffing
Breathing			
Initial slow breaths	Two	Two	Two
Circulation			
Pulse check	Brachial or femoral	Carotid	Carotid
Landmark	One finger-breadth below nipple line	One finger-breadth above xiphisternum	Two finger-breadths above xiphisternum
Technique	Two fingers or two thumbs	One hand	Two hands
Cardiopulmonary resuscitation			
ratio	5:1	5:1	15:2

Mechanical adjuncts for chest compression

Mechanical devices to compress the sternum are currently not recommended for paediatric patients. They were designed and tested for use in adults and there is no information on safety and efficacy in childhood.

Similarly, active compression–decompression CPR, considered an optional technique in adults, has not been studied and is therefore not recommended in children.

Automatic External Defibrillators (AEDs) in children

The use of the AED is now included in basic life support teaching for adults. In this text there is a discussion of the use of AEDs with regard to children in the chapter on The Management of Cardiac Arrest (Chapter 6).

Recovery position

No specific recovery position has been identified for children. The child should be placed in a position that ensures maintenance of an open airway, ability to monitor and gain access to the patient, security of the cervical spine and attention to pressure points.

Audio-prompts

The use of audio-prompts such as a metronome set at 100 beats per minute appears to help in both training and performance of CPR to keep chest compressions at the recommended rate.

BASIC LIFE SUPPORT AND INFECTION RISK

There have been a few reports of transmission of infectious diseases from casualties to rescuers during mouth-to-mouth resuscitation. The most serious concern in children is meningococcus, and rescuers involved in the resuscitation of the airway in such patients should take standard prophylactic antibiotics (usually rifampicin).

There have been no reported cases of transmission of either hepatitis B or human immunodeficiency virus (HIV) through mouth-to-mouth ventilation. Blood-to-blood contact is the single most important route of transmission of these viruses, and in nontrauma resuscitations the risks are negligible. Sputum, saliva, sweat, tears, urine, and vomit are low-risk fluids. Precautions should be taken, if possible, in cases where there might be contact with blood, semen, vaginal secretions, cerebrospinal fluid, pleural and peritoneal fluids, and amniotic fluid. Precautions are also recommended if any bodily secretion contains visible blood. Devices that prevent direct contact between the rescuer and the victim (such as resuscitation masks) can be used to lower risk; gauze swabs or any other porous material placed over the victim's mouth is of no benefit in this regard.

The number of children in the UK with AIDS or HIV-l infection in June 1992 was estimated at 501, whereas the number of adults similarly affected was estimated at 23 806 (a ratio of 1:47). If transmission of HIV-l does occur in the UK, it is therefore much more likely to be from adult rescuer to child rather than the other way around.

Although practice manikins have not been shown to be a source of infection, regular cleaning is recommended and should be carried out as shown in the manufacturer's instructions. Infection rates vary from country to country and rescuers must be aware of the local risk.

THE CHOKING CHILD

Introduction

The vast majority of deaths from foreign body aspiration occur in pre-school children. Virtually anything may be inhaled. The diagnosis is very rarely clear-cut, but should be suspected if the onset of respiratory compromise is sudden and is associated with coughing, gagging, and stridor. Airway obstruction may also occur with infections such as acute epiglottitis and croup. In such cases, attempts to relieve the obstruction using the methods described below are dangerous. Children with known or suspected infectious causes of obstruction, and those who are still breathing and in whom the cause of obstruction is unclear, should be taken to hospital urgently. The treatment of these children is dealt with in Chapter 9.

The physical methods of clearing the airway, described below, should therefore only be performed if:

1 The diagnosis of foreign body aspiration is clear-cut (witnessed or strongly suspected) and ineffective coughing and increasing dyspnoea, loss of consciousness or apnoea have occurred.
2 Head tilt/chin lift and jaw thrust have failed to open the airway of an apnoeic child. The sequence of instructions is shown in Figure 4.12.

If the child is coughing he should be encouraged. No intervention should be made unless the cough becomes ineffective (quieter) or the child loses consciousness. A spontaneous cough is more effective than any manoeuvre.

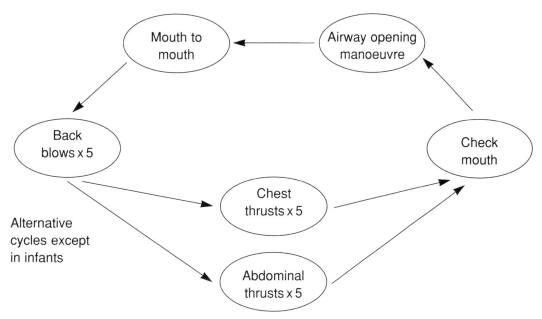

Figure 4.12. The sequence of actions in a choking child

Infants

Abdominal thrusts may cause intra-abdominal injury in infants. Therefore a combination of back blows and chest thrusts is recommended for the relief of foreign body obstruction in this age group.

The baby is placed along one of the rescuer's arms in a head-down position. The rescuer then rests his or her arm along the thigh, and delivers five back blows with the heel of the free hand.

If the obstruction is not relieved the baby is turned over and laid along the rescuer's thigh, still in a head-down position. Five chest thrusts are given – using the same landmarks as for cardiac compression but at a rate of one per second. If an infant is too large to allow the single-arm technique described above to be used, then the same manoeuvres can be performed by lying the baby across the rescuer's lap. These techniques are shown in Figures 4.13 and 4.14.

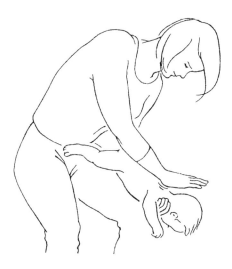

Figure 4.13. Back blows in an infant

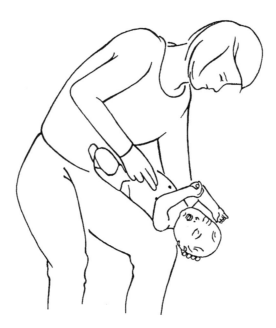

Figure 4.14. Chest thrusts in an infant

Children

Back blows and chest thrusts can be used as in infants (Figure 4.15). In the child the Heimlich manoeuvre can also be used. This can be performed with the victim either standing, sitting, kneeling, or lying.

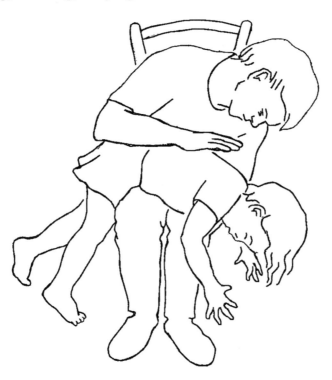

Figure 4.15. Back blows in a small child

If this is to be attempted with the child standing, kneeling, or sitting, the rescuer moves behind the victim and passes his or her arms around the victim's body. Due to the height of children, it may be necessary for an adult to raise the child or kneel behind them to carry out the standing manoeuvre effectively. One hand is formed into a fist and placed against the child's abdomen above the umbilicus and below the xiphisternum. The other hand is placed over the fist, and both hands are thrust sharply upwards into the abdomen. This is repeated five times unless the object causing the obstruction is expelled before then. This technique is shown in Figure 4.16.

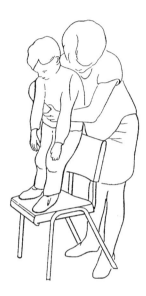

Figure 4.16.   Heimlich manoeuvre in a standing child

To carry out the Heimlich manoeuvre in a supine child, the rescuer kneels at his or her feet (Figure 4.17). If the child is large it may be necessary to kneel astride him or her. The heel of one hand is placed against the child's abdomen above the umbilicus and below the xiphisternum. The other hand is placed on top of the first, and both hands are thrust sharply upwards into the abdomen with care being taken to direct the thrust in the midline. This is repeated five times unless the object causing the obstruction is expelled before then.

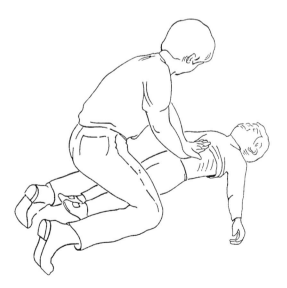

Figure 4.17.   Abdominal thrusts

33

5

Advanced support of the airway and ventilation

Management of airway and breathing has priority in the resuscitation of patients of all ages; the rate at which respiratory function can deteriorate in children is particularly rapid. It is vital that effective resuscitation techniques can be applied quickly and in order of priority. To do so, it is useful to appreciate the differences between adults and children, and essential to be familiar with commonly used equipment. Techniques for obtaining a patent and protected airway, and of achieving adequate ventilation and oxygenation, must be learned and practised. Finally, these techniques must be integrated into a prioritised system of care, planned in advance, to avoid delays and uncertainties in emergency situations.

EQUIPMENT FOR MANAGING THE AIRWAY

The airway equipment indicated in the box should be available in designated resuscitation areas. It is crucial that familiarity with it is gained before it is needed in an emergency situation.

Necessary airway equipment

Pharyngeal airways
Laryngoscopes
Tracheal tubes, introducers, and connectors
Magill's forceps
Suction devices and catheters
Cricothyroidotomy cannulae
Ventilation systems

Suction devices

In the resuscitation room, the usual suction device is the pipeline vacuum unit. It consists of a suction hose inserted into a wall terminal outlet, a controller (to adjust the vacuum pressure), a reservoir jar, suction tubing, and a suitable sucker nozzle or catheter. In order to aspirate vomit effectively, it should be capable of producing a high negative pressure and a high flow rate, although these can be reduced in non-urgent situations, so as not to cause mucosal injury.

The most useful suction ending is the Yankauer sucker, which is available in both adult and paediatric sizes. The paediatric size has a side hole which can be occluded by a finger, allowing greater control over vacuum pressure. In small infants, a suction catheter and a Y-piece are often preferred, but are less capable of removing vomit.

Portable suction devices are required for resuscitation in remote locations, and for transport to and from the resuscitation room. These are commonly operated by a hand or foot pump.

Pharyngeal airways

There are two main types of pharyngeal airway:

1. Oropharyngeal.
2. Nasopharyngeal.

The oropharyngeal or Guedel airway is used in the obtunded patient to provide a patent airway channel between the tongue and the posterior pharyngeal wall. It may also be used to stabilise the position of an oral tracheal tube. In the awake patient with an intact gag reflex, it may not be tolerated and may stimulate vomiting. The oropharyngeal airway is available in a variety of sizes. A suitably sized airway reaches from the centre of the incisors to the angle of the mandible when laid on the face concave side up. An inappropriate size may cause laryngospasm, mucosal trauma or may worsen the airway obstruction. Two techniques for insertion are described in Chapter 22.

The nasopharyngeal airway is often better tolerated than the Guedel airway. It is contraindicated in fractures of the anterior base of the skull. It may also cause significant haemorrhage from the friable, vascular, nasal mucosa. A suitable length can be estimated by measuring from the tip of the nose to the tragus of the ear. An appropriate diameter is one that just fits into the nostril without causing sustained blanching of the alae nasi. As small-sized nasopharyngeal airways are not commercially available, shortened tracheal tubes may be used.

Laryngoscopes

There are two principal designs of laryngoscope for use in children: the straight-blade and the curved-blade laryngoscope. In general the straight-blade laryngoscope is designed to lift the epiglottis under the tip of the blade, whereas the curved-blade laryngoscope is designed to rest in the vallecula. The straightblade device can also be placed short of the epiglottis in the vallecula. The advantage of taking the epiglottis is that it cannot then obscure the view of the vocal cords (vocal folds). The advantage of stopping short of the epiglottis is that it causes less stimulation, and is less likely to cause laryngospasm. The blade length should be varied according to age. It should be noted that it is possible to intubate successfully with a blade that is too long, but not with one that is too short. In general, straight blades are preferred up to the age of 1 year, and many prefer to use them up to the age of 5 years.

It is important to have a spare laryngoscope available, together with spare bulbs and batteries, to overcome equipment failure. In fibreoptic designs, the bulbs are set in the top of the blade handle rather than in the blade itself. This has advantages in terms of bulb protection and the ability to clean the blade after use.

The essential parts of these laryngoscopes are shown in Figures 5.1 and 5.2. The blade is designed to displace the tongue to the left in order to optimise the view of the larynx. Failure to control the tongue adequately in the haste to see the vocal cords may leave a portion of the tongue overhanging the blade. It may still be possible to see the larynx at first, but as soon as the tracheal tube is placed in the mouth, the view is obscured.

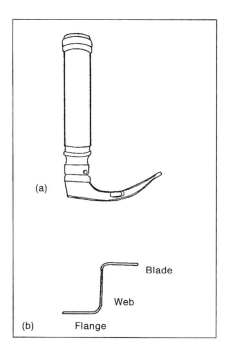

Figure 5.1. (a) Mackintosh curved-blade laryngoscope; (b) blade cross-section

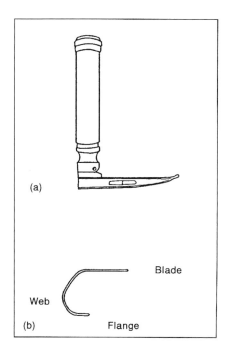

Figure 5.2. (a) Straight-blade laryngoscope; (b) blade cross-section

Tracheal tubes

Tracheal tubes come in a variety of designs, the most useful for resuscitation being the plain plastic tube. Uncuffed tubes are preferred up until approximately eight years of age so as not to cause oedema at the cricoid ring.

The Cole tube, with its shouldered tip, has been widely used in neonatal resuscitation. The shoulder increases turbulent flow and therefore airway resistance, and may also exacerbate tracheal oedema. These tubes should no longer be used.

Estimating the appropriate size of an tracheal tube is carried out as follows:

$$\text{Internal diameter (mm)} = (\text{Age}/4) + 4$$
$$\text{Length (cm)} = (\text{Age}/2) + 12 \text{ for an oral tube}$$
$$\text{Length (cm)} = (\text{Age}/2) + 15 \text{ for nasal tube}$$

These formulae are appropriate for ages over 1 year. Neonates usually require a tube of internal diameter 3–3·5 mm, although pre-term infants may need one of diameter 2·5 mm. Another useful guideline is to use a tube of such a size that will just fit into the nostril. Tracheal tubes are measured in sizes by their internal diameter in millimetres. They are provided in whole and half millimetre sizes. The clinician should select a tube of appropriate size but also prepare one a size smaller and one a size larger. The correct size is that which passes easily between the vocal cords but still allows a small air leak.

Tracheal tube introducers

A difficult intubation can be facilitated by the use of a stylet or introducer, placed through the lumen of the tracheal tube. These are of two types: soft and flexible or firm and malleable. The former can be allowed to project out of the tip of the tube, as long as it is handled very gently. The latter is used to alter the shape of the tube, but can easily damage the tissues if allowed to protrude from the end of the tracheal tube. Tracheal tube introducers should not be used to force a tracheal tube into position.

Tracheal tube connectors

In adults, the proximal end of the tube connectors is of standard size, based on the 15–22 mm system, ensuring that they can be connected to a standard self-inflating bag. The same standard Portex system exists for children, including neonates. However, many prefer to use smaller connectors in infants. Breathing systems based on smaller connectors are no longer generally recommended for use in the emergency situation, especially as a resuscitation kit containing both sets of sizes is confusing and dangerous.

Magill's forceps

Magill's forceps are used to grasp a tracheal tube, particularly one inserted through the nose, and pass it through the vocal cords. They are also suitable for removing foreign bodies in the upper airway under direct vision, and are designed to pass into the mouth with the handle at an angle so as not to obscure the view.

Tracheal suction catheters

These may be required after intubation to remove bronchial secretions or aspirated fluids. In general, the appropriate size in French gauge is numerically twice the internal diameter in millimetres, e.g. for a tracheal tube size $3\cdot0$ mm the correct suction catheter is a French gauge 6.

Cricothyroidotomy cannulae and ventilation systems

Purpose-made cricothyroidotomy cannulae are available, usually in three sizes: 12-gauge for an adult, 14-gauge for a child, and 18-gauge for a baby. They are less liable to kinking than intravenous cannulae and have a flange for suturing or securing to the neck.

In an emergency a 14-gauge intravenous cannula can be inserted through the cricothyroid membrane, and oxygen insufflated at 1 l/min/year of age to provide some oxygenation (but no ventilation). A side hole can be cut in the oxygen tubing or a Y-connector can be placed between the cannula and the oxygen supply, to allow intermittent occlusion and achieve partial ventilation as described in Chapter 22.

EQUIPMENT FOR PROVIDING OXYGEN AND VENTILATION

The equipment for oxygenation and ventilation indicated in the box should be readily available.

Necessary equipment for oxygenation and ventilation

Oxygen source and masks for spontaneous breathing
Face masks (for artificial ventilation)
Self-inflating bags
T-piece and open-ended bag
Mechanical ventilators
Chest tubes
Gastric tubes

Oxygen source and masks for spontaneous breathing

A wall oxygen supply (at a pressure of 4 atmospheres, 400 kPa or 60 p.s.i.) is provided in most resuscitation rooms. A flowmeter capable of delivering at least 15 l/min should be fitted.

A mask with a reservoir bag should be used in the first instance so that a high concentration of oxygen is delivered. A simple mask or other device such as a head box may be used later on if a high oxygen concentration is no longer required. Nasal prongs are often well tolerated in pre-school age, but they cause drying of the airway, may cause nasal obstruction in infants, and provide an unreliable oxygen concentration.

Younger children are more susceptible to the drying effect of a non-humidified oxygen supply.

Although the pre-term infant is vulnerable to retrolental fibroplasia caused by high-concentration oxygen, high concentrations should never be withheld for immediate resuscitation.

Face masks (for artificial ventilation)

Face masks for mouth-to-mask or bag-valve-mask ventilation in infants are of two main designs. Some masks conform to the anatomy of the child's face and have a low deadspace. Circular soft plastic masks give an excellent seal and are preferred by many. Children's masks should be clear to allow the child's colour or the presence of vomit to be seen.

The Laerdal pocket mask is a single-size clear plastic mask with an air-filled cushion rim designed for mouth-to-mask resuscitation. It can be supplied with a port for attaching to the oxygen supply and can be used in adults and children. By using it upside-down it may be used to ventilate an infant.

Self-inflating bags

Self-inflating bags come in three sizes: 250 ml, 500 ml, and 1500 ml. The smallest bag is ineffective except in very small babies. The two smaller sizes generally have a pressure-limiting valve set at 4·41 kPa (45 cm H_2O), which may (rarely) need to be overridden for high resistance/low compliance lungs, but which protects the normal lungs from inadvertent barotrauma. The patient end of the bag connects to a one-way valve of a fish-mouth or leaf-flap design. The opposite end has a connection to the oxygen supply, and to a reservoir attachment. The reservoir enables high oxygen concentrations to be delivered. Without a reservoir bag it is difficult to supply more than 50% oxygen to the patient, whatever the fresh gas flow, whereas with it an inspired oxygen concentration of 98% can be achieved.

T-piece and open-ended bag

This equipment should only be used in children up to about 20 kg. It is used frequently by anaesthetists, but requires a "knack" to use it effectively. The open end of the bag is grasped by the ring and little fingers to regulate escape of the gas, while the rest of the hand squeezes the bag as shown in Figure 5.3. In experienced hands, it gives a reliable "feel" of the state of the lungs and allows some positive end-expiratory pressure (PEEP) to be applied manually. It requires a reliable and controllable oxygen supply, and is totally ineffective if the supply fails. For this reason, self-inflating bags are generally preferred for initial resuscitation.

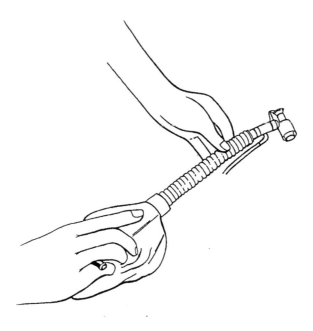

Figure 5.3. T-piece and open-ended bag

Mechanical ventilators

A detailed discussion of individual mechanical ventilators is beyond the scope of this book. Although clearly important in providing ventilation after initial resuscitation, they can give a false sense of security during inadequate or excessive ventilation. Continual re-evaluation with monitoring of expired CO_2 is mandatory.

Chest tubes

These are included because haemothorax or pneumothorax may severely limit ventilation. They are described elsewhere.

Gastric tubes

Children are prone to air swallowing and vomiting. Air may also be inadvertently forced into the stomach during bag and mask ventilation. This may cause vomiting, vagal stimulation or diaphragmatic splinting. A gastric tube will decompress the stomach and significantly improve both breathing and general well-being. Withholding the procedure "to be kind to the child" may cause more distress than performing it.

PRACTICAL SKILLS

The following practical skills are described in detail in Chapter 22:

- Oropharyngeal airway insertion:
  small child
  older child.
- Nasopharyngeal airway insertion.
- Orotracheal intubation:
  infant/small child
  older child.
- Surgical airway:
  needle cricothyroidotomy
  surgical cricothyroidotomy.
- Ventilation without intubation:
  mouth-to-mask ventilation
  bag-and-mask ventilation.

The basic skills of head and neck positioning, chin lift and jaw thrust are discussed in Chapter 4.

Ventilation with a mechanical ventilator

A full description is beyond the scope of this book. In general, in small children, pressure-controlled ventilation is preferred. In this mode, gas flow is supplied to the child at a set pressure during inspiration, e.g. 1.50–2.0 kPa (15–20 cmH$_2$O). In the child with very stiff lungs, pressures of up to 3.0 kPa (30 cmH$_2$O) may be required. During expiration, a positive end-expiratory pressure (PEEP) is generally used, typically 0.3–0.5 kPa (3–5 cmH$_2$O). Pressure control partially compensates for any leak around the tracheal cuff.

In the older child, controlled minute ventilation is a common mode of ventilation. The child receives a set volume of gas at a constant flow rate during inspiration, typically about 10 ml/kg tidal volume. Respiratory rate should be set according to the child's age. In both the above modes, inspiratory and expiratory times are fixed. The inspiratory to expiratory (I:E) ratio is generally less than 1.

Other modes include synchronised intermittent mandatory volume (SIMV), pressure support, and continuous positive airway pressure (CPAP), but these are not discussed further.

Tracheal tube placement check

Following the placement of the tracheal tube into the trachea its position must be verified by:

- Observing bilateral and symmetrical movement of the chest.
- Ausculation of chest and abdomen.
- Monitoring expired carbon dioxide in the exhaled air by either colour change capnometry or carbon dioxide capnography.

The continued monitoring of expired carbon dioxide is a good indicator of effective ventilation, but it must be remembered that carbon dioxide will not be detected in the absence of a circulation (cardiac arrest) or where the lungs have not been inflated (at birth).

Laryngeal mask airway

The laryngeal mask airway (LMA) is an airway device that has become widely advocated in adult anaesthesia and resuscitation. Although it is available in smaller sizes for infants and children, it is difficult to position and can become dislodged easily. The device sits over the glottic opening and the user must be aware that the LMA does not guarantee the airway to the same extent as tracheal intubation. Neither does it protect against aspiration. The use of the LMA for resuscitation of infants and children is not recommended currently although it may be employed by those proficient in its use.

PUTTING IT TOGETHER: AIRWAY-BREATHING MANAGEMENT

In order to respond urgently and yet retain thoroughness, effective emergency management demands a systematic, prioritised approach. Care can be structured into the following phases.

Primary assessment

This consists of a rapid "physiological" examination to identify immediately life-threatening emergencies. It should be completed in less than a minute. It is prioritised as shown in the box.

Airway
Breathing
Circulation
Disability (nervous system)
Exposure

From the respiratory viewpoint, do the following:

- Look, listen and feel for airway obstruction, respiratory arrest, depression, or distress.
- Assess the effort of breathing.
- Count the respiratory rate.
- Listen for stridor and/or wheeze.
- Auscultate for breath sounds.
- Assess skin colour.

If a significant problem is identified, management should be started immediately. After appropriate interventions have been performed, primary assessment can be resumed or repeated.

Resuscitation

During this phase, life-saving interventions are performed. These include such procedures as intubation, ventilation, cannulation, and fluid resuscitation. At the same time, oxygen is provided, vital signs are recorded, and essential monitoring is established.

From the respiratory viewpoint, do the following:

- Consider jaw- and neck-positioning manoeuvres.
- Administer oxygen.
- Consider suction and foreign body removal.
- Consider mask ventilation, and pharyngeal or tracheal intubation.
- Consider chest decompression.
- Consider needle cricothyroidotomy, if unable to oxygenate by alternative means.
- Initiate pulse oximetry and other monitoring at this time.

Secondary assessment

This consists of a thorough physical examination, together with appropriate investigations. Conventionally, examination is from head to toe, and represents an "anatomical" assessment. Before embarking on this phase, it is important that the resuscitative measures are fully under way.

From the respiratory viewpoint, do the following:

- Perform a detailed examination of the airway, neck, and chest.
- Identify any swelling, bruising, or wounds.
- Re-examine for symmetry of breath sounds and movement.
- Do not forget to inspect and listen to the back of the chest.

Emergency treatment

All other urgent interventions are included in this phase.

If at any time the patient deteriorates, care returns to the primary assessment, and recycles through the system.

In the very sick or critically injured child, the primary assessment and resuscitation phases become integrally bound together. As a problem is identified, care shifts to the relevant intervention, before returning to the next part of the primary assessment. The simplified airway and breathing management protocol illustrates how this integration can be achieved.

Airway and breathing management protocol

Begin primary assessment. . . .
Assess the airway. . .
    If evidence of blunt trauma
        then protect the cervical spine from the outset
    If any evidence of obstruction and altered consciousness
        then optimise the head and neck positioning
        and administer oxygen
        and consider chin lift, jaw thrust, suction, foreign body removal
    If obstruction persists
        then consider oro- or nasopharyngeal airway
    If obstruction still persists
        then consider intubation and check the position of the tracheal tube
    If intubation impossible or unsuccessful
        then consider cricothyroidotomy

If stridor but relatively alert
   then allow self-ventilation whenever possible
   and encourage oxygen but do not force to wear mask
   and do not force to lie down
   and do not inspect the airway (except as a definitive procedure under controlled conditions)
   and assemble expert team and equipment
Assess the breathing . . .
  If respiratory arrest or depression
    then administer oxygen by bag-valve-mask
    and consider intubation and check the position of the tracheal tube
  If sedative or paralysing drugs possible
    then administer reversal agent
  If respiratory distress or tachypnoea
    then administer oxygen
  If lateralised ventilatory deficit
    then consider haemopneumothorax and inhaled foreign body
    and also consider lung consolidation, collapse, or pleural effusion
  If chest injury
    then consider tension pneumothorax and massive haemothorax
    and consider flail segment and open pneumothorax
  If evidence of tension pneumothorax
    then perform immediate needle decompression
    and follow up with chest drain
  If evidence of massive haemothorax
    then consider simultaneous chest drain
    and blood volume replacement
  If wheeze or crackles
    then consider asthma, bronchiolitis, pneumonia, and heart failure
    but remember inhaled foreign body as a possible cause
  If evidence of acute severe asthma
    then consider inhaled or intravenous β-agonists
    and consider intravenous steroids and aminophylline
Continue the primary assessment . . . .
    . . . . proceed to assess the circulation and nervous system
If deteriorating from whatever cause
    then reassess the airway and breathing
    and be prepared to intubate and ventilate

CHAPTER 6

The management of cardiac arrest

INTRODUCTION

Cardiac arrest has occurred when there are no palpable central pulses. Before any specific therapy is started effective basic life support must be established as described in Chapter 4.

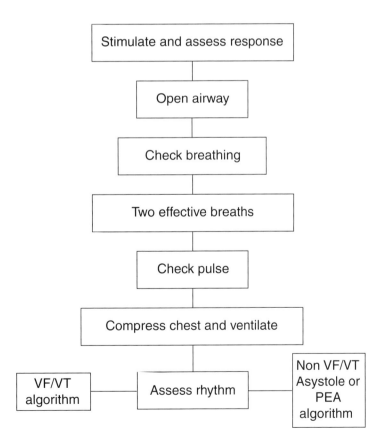

Figure 6.1. Initial approach to cardiac arrest

Three cardiac arrest rhythms will be discussed in this chapter:

1. Asystole.
2. Ventricular fibrillation and pulseless ventricular tachycardia.
3. Pulseless electrical activity (including electro mechanical dissociation).

The initial approach to cardiac arrest is shown in Figure 6.1 but for the purpose of teaching the arrest rhythms will be discussed separately.

ASYSTOLE

This is the most common arrest rhythm in children, because the response of the young heart to prolonged severe hypoxia and acidosis is progressive bradycardia leading to asystole.

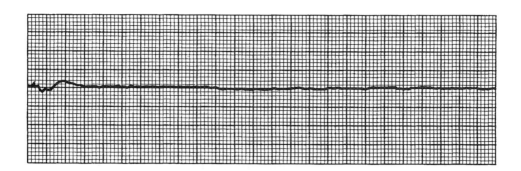

Figure 6.2. Asystole

The ECG will distinguish asystole from ventricular fibrillation, ventricular tachycardia and pulseless electrical activity. The ECG appearance of ventricular asystole is an almost straight line; occasionally P-waves are seen. Check that the appearance is not caused by an artifact, e.g. a loose wire or disconnected electrode. Turn up the gain on the ECG monitor.

Drugs in asystole

Before the administration of any drugs the patient must be receiving continuous and effective basic life support and ventilation with oxygen.

The protocol for drug use in asystole is shown in Figure 6.3.

Epinephrine (Adrenaline)
Epinephrine is the first line drug for asystole. Through adrenergic-mediated vaso-constriction, its action is to increase aortic diastolic pressure during chest compressions and thus coronary perfusion pressure and the delivery of oxygenated blood to the heart. It also enhances the contractile state of the heart and stimulates spontaneous contractions. The initial intravenous or intraosseous dose is 10 micrograms/kg (0·1 ml of 1:10 000 solution). This is best given through a central line but if one is not in place it may be given through a peripheral line.

In the child with no existing intravenous access the intraosseous route is recommended as the route of choice as it is rapid and effective. In each case the epinephrine is followed by a normal saline flush (2–5 ml). If circulatory access cannot be gained, the tracheal tube can be used. Ten times the intravenous dose (100 micrograms/kg) should

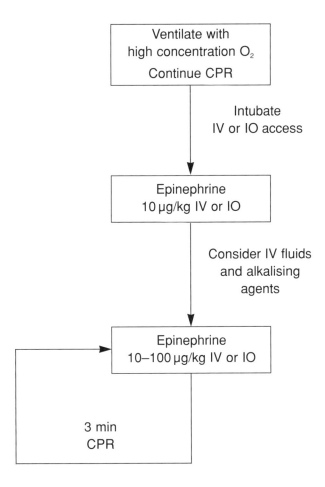

Figure 6.3. Protocol for drugs in asystole. CPR = cardiopulmonary resuscitation; IO = intraosseous; IV = intravenous

be given via this route. The drug should be injected quickly down a narrow bore suction catheter beyond the tracheal end of the tube and then flushed in with 1 or 2 ml of normal saline. In patients with pulmonary disease or prolonged asystole pulmonary oedema and intrapulmonary shunting may make the tracheal route poorly effective. If there has been no clinical effect, further doses should be given intravenously as soon as circulatory access has been secured.

Alkalising agents

Children with asystole will be acidotic as cardiac arrest has usually been preceded by respiratory arrest or shock. However, the routine use of alkalising agents has not been shown to be of benefit. Sodium bicarbonate therapy increases intracellular carbon dioxide levels so administration, if used at all, should follow assisted ventilation with oxygen, and effective BLS.

Once ventilation is ensured and epinephrine plus chest compressions are provided to maximize circulation, use of sodium bicarbonate may be considered for the patient with prolonged cardiac arrest or cardiac arrest associated with documented severe metabolic acidosis. These agents should be administered only in cases where profound acidosis is likely to adversely affect the action of epinephrine. An alkalising agent is usually considered if spontaneous circulation has not returned after the first or second dose of epinephrine. In addition sodium bicarbonate is recommended in the treatment of patients with hyperkalaemia (see Appendix B) and tricyclic antidepressant overdose (see Chapter 14).

In the arrested patient arterial pH does not correlate well with tissue pH. Mixed venous or central venous pH should be used to guide any further alkalising therapy and it should always be remembered that good basic life support is more effective than alkalising agents at raising myocardial pH.

Bicarbonate is the most common alkalising agent currently available, the dose being 1 mmol/kg (1 ml/kg of an 8·4% solution). Certain caveats must be kept in mind.

- Bicarbonate must not be given in the same intravenous line as calcium because precipitation will occur.
- Sodium bicarbonate inactivates epinephrine and dopamine and therefore the line must be flushed with saline if these drugs are subsequently given.
- Bicarbonate may not be given by the intra-tracheal route.

Intravenous fluids

In some situations, where the cardiac arrest has resulted from circulatory failure, a standard (20 ml/kg) bolus of crystalloid fluid should be given if there is no response to the initial dose of epinephrine.

Second epinephrine dose

There is no convincing evidence that a tenfold increase in epinephrine dose is beneficial in children and in some adult studies a deleterious effect was observed. However, there are some anecdotal cases of return of spontaneous circulation with large doses of epinephrine and therefore it can still be used for second and subsequent doses in patients where cardiac arrest is thought to have been secondary to circulatory collapse. It is clear that patient response to epinephrine is very variable, therefore if the patient has continuous intra-arterial monitoring the epinephrine dose can be titrated to best effect.

Vasopressin

Vasopressin is now being used in adult cardiac arrest as an alternative to epinephrine in shock resistant ventricular fibrillation. There is currently no evidence for its efficacy in children so it is not recommended.

Calcium

In the past, calcium was recommended in the treatment of electromechanical dissociation and asystole, but there is no evidence for its efficacy and there is evidence for harmful effects as calcium is implicated in cytoplasmic calcium accumulation in the final common pathway of cell death. This results from calcium entering cells following ischaemia and during reperfusion of ischaemic organs. Administration of calcium in resuscitation of asystolic patients is not recommended Calcium is indicated for treatment of documented hypocalcaemia and hyperkalaemia, and for the treatment of hypermagnesaemia and of calcium channel blocker overdose.

VENTRICULAR FIBRILLATION AND PULSELESS VENTRICULAR TACHYCARDIA

ECGs showing ventricular fibrillation and ventricular tachycardia are shown in Figures 6.4 and 6.5 respectively.

These arrhythmias are uncommon in children but may be expected in those suffering from hypothermia, poisoning by tricyclic antidepressants and with cardiac disease. The protocol for ventricular fibrillation and pulseless ventricular tachycardia is shown in Figure 6.6.

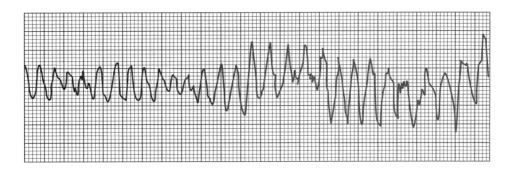

Figure 6.4. Ventricular fibrillation

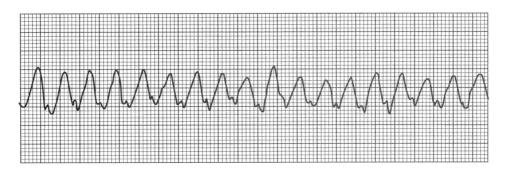

Figure 6.5. Ventricular tachycardia

Asynchronous electrical defibrillation should be carried out immediately. A precordial thump may be given in monitored children in whom the onset of the arrhythmia is witnessed and if the defibrillator is not immediately to hand. Paediatric paddles (4·5 cm) should be used for children under 10 kg. One electrode is placed over the apex in the mid axillary line, whilst the other is put immediately below the clavicle just to the right of the sternum. If only adult paddles are available for an infant under 10 kg one may be placed on the infant's back and one over the left lower part of the chest at the front.

The first two shocks are given at 2 J/kg. If these two attempts are unsuccessful the third shock should be at 4 J/kg. If three shocks fail to produce defibrillation attention must turn to supporting coronary and cerebral perfusion as in asystole. The airway should be secured and the patient ventilated with high flow oxygen. Epinephrine is given either as 10 micrograms/kg intravenously or intraosseously or as 100 micrograms/kg via the tracheal route, then three further shocks of 4 J/kg are administered. In between the shocks basic life support should not be interrupted for any cause.

After each shock the clinician should observe the ECG monitor. If the rhythm has altered, a pulse check should be carried out. If the rhythm has not altered, a pulse check should be carried out at the end of each set of three shocks.

Anti-arrhythmic drugs

Amiodarone is now the treatment of choice in shock resistant ventricular fibrillation and pulseless ventricular tachycardia. This is based on evidence from adult cardiac arrest and experience with the use of amiodarone in children in the catheterisation laboratory setting. The dose of amiodarone for VF/pulseless VT is 5 mg/kg via rapid IV/IO bolus followed by continued basic life support and a further defibrillation attempt within 60 seconds.

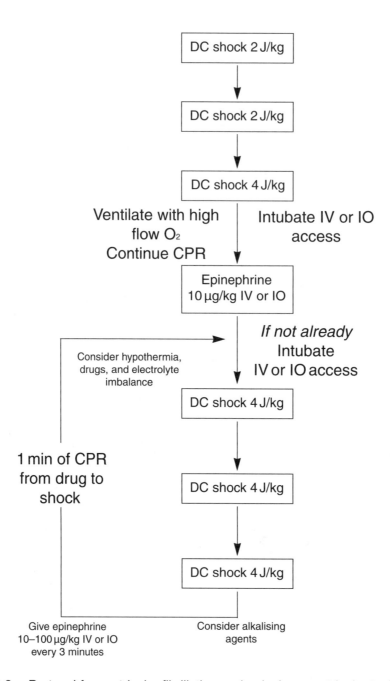

Figure 6.6. Protocol for ventricular fibrillation and pulseless ventricular tachycardia

Further doses of epinephrine (usually at low dose unless specifically indicated by the clinical situation) should be given every 3–5 minutes.

Lignocaine may still be considered but bretylium is no longer thought to be an appropriate agent in children.

After each drug CPR should continue for a minute to allow the drug to reach the heart before a further defibrillation attempt. It is DC shock that converts the heart back to a perfusing rhythm not the drug. The purpose of the anti-arrhythmic drug is to stabilise the converted rhythm and the purpose of epinephrine is to improve myocardial oxygenation by increasing coronary perfusion pressure. Epinephrine also increases the vigour and intensity of ventricular fibrillation which increases the success of defibrillation.

During the resuscitation the underlying cause of the arrhythmia should be considered. If the VF/VT is due to hypothermia then defibrillation may be resistant until core temperature is increased. Active rewarming should be commenced. If the VF has been caused by an overdose of tricyclic antidepressants then the patient should be alkalised (see Chapter 14) and anti-arrhythmic drugs avoided except under expert guidance. The possibility of hyperkalaemia should be considered and treated if identified with bicarbonate, insulin and glucose (see Appendix B).

If there is still resistance to defibrillation, different paddle positions or another defibrillator may be tried. In the infant in whom paediatric paddles have been used, larger paddles applied to the front and back of the chest may be an alternative.

If the rhythm initially converts and then deteriorates back to ventricular fibrillation or pulseless ventricular tachycardia then the lower defibrillation dose should be started following the giving of stabilising medication such as amiodarone.

Automatic External Defibrillators (AEDs)

The introduction of automatic external defibrillators in the pre-hospital setting and especially for public access is likely to significantly improve the outcome for VF cardiac arrest in adults. Current models have a fixed initial dose of electricity of 150–200 J which significantly exceeds the recommended dose of 2–4 J/kg in young children and infants.

In the prehospital setting, automatic external defibrillators (AEDs) are commonly used in adults to assess cardiac rhythm and to deliver defibrillation. In children AEDs can accurately detect ventricular fibrillation at all ages, but there is concern over their ability to identify correctly tachycardic rhythms in infants. At present, therefore, AEDs can be used to identify rhythms in children but not in infants.

The energy dose delivered by both monophasic and biphasic AEDs exceeds the recommended dose of 2–4 J/kg in most children < 8 years of age. The average weight of children > 8 years old is usually more than 25 kg. Therefore the initial dose from an AED (150–200 J) will be less than 10 J/kg. Children appear tolerant of high doses so this is a safe dose for the over 8 year old in VF/pulseless VT. Defibrillation of VF/pulseless VT detected by an AED may be considered in these older children. Defibrillation of children younger than approximately 8 years of age with energy doses typical of AEDs cannot be recommended. However, if an AED were the only defibrillator available to a clinician confronted with a child in VF/pulseless VT the majority opinion would be to use the device.

Institutions must be advised that AEDs are not suitable for the treatment of children under the age of 8 years and that alternative defibrillators must continue to be provided until suitable equipment is widely available.

Biphasic waveforms

Biphasic waveforms for transthoracic defibrillation appears to be as effective at lower energy doses than conventional waveforms in adults. There are currently inadequate data to recommend its use for treatment of VF/VT in children. However, if a biphasic waveform defibrillator was the only machine available to a clinician confronted with a child in VF/pulseless VT the majority opinion would be to use the device.

PULSELESS ELECTRICAL ACTIVITY (PEA)

This is the absence of a palpable pulse despite the presence of recognisable complexes on the ECG monitor. This is often a pre-asystolic state and is treated in the same way as asystole.

Sometimes, pulseless electrical activity is due to an identifiable and reversible cause. In children this is most often associated with trauma. In the trauma setting PEA may be caused by severe hypovolaemia, tension pneumothorax and pericardial tamponade.

PEA is also seen in hypothermic patients and in patients with electrolyte abnormalities, including hypocalcaemia from calcium channel blocker overdose. Rarely in children it may be seen after massive pulmonary thromboembolus.

It is appropriate to give an early bolus of 20 ml/kg of crystalloid as this will be supportive in cases related to trauma. In addition, however, a tension pneumothorax and/or pericardial tamponade requires definitive treatment. Continuing fluid replacement and the stemming of exsanguination may be required.

Rapid identification and treatment of reversible causes such as trauma, hypothermia, electrolyte and acid–base disturbance is vital.

Post-resuscitation management

Once spontaneous cardiac output has returned, frequent clinical reassessment must be carried out to detect deterioration or improvement with therapy. In the emergency department or ward situation, invasive monitoring may not be available. However, all patients should be monitored for:

- Pulse rate and rhythm — ECG monitor.
- Oxygen saturation — pulse oximeter.
- Core temperature — low reading thermometer.
- Skin temperature
- Blood pressure — non-invasive monitor.
- Urine output — urinary catheter.
- Arterial pH and gases — arterial blood sample.
- CO_2 monitoring — capnography.

Additionally some patients will require:

- Invasive BP monitoring — arterial cannula with pressure transducer.
- Central venous pressure monitoring — femoral, brachial or jugular catheter.
- Intracranial pressure monitoring — subarachnoid, subdural, or intraventricular devices.

These facilities may not be available until transfer to an intensive care setting.

The investigation shown in the box should be performed immediately following successful resuscitation:

Post-resuscitation investigations
• Chest radiograph
• Arterial and central venous blood gases
• Haemoglobin, haematocrit, and platelets
• Group and save serum for cross-match
• Na^+, K^+, urea, and creatinine
• Clotting screen
• Blood glucose
• Liver function tests
• 12-lead ECG

Often children who have been resuscitated from cardiac arrest die hours or days later from multiple organ failure. In addition to the cellular and homeostatic abnormalities that occur during the preceding illness, and during the arrest itself, cellular damage continues after spontaneous circulation has been restored. This is called reperfusion injury and is caused by the following:

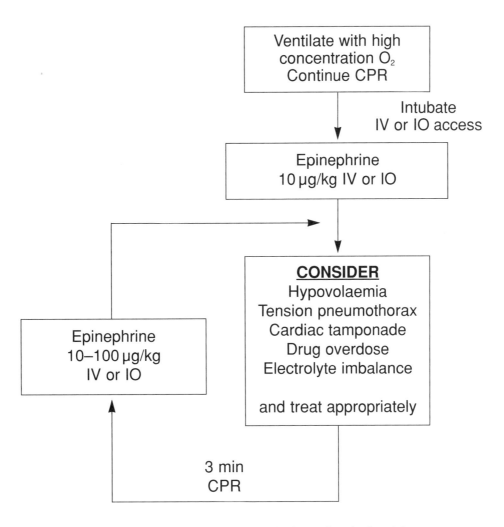

Figure 6.7. Protocol for pulseless electrical activity

- Depletion of ATP.
- Entry of calcium into cells.
- Free fatty acid metabolism activation.
- Free-radical oxygen production.

Post-resuscitation management aims to achieve and maintain homeostasis in order to optimise the chances of recovery. Management should be directed in a systematic way.

Airway and breathing

Most recently resuscitated patients will have an impaired conscious level or depressed gag reflex. These children should remain intubated, and should be ventilated with a fractional concentration of inspired oxygen (FIO_2) which is sufficient to keep oxygen saturation above 95%; other ventilation parameters should be set to keep blood gases as normal as possible.

Circulation

Following cardiac arrest from any cause there will usually be poor cardiac output. This may be due to any combination of the following factors:

- Underlying cardiac abnormality.
- Effects on myocardium of hypoxia, acidosis, and toxins, preceding and during arrest.
- Continuing acid–base or electrolyte disturbance.
- Hypovolaemia.

The following steps should be taken if there are signs of poor perfusion:

- Assess cardiac output clinically.
- Ensure normal arterial pH and oxygenation.
- Support ventilation.
- Identify and start to correct electrolyte abnormality or hypoglycaemia.
- Infuse crystalloid or colloid 20 ml/kg and reassess cardiac output clinically.
- Normalise body temperature to about 34°C if initially below 33°C and reduce hyperthermic temperatures to normal.

At this stage, there may be a need for:

- Further circulatory expansion.
- Inotropic drug support of the myocardium.
- Vasodilatation of the circulatory system.

A central venous pressure line will give useful information about systemic venous pressure which will assist in the decisions about fluid infusion or inotropic support. The central venous pressure measures right ventricular function and the effect of venous return on preload.

The central venous pressure is best used in assessing the response to a fluid challenge. In hypovolaemic patients, central venous pressure alters little with a fluid bolus, but in euvolaemia or hypervolaemia it shows a sustained rise.

Kidney

It is important both to maximise renal blood flow and to maintain renal tubular patency by maintaining urine flow. To achieve this the following are necessary:

- Maintenance of good oxygenation.
- Maintenance of good circulation using inotropes and fluids as required.
- Judicious use of diuretics (e.g. frusemide 1 mg/kg) to maintain urine output at or above 1 ml/kg/h.
- Monitoring and normalisation of electrolytes (Na^+, K^+, urea, creatinine) and acid–base balance in blood and urine.

Liver

Hepatic cellular damage can become manifest up to 24 hours following an arrest. Among other things coagulation factors can become depleted, and bleeding may be worsened by concomitant, ischaemia-induced, intravascular coagulopathy. The patient's clotting profile should be monitored and corrected as indicated with fresh frozen plasma.

Brain

The aim of therapy is to protect the brain from further (secondary) damage. To achieve this the cerebral blood flow must be maintained, normal cellular homeostasis must be achieved, and cerebral metabolic needs must be reduced.

Adequate cerebral blood flow can only be achieved if the cerebral perfusion pressure *(mean arterial pressure – intracranial pressure)* is kept about 5 mmHg. Cellular homeostasis is helped by normalisation of acid–base and electrolyte balances. Cerebral metabolic needs can be reduced by sedating the child and by controlling convulsions. Although barbiturate coma does reduce cerebral metabolism, it has not been shown to improve neurological outcome.

Practical steps to minimise secondary brain injury are:

· Maintenance of good oxygenation.
· Maintenance of good circulation using inotropes and fluids as required.
· Monitoring and normalisation of electrolytes (Na$^{]}$, K$^{]}$, urea, creatinine) and acid–base balance.
· Normalisation of blood glucose.
· Normalise body temperature to about 34°C if initially below 33°C and reduce hyperthermic temperatures to normal.
· Maintenance of adequate analgesia and sedation.
· Control of seizures.
· Reduction of intracranial pressure (see Chapter 18).

Drugs used to maintain perfusion following cardiac arrest

There are no research data comparing one drug to another that shows an advantage of any specific drug on outcome. In addition, the pharmacokinetics of these drugs vary from patient to patient and even from hour to hour in the same patient. Factors that influence, in an unmeasurable manner, the effects of these drugs include the child's age and maturity, underlying disease process, metabolic state, acid–base balance, the patient's autonomic and endocrine response, and liver and renal function. Therefore, the recommended infusion doses are starting points: the infusions must be adjusted according to patient response.

Dobutamine

Dobutamine increases myocardial contractility and has some vasodilating effect by decreasing peripheral vascular tone. Dobutamine is therefore particularly useful in the treatment of low cardiac output secondary to poor myocardial function for example in septic shock and following cardiac arrest. It is infused in a dose range of 2–20 micrograms/kg per minute. Higher infusion rates may produce tachycardia or ventricular ectopy. Pharmacokinetics and clinical response vary widely so the drug must be titrated according to individual patient response.

Infusion concentration: 15 mg/kg in 50 ml of 5% dextrose or normal saline will give 5 micrograms/kg/min if run at 1 ml/h.
To give 2–20 micrograms/kg/min give 0·4–4 ml/h of the above dilution.

Dopamine

Dopamine is an endogenous catecholamine with complex cardiovascular effects. At low infusion rates (0·5–2 micrograms/kg per minute), dopamine increases renal perfusion with little effect on systemic haemodynamics. At infusion rates greater than 5 micrograms/kg per minute, dopamine directly stimulates cardiac ß-adrenergic receptors and releases norepinephrine from cardiac sympathetic nerves. Myocardial norepinephrine stores are low in chronic congestive heart failure and in infants so the drug is less effective in those groups. Dopamine can be used instead of dobutamine in the treatment of circulatory shock following resuscitation or when shock is unresponsive to fluid administration. It can also be used with dobutamine but at the lower renal perfusion dose. Infusions are usually begun at 2–5 micrograms/kg per minute and may be increased to 10–20 micrograms/kg per minute

Dopamine infusions may produce tachycardia, vasoconstriction, and ventricular ectopy. Infiltration of dopamine into tissues can produce local tissue necrosis. Dopamine and other catecholamines are partially inactivated in alkaline solutions and therefore should not be mixed with sodium bicarbonate.

Infusion concentration: 15 mg/kg in 50 ml of 5% dextrose or normal saline will give 5 micrograms/kg/min if run at 1 ml/h.

To give 2–20 micrograms/kg/min give 0·4–4 ml/h of the above dilution.

Epinephrine

An epinephrine infusion is used in the treatment of shock with poor systemic perfusion from any cause that is unresponsive to fluid resuscitation. Epinephrine may be preferable to dobutamine or dopamine in patients with severe, hypotensive shock, and in very young infants in whom other inotropes may be ineffectual The infusion is started at 0·1–0·3 microgram/kg per minute and increased to 1 microgram/kg per minute depending on clinical response. Epinephrine should be infused only into a secure intravenous line because tissue infiltration may cause local ischaemia and ulceration.

Infusion concentration: 0·3 mg/kg in 50 ml of 5% dextrose or normal saline will give 0·1 microgram/kg/min if run at a rate of 1 ml/h.

To give 0·1–2·0 micrograms/kg/h give 1-20 ml/h of the above dilution.

3 mg/kg in 50 ml of 5% dextrose or normal saline will give 1 microgram/kg/min if run at a rate of 1ml/h.

To give 0·5–2·0 micrograms/kg/h give 0·5–2 ml/h of the above dilution.

Hypothermia

Recent data suggest that there is some evidence that post-arrest hypothermia (core temperatures of 33 to 36°C) may have beneficial effects on neurological recovery but there is insufficient evidence to recommend the routine use of hypothermia. Current recommendations are that post-arrest patients with core temperatures less than 37.5°C should not be actively rewarmed, unless the core temperature is < 33°C when they should be rewarmed to 34°C. Conversely, increased core temperature increases metabolic demand by 10–13% for each degree Centigrade increase in temperature above normal. Therefore in the post-arrest patient with compromised cardiac output, hyperthermia should be treated with active cooling to achieve a normal core temperature. Shivering should be prevented, since it will increase metabolic demand. Sedation may be adequate to control shivering, but neuromuscular blockade may be needed.

Hypoglycaemia

All children, especially infants can become hypoglycaemic when seriously ill. Blood glucose should be checked frequently and hypoglycaemia corrected carefully. It is important not to cause hyperglycaemia as this will promote an osmotic diuresis and also hyperglycaemia is associated with worse neurological outcome in animal models of cardiac arrest.

WHEN TO STOP RESUSCITATION

Resuscitation efforts are unlikely to be successful and can be discontinued if there is no return of spontaneous circulation at any time with up to 30 min of cumulative life support and in the absence of recurring or refractory VF/VT. Exceptions are patients with a history of poisoning or a primary hypothermic insult in whom prolonged attempts may occasionally be successful. Seek expert help from a toxicologist or paediatric intensivist.

CHAPTER

7

Resuscitation at birth

INTRODUCTION

The resuscitation of babies at birth is different from the resuscitation of all other age groups and knowledge of the relevant physiology and pathophysiology is essential. However, the majority of newly born babies will establish normal respiration and circulation spontaneously.

NORMAL PHYSIOLOGY

After the delivery of a healthy term baby the first breath usually occurs within 60–90 seconds of clamping or obstructing the umbilical cord. Clamping of the cord leads to the onset of asphyxia, which is the major stimulant to start respiration. Physical stimuli such as cold air or physical discomfort may also provoke respiratory efforts. The first breaths are especially important, as the lungs are initially full of fluid.

Labour causes the fluid producing cells within the lung to cease secretion and begin reabsorption of that fluid. During vaginal delivery up to 35 ml of fluid is expelled from the baby by uterine contraction. In a healthy baby the first spontaneous breaths generate a negative pressure of between -40 cm H_2O and -100 cm H_2O ($-3 \cdot 9$ and $-9 \cdot 8$ kPa), which inflate the lungs for the first time. This pressure is 10–15 times greater than that needed for later breathing when the lungs are aerated but is necessary to overcome the viscosity of fluid filling the airways, the surface tension of the fluid-filled lungs and the elastic recoil and resistance of the chest wall, lungs and airways. These powerful chest movements cause fluid to be displaced from the airways into the lymphatics.

In a 3 kg baby up to 100 ml of fluid are cleared from the airways following the initial breaths, a process aided by full inflation and prolonged high pressure on expiration, i.e. crying. Bypassing labour and vaginal delivery by caesarian section before the onset of labour may slow the clearance of pulmonary fluid from the lungs and reduce the initial functional reserve capacity.

The first breaths produce the baby's functional residual capacity. This is less likely to occur following caesarean delivery performed before the onset of labour. Neonatal circulatory adaptation commences with the detachment of the placenta but lung inflation and alveolar distension releases mediators, which affect the pulmonary vasculature as well as increasing oxygenation.

Surfactant (which is 85% lipid) is made by type II (granular) pneumocytes in the alveolar epithelium. Surfactant reduces alveolar surface tension and prevents alveolar collapse on expiration. Surfactant can be demonstrated from 20 weeks gestation, but the increase is slow until a surge in production at 30–34 weeks. Surfactant is released at birth due to aeration and distension of the alveoli. The half-life of surfactant is approximately 12 hours. Production is reduced by hypothermia (<35°C), hypoxia and acidosis (pH <7·25).

Pathophysiology

Our knowledge of the pathophysiology of fetal asphyxia is based on pioneering animal work in the early 1960s. The results of these experiments which followed the physiology of newborn animals during prolonged asphyxia and subsequent resuscitation are summarised in Figure 7.1.

When the placental oxygen supply is interrupted the foetus initiates breathing movements. Should these fail to provide an alternative oxygen supply (as they will obviously fail to do in utero) the baby loses consciousness. If hypoxia continues then the respiratory centre becomes unable to continue initiating breathing and breathing stops, usually within 2–3 minutes (primary apnoea). Babies have a number of automatic reflex responses to such a situation, conserving energy by shutting down the circulation to non-vital organs. Bradycardia ensues but blood pressure is maintained primarily by peripheral vasoconstriction but also an increased stroke volume. After a latent period of apnoea (primary), which may vary in duration, primitive spinal centres no longer suppressed by the respiratory centre exert an effect by initiating primitive gasping breaths. These deep spontaneous gasps are easily distinguishable from normal respirations as they occur 6–12 times per minute and involve all accessory muscles in a maximal inspiratory effort. After a while, if hypoxia continues, even this activity ceases (terminal apnoea). The time taken for such activity to cease is longer in the newly born baby than in later life, taking up to 20 minutes.

The circulation is almost always maintained until all respiratory activity ceases. This resilience is a feature of all newborn mammals at term, largely due to the reserves of glycogen in the heart. Resuscitation is therefore relatively easy if undertaken before all respiratory activity has stopped. Once the lungs are inflated, oxygen will be carried to the heart and then to the brain. Recovery will then be rapid. *Most* infants who have not progressed to terminal apnoea, will resuscitate themselves if their airway is patent.

Once gasping ceases, however, the circulation starts to fail and these infants are likely to need extensive resuscitation.

Meconium

Hypoxia in utero in the term infant (>37 weeks), leads to gut vessel vasoconstriction, increased peristalsis, and a relaxation of the sphincters. This can result in passage of meconium in utero. In addition, fetal hypoxia as described above, if severe enough, may lead to gasping and aspiration of amniotic fluid with meconium before birth.

Once the baby is delivered, meconium causes problems related to complete or partial airway obstruction. With the asphyxial insult this combines to produce a multi-organ problem, which is fortunately relatively uncommon in the UK.

Slight coloration of liquor with meconium is not significant.

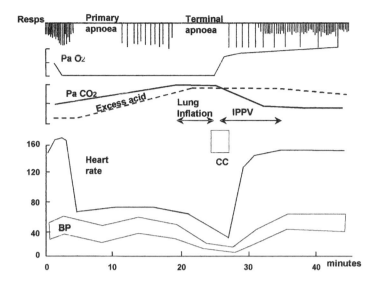

Figure 7.1. Effects of asphyxia (reproduced with permission from the Northern Neonatal Network)

Practical aspects of neonatal resuscitation

Most babies, even those born apnoeic, will resuscitate themselves given a clear airway. However, the basic approach to resuscitation is **A**irway, **B**reathing and **C**irculation but there are a number of additions to the formula:

- Get help
- Start the clock
- Dry, wrap and keep baby warm
- Assess baby

Call for help

Airway
Breathing (Lung inflation and ventilation)
Circulation

Ask for help if you expect or encounter any difficulty.

Start clock

If available or note the time.

Temperature control

Dry the baby off immediately and then wrap in a dry towel. A cold baby has an increased oxygen consumption and cold babies are more likely to become hypoglycaemic and acidotic, they also have an increased mortality. If this is not addressed at the beginning of resuscitation it is often forgotten. Most of the heat loss is by latent heat of

61

evaporation – hence the need to dry the baby and then to wrap the baby in a dry towel. Babies also have a large surface area to weight ratio – thus heat can be lost very quickly. Ideally delivery should take place in a warm room and an overhead heater should be switched on. However, drying effectively and wrapping the baby in a warm dry towel is the most important factor in avoiding hypothermia. A naked wet baby can still become hypothermic despite a warm room and a radiant heater, especially if there is a draught.

Assessment of the newborn

The Apgar score was proposed as tool for evaluating a baby's condition at birth. Although the score, calculated at 1 and 5 minutes, may be of some use retrospectively, it is almost always recorded very subjectively and it is not used to guide resuscitation. Acute assessment is made by assessing:

- Colour   (pink, blue, white)
- Respiration   (rate and quality)
- Heart rate   (fast, slow, absent)
- Tone   (unconscious, apnoeic babies are floppy)

This will categorise the baby into one of the three following groups:

1. *Pink, regular respirations, heart rate fast (more than 100/min)*
   These are healthy babies and they should be kept warm and given to their mothers.
2. *Blue, irregular or inadequate respirations, heart rate slow (60/min or less)*
   If gentle stimulation does not induce effective breathing, the airway should be opened and cleared. If the baby responds then no further resuscitation is needed. If not progress to lung inflation.
3. *Blue or white, apnoeic, heart rate slow (less than 60/min) or absent*
   Whether an apnoeic baby is in primary or secondary apnoea (Figure 7.1) the initial management is the same. Open the airway and then inflate the lungs. A reassessment of any heart rate response then directs further resuscitation. Reassess heart rate and respiration at regular intervals throughout.
   White colour, apnoea and low or absent heart rate suggest terminal apnoea. However initial management of such babies is unchanged but resuscitation may be prolonged.

Depending upon the assessment, resuscitation follows:

- Airway
- Breathing
- Circulation
- With the use of drugs in selected cases

Airway

The baby should be positioned with the head in the neutral position. Overextension may collapse the newborn baby's pharyngeal airway just as flexion will. Beware the large, often moulded, occiput. A folded towel placed under the neck and shoulders may help to maintain the airway in a neutral position and a jaw thrust may be needed to bring the tongue forward and open the airway, especially if the baby is floppy. Gentle suction of nares and oropharynx with a soft suction catheter may stimulate respiration. Blind deep pharyngeal suction should be avoided as it may cause vagally induced bradycardia and laryngospasm.

NEWBORN LIFE SUPPORT
Dry the baby, remove any wet cloth & cover

Initial Assessment at birth
Start the clock or note the time
Assess: COLOUR, TONE, BREATHING, HEART RATE

If not breathing...

Control the airway
Head in the neutral position

Support the breathing
If not breathing – FIVE INFLATION BREATHS (each 2–3 seconds duration)
Confirm a response: visible CHEST MOVEMENT or Increase in HEART RATE

If there is no response
Double check head position and apply JAW THRUST
5 inflation breaths
Confirm a response: visible CHEST MOVEMENT or increase in HEART RATE

If there is still no response
a) use a second person (if available) to help with airway control and repeat inflation breaths
b) inspect the oropharynx under direct vision and repeat inflation breaths
c) insert an oro-pharyngeal airway and repeat Inflation breaths
Consider intubation
Confirm a response: visible CHEST MOVEMENT or increase in HEART RATE

When the chest is moving
Continue with ventilation breaths if no spontaneous breathing

Check the heart rate
If the heart rate is not detectable or slow (less than around 60 bpm) and NOT rising

Start chest compressions
First confirm chest movement – if not moving return to airway
Cycles of 3 chest compressions to 1 breath for 30 seconds

Reassess pulse
If improving – stop chest compressions, if not breathing – continue ventilation
If heart rate still slow – continue ventilation and chest compressions
consider venous access and drugs at this stage

AT ALL STAGES, ASK... DO YOU NEED HELP??

Figure 7.2. Alogorithm for resuscitation at birth

Meconium aspiration

Meconium stained liquor in various guises is relatively common. Happily meconium aspiration is a rare event. Meconium aspiration usually happens in utero before delivery. It may be helpful to aspirate any meconium from the mouth and nose on the perineum. If the baby is vigorous a randomised trial has shown that no specific action (other than drying and wrapping the baby) is needed. If the baby is not vigorous inspect the oropharynx with a laryngoscope and aspirate any particulate meconium seen using a wide bore catheter. Suction should not exceed –100 mmHg (9·8 kPa). If intubation is possible and the baby is still unresponsive aspirate the trachea using the tracheal tube as a suction catheter. However, if intubation cannot be achieved immediately, clear the oropharynx and start mask inflation. If, while attempting to clear the airway, the heart rate falls to less than 60 bpm then stop airway clearance and start inflating the chest.

Breathing (Inflation Breaths and Ventilation)

The first five breaths should be inflation breaths. These should be 2–3 second sustained breaths using a continuous gas supply, a pressure-limiting device and a mask. Use a transparent, circular, soft mask big enough to cover the nose and mouth of the baby. If no such system is available then a 500 ml self-inflating bag and a blow off valve set at 30–40 cms H_2O can be used.

The chest may not move during the first 1–3 breaths as fluid is displaced. Once the chest is inflated reassess the heart rate. Assess air entry by chest movement not by auscultation. In fluid-filled lungs, breath sounds may be heard without lung inflation. However, it is safe to assume the chest has been inflated successfully if the heart rate responds.

Once the chest is inflated, ventilation is continued at a rate of 30-40 per minute.

Circulation

If the heart rate remains slow (less than 60 per minute) once the lungs are inflated, cardiac compressions must be started. The most efficient way of doing this in the neonate is to encircle the chest with both hands, so that the fingers lie behind the baby and the thumbs are apposed on the sternum just below the inter-nipple line. Compress the chest briskly, *by one third of its depth*. Current advice is to perform three compressions for each inflation of the chest.

The purpose of cardiac compression is to move oxygenated blood or drugs to the coronary arteries in order to initiate cardiac recovery. Thus there is no point in cardiac compression before the lungs have been inflated. Similarly, compressions are ineffective unless interposed breaths are of good quality and inflate the chest. The emphasis must be upon good quality breaths followed by effective compressions.

Once the heart rate is above 60/minute and rising, cardiac compression can be discontinued.

Drugs

If after adequate lung inflation and cardiac compression, the heart rate has not responded, drug therapy should be considered. However, the commonest reason for failure of the heart rate to respond is failure to achieve lung inflation. Airway and breathing must be reassessed as adequate before proceeding to drug therapy. Venous access will be required via an umbilical venous line as drugs should be given centrally. The outcome is poor if drugs are required for resuscitation.

Epinephrine (Adrenaline)

In the presence of profound unresponsive bradycardia or circulatory standstill, 10 micrograms/kg (0·1 ml/kg 1:10 000) epinephrine may be given intravenously or tracheally. Further doses of 10–30 micrograms/kg (0·1–0·3 ml 1:10 000) may be tried at 3–5 minute intervals if there is no response. For this drug the tracheal route is accepted but effectiveness is unproven in resuscitation at birth.

Bicarbonate

Any baby who is in terminal apnoea will have a significant metabolic acidosis. Acidosis depresses cardiac function and, in a highly acidotic environment epinephrine does not bind to receptors. Bicarbonate 1 mmol/kg (2 ml/kg of 4·2% solution) is used to raise the pH and enhance the effects of oxygen and epinephrine.

Bicarbonate remains controversial and should only be used in the absence of discernible cardiac output or in profound and unresponsive bradycardia.

Dextrose

Hypoglycaemia is a potential problem for all stressed or asphyxiated babies. It is treated by using a slow bolus of 5 ml/kg of 10% dextrose intravenously, and then providing a secure intravenous dextrose infusion at a rate of 100 ml/kg/day 10% dextrose. BM stix are not reliable in neonates when reading less than 5 mmol/l.

Fluid

Very occasionally hypovolaemia may be present because of known or suspected blood loss (antepartum haemorrhage, placenta or vasa praevia, unclamped cord) or be secondary to loss of vascular tone following asphyxia. Volume expansion, initially with 10 ml/kg, may be appropriate. Normal saline can be used; alternatively Gelofusine has been used safely and if blood loss is acute and severe, non-cross-matched O-negative blood should be given immediately. However, most newborn or neonatal resuscitations do not require fluid unless there has been known blood loss or septicaemic shock.

Naloxone

This is not a drug of resuscitation. Occasionally a baby who has been effectively resuscitated, is pink with a heart rate over 100 per minute, may not breathe because of the effects of maternal opiates. If respiratory depressant effects are suspected the baby should be given naloxone intramuscularly (200 micrograms in a full term baby). Smaller doses of 10 micrograms/kg will also reverse the sedation but the effect will only last a short time (20 minutes IV or a few hours IM).

Atropine and calcium gluconate

Atropine and calcium gluconate have no place in newborn resuscitation. Atropine may, rarely, be useful in the neonatal unit, when vagal stimulation has produced resistant bradycardia or asystole (see bradycardia protocol).

RESPONSE TO RESUSCITATION

Often the first indication of success will be an increase in heart rate. Recovery of respiratory drive may be delayed. Babies in terminal apnoea will tend to gasp first as they recover before starting normal respirations. Those who were in primary apnoea are likely to start with normal breaths, which may commence at any stage of resuscitation.

Tracheal intubation

Most babies can be resuscitated using a mask system. Swedish data suggests that if this is applied adequately, only 1:500 babies actually need intubation. However, tracheal intubation remains the gold standard in airway management. It is especially useful in prolonged resuscitations, preterm babies and meconium aspiration. It should be considered if mask ventilation has failed, although the most common reason for failure with mask inflation is poor positioning of the head with consequent failure to open the airway.

The technique of intubation is the same as for infants and is described in Chapter 22. A normal full term newborn usually needs a 3·5 mm tracheal tube, but 3·0 and 2·5 mm tubes should also be available.

Preterm babies

The more preterm a baby the less likely it is to establish adequate respirations. Preterm babies (<32 weeks) are likely to be deficient in surfactant. Effort of respiration will be increased although musculature will be less developed. One must anticipate that babies born before 32 weeks may need help to establish prompt aeration and ventilation.

Preterm babies with surfactant deficiency may need *relatively* higher inflation pressures than term babies. It is appropriate to start with a pressure of 2·0–2·5 kPa (20–25 cm H_2O) but to increase this if there is no heart rate response and chest movement is inadequate after initial breaths.

Preterm babies are more likely to get cold (higher surface area to mass ratio), more likely to be hypoglycaemic (fewer glycogen stores).

Actions in the event of poor initial response to resuscitation

1. Check airway and breathing
2. Check for a technical fault
    (a) Is oxygen connected?
    (b) Is mask ventilation effective? Auscultate both axillae and observe movement
    (c) Is tracheal tube in the trachea? Auscultate both axillae and observe movement
    (d) Is tracheal tube in the right bronchus? Auscultate both axillae and observe movement
    (e) Is tracheal tube blocked?
        If there is doubt about the position or patency of the tracheal tube replace it.
    (f) Is a longer inflation time required?
3. Does the baby have a pneumothorax? This occurs spontaneously in up to 1% of newborns but those needing action in the delivery unit are exceptionally rare. Auscultate the chest for asymmetry of breath sounds. A cold light source can be used to transilluminate the chest – a pneumothorax may show as a hyper-illuminating area. If a tension pneumothorax is thought to be present clinically, a 21 gauge butterfly needle should be inserted through the second intercostal space in the mid-clavicular line. Alternatively, a 22 gauge cannula may be used connected to a three-way tap. Remember that you may well cause a pneumothorax during this procedure.
4. Does the baby remain cyanosed despite breathing with a good heart rate? There may be a congenital heart malformation, which may be duct dependent (Chapter 10) or persistent pulmonary hypertension of the newborn.

5. If the baby is pink with a good heart rate but not breathing effectively it may be suffering the effects of maternal opiates. In this situation naloxone 200 micrograms IM may be given. This should outlast the opiate effect.
6. Is there severe anaemia or hypovolaemia? In the face of large blood loss, 20 ml/kg O-negative blood or a volume expander should be given.

DISCONTINUATION OF RESUSCITATION

Such a decision should be taken be taken by a senior member of the team, ideally a consultant. This means that help must have been called. The outcome for a baby with no cardiac output after 15 minutes of resuscitation is likely to be very poor.

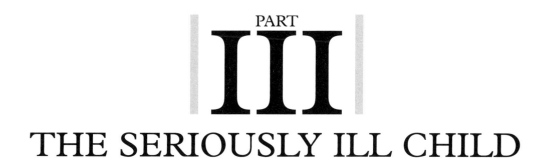

III

THE SERIOUSLY ILL CHILD

CHAPTER

8

The structured approach to the seriously ill child

INTRODUCTION

Treatment of a child in an emergency requires rapid assessment and urgent intervention. The structured approach includes:

> - Primary assessment
> - Resuscitation
> - Secondary assessment
> - Emergency treatment
> - Definitive care

Primary assessment and resuscitation involves management of the vital ABC functions and assessment of disability (CNS function). This assessment and stabilisation occurs before any illness-specific diagnostic assessment or treatment takes place. Once the patient's vital functions are supported, *secondary assessment and emergency treatment* begins. Illness-specific pathophysiology is sought and emergency treatments are instituted. During the secondary assessment vital signs should be checked frequently to detect any change in the child's condition. If there is deterioration then primary assessment and resuscitation should be repeated.

A discussion of *definitive* care is outside the scope of this text.

PRIMARY ASSESSMENT AND RESUSCITATION

In a severely ill child, a rapid examination of vital functions is required. The physical signs described in Chapter 3 are used in an ABC approach. This primary assessment and any necessary resuscitation must be completed before the more detailed secondary assessment is performed.

Airway

Primary assessment

Patency of the airway must be assessed. It is important to remember that the "look, listen, and feel" method of assessing airway patency is only effective if there is some spontaneous ventilation present.

- If the child can speak, this indicates that the airway is patent, that breathing is occurring and there is adequate circulation. The child may not respond to a health professional but may be induced to speak by the accompanying adult.
- If the child is too young or frightened to give a response then he or she may cry: this is an equally adequate indication that the airway is patent.
- If there is no evidence of air movement then chin lift or jaw thrust manoeuvres should be carried out and the airway reassessed. If there continues to be no evidence of air movement then airway patency can be assessed by performing an opening manoeuvre and giving rescue breaths (see Basic Life Support, Chapter 4).
- If there is stridor, upper airway pathology is implicated.

Resuscitation

If the airway is not patent when assessed by the "look, listen, and feel" technique, but patency can be secured by a chin lift or jaw thrust, then an airway adjunct may be required to maintain it. Intubation should be considered.

Breathing

Primary assessment

A patent airway does not ensure adequate ventilation. The latter requires an intact respiratory centre and adequate pulmonary function augmented by coordinated movement of the diaphragm and chest wall. The adequacy of breathing can be assessed as shown in the box.

Assessment of the adequacy of breathing

- *The effort of breathing*
    Recession
    Respiratory rate
    Inspiratory or expiratory noises
    Grunting
    Accessory muscle use
    Flare of the alae nasi
- *Effectiveness of breathing*
    Breath sounds
    Chest expansion
    Abdominal excursion
- *Effects of inadequate respiration*
    Heart rate
    Skin colour
    Mental status

The normal range of respiratory rate by age is given in Table 8.1.

Table 8.1.   Respiratory rate by age

Age (years)	Respiratory rate (breaths per minute)
<1	30–40
1–2	25–35
2–5	25–30
5–12	20–25
>12	15–20

A pulse oximeter should be put in place and the oxygen saturation while breathing air noted. A saturation of less than 90% while breathing air or less than 95% while breathing oxygen is very low.

Resuscitation

High-flow oxygen should be given to all children with respiratory difficulty or hypoxia. In the non-intubated patient the high-flow oxygen should be delivered via a non re-breathing mask with a reservoir bag.

In the child with inadequate breathing, this should be supported either with bag-valve-mask oxygenation or intubation and intermittent positive pressure ventilation.

Circulation

Primary assessment

Circulation is assessed as shown in the box. Circulation is more difficult to assess than breathing and individual measurements must not be over-interpreted.

Assessment of the adequacy of circulation

- *Cardiovascular status*
    Heart rate
    Pulse volume
    Capillary refill
    Blood pressure
- *Effects of circulatory inadequacy on other organs*
    Respiratory rate and character
    Skin appearance and temperature
    Mental status
    Urinary output
- *Signs of heart failure*
    Raised JVP
    Gallop rhythm
    Crepitations in lungs
    Enlarged liver

The normal circulatory parameters are as shown in Table 8.2.

Table 8.2.   Heart rate and systolic blood pressure by age

Age (years)	Heart rate (beats per minute)	Systolic blood pressure (mmHg)
<1	110–160	70–90
2–5	95–140	80–100
5–12	80–120	90–110
>12	60–100	100–120

The child's heart rate and pulse volume should be assessed by palpating both central and peripheral pulses. Capillary refill time (CRT) should be assessed with due allowance for ambient temperature. Normal CRT is less than 2 seconds.

The blood pressure should be measured using an appropriately sized cuff.

Resuscitation

Every child with an inadequate circulation (shock) should have oxygen at a high flow rate through a non re-breathing mask with a reservoir bag or via an tracheal tube if intubation has been necessary for airway control.

Venous or intraosseous access should be gained and an immediate infusion of crystalloid or colloid (20 ml/kg) given. Urgent blood samples may be taken at this point.

Disability (neurological evaluation)

Primary assessment

Both hypoxia and shock can cause a decrease in conscious level. Any problem with ABC must be addressed before assuming that a decrease in conscious level is due to a primary neurological problem.

The assessment proceeds as follows:

- The level of consciousness should be recorded using the AVPU scale.
  - **A** ALERT
  - **V** Responds to VOICE
  - **P** Responds to PAIN
  - **U** UNRESPONSIVE
- Pupillary size and reaction should be noted as a baseline.
- The presence of convulsive movements should be noted.
- Any patient with a decreased conscious level or convulsions must have an initial glucose stick test performed.

Resuscitation

In a child with a conscious level recorded as P or U (only responding to painful stimuli or unresponsive), consideration should be given to intubation to stabilise the airway.

Hypoglycaemia should be treated with 0·5 g/kg of dextrose (i.e. 5 ml/kg of 10% dextrose). Before the dextrose is given, blood must be taken for glucose measurement in the laboratory and a clotted sample for further studies.

Prolonged or recurrent fits require active intervention. Intravenous lorazepam or rectal diazepam should be given.

SECONDARY ASSESSMENT AND EMERGENCY TREATMENT

The secondary assessment takes place once vital functions have been assessed and the initial treatment of life threat to those vital functions has been started. It includes a medical history, a clinical examination and specific investigations. It differs from a standard medical history and examination in that it is designed to establish which emergency treatments might benefit the child. Time is limited and a focused approach is essential. At the end of secondary assessment, the practitioner should have a better understanding of the illness affecting the child and may have formulated a differential diagnosis. Emergency treatments will be appropriate at this stage – either to treat specific conditions (such as asthma) or processes (such as raised intracranial pressure). The establishment of a definite diagnosis is part of definitive care.

The history often provides the vital clues that help the practitioner identify the disease process and provide the appropriate emergency care. In the case of children, the history is often obtained from an accompanying parent, although a history should be sought from the child if possible. Do not forget to ask the paramedic about the child's initial condition and about treatments and response to treatments that have already been given.

Some children will present with an acute exacerbation of a known condition such as asthma or epilepsy. Such information is helpful in focusing attention on the appropriate system but the practitioner should be wary of dismissing new pathologies in such patients. The structured approach prevents this problem. Unlike trauma (which is dealt with later), illness affects systems rather than anatomical areas. The secondary assessment must reflect this and the history of the complaint should be sought with special attention to the presenting system or systems involved. After the presenting system has been dealt with, all other systems should be assessed and any additional emergency treatments commenced as appropriate.

The secondary assessment is not intended to complete the diagnostic process, but rather is intended to identify any problems that require emergency treatment.

The following gives an outline of a structured approach in the first hour of emergency management. It is not exhaustive but addresses the majority of emergency conditions which are amenable to specific emergency treatments in this time period.

The symptoms, signs and treatments relevant to each emergency condition are elaborated in the relevant chapters of Part III.

Respiratory

Secondary assessment

The box below gives common symptoms and signs which should be sought in the respiratory system. Emergency investigations are suggested.

Symptoms	Signs
Breathlessness	Tachypnoea
Coryza	Recession
Cough	Grunting
Noisy breathing (grunting, stridor, wheeze)	Flaring of alae nasi
	Stridor
Hoarseness	Wheeze
Drooling and inability to drink	Chest wall crepitus
Abdominal pain	Tracheal shift
Cyanosis	Abnormal percussion note
Recession	Crepitations on auscultation
Chest pain	
Apnoea	
Feeding difficulties	
Acidotic breathing	

Investigations

Peak flow if asthma suspected, chest X-ray (selective), arterial blood gases (selective), oxygen saturation

Emergency treatment
- If "bubbly" noises are heard, the airway is full of secretions requiring clearance by suction.
- If there is a harsh stridor associated with a barking cough and severe respiratory distress, upper airway obstruction due to severe croup should be suspected and the child given nebulised adrenaline (5 ml of 1:1000 nebulised in oxygen).

- If there is a quiet stridor in a sick-looking child, consider epiglottitis. (Rare but not gone!) Intubation may be required. Contact a senior anaesthetist urgently. Do not jeopardise the airway by unpleasant or frightening interventions.
- With a sudden onset and significant history of inhalation, consider a laryngeal foreign body. If the "choking child" procedure has been unsuccessful, the patient may require laryngoscopy. Do not jeopardise the airway by unpleasant or frightening interventions but contact a senior anaesthetist/ENT surgeon urgently. However, in extreme cases of life threat immediate direct laryngoscopy to remove a visible foreign body with Magill's forceps may be necessary.
- Stridor following ingestion/injection of a known allergen suggests anaphylaxis. Children in whom this is likely should receive IM epinephrine (10 µg/kg).
- Children with a history of asthma or with wheeze and significant respiratory distress, depressed peak flow and/or hypoxia should receive nebulised ß$_2$ agonists and ipratropium driven with oxygen. Infants are likely to have bronchiolitis and require only oxygen.
- In acidotic breathing, take arterial blood sample for acid–base balance and blood sugar. Treat diabetic ketoacidosis with IV normal (physiological) saline and insulin.

Cardiovascular (circulation)

Secondary assessment

The box below gives common symptoms and signs which should be sought in the cardiovascular system. Emergency investigations are suggested.

Symptoms	Signs
Breathlessness	Tachycardia
Fever	Bradycardia
Palpitations	Abnormal pulse volume or rhythm
Feeding difficulties	Abnormal skin perfusion or colour
Cyanosis	Hypotension
Pallor	Hypertension
Hypotonia	Abnormal ventilation rate or depth
Drowsiness	Hepatomegaly
Fluid loss	Auscultatory crepitations
Oliguria	Cardiac murmur
	Peripheral oedema
	Raised jugular venous pressure

Investigations
Urea and electrolytes, arterial blood gas, ECG, chest X-ray (selective), full blood count, blood culture (selective)

Emergency treatment
- Further boluses of fluid should be given to shocked children who have not had a sustained improvement to the first bolus given at resuscitation. Consider inotropes and intubation with the third bolus.
- Consider IV antibiotics in shocked children with no obvious fluid loss. Sepsis is likely.
- If a patient has a cardiac arrhythmia the appropriate protocol should be followed.
- If anaphylaxis is suspected in a shocked patient adrenaline should be given intramuscularly in a dose 10 micrograms/kg, in addition to fluid boluses.
- Consider duct-dependent congenital heart disease in infants with unresponsive shock. Give alprostadil.

Neurological (disability)

Secondary assessment

The box below gives common symptoms and signs which should be sought in the nervous system.

Symptoms	Signs
Headache	Altered conscious level
Convulsions	Convulsions
Change in behaviour	Altered pupil size and reactivity
Change in conscious level	Abnormal posture
Weakness	Abnormal oculo-cephalic reflexes
Visual disturbance	Meningism
Fever	Papilloedema or retinal haemorrhage
	Altered deep tendon reflexes
	Hypertension
	Slow pulse

Investigations
Urea and electrolyte, blood sugar, blood culture (selective)

Emergency treatment
- If convulsions persist, continue the status epilepticus protocol.
- If there is evidence of raised intracranial pressure, that is, an acutely unconscious patient with a decreasing conscious level and abnormal posturing and/or abnormal ocular motor reflexes, then the child should be intubated and ventilated. Consider giving mannitol 0·5 g/kg IV.
- In a child with a depressed conscious level or convulsions, consider meningitis/-encephalitis. Give cefotaxime/acyclovir.
- In drowsiness with sighing respirations check blood sugar, acid–base balance or salicylate level. Treat diabetic ketoacidosis with IV normal saline and insulin.
- In unconscious children with pin-point pupils, consider opiate poisoning. A trial of naloxone should be given.

External (exposure)

Secondary assessment

The box below gives common symptoms and signs which should be sought externally.

Symptoms	Signs
Rash	Purpura
Swelling of lips/tongue	Urticaria
Fever	Angio-oedema

Emergency treatment
- In a child with circulatory or neurological symptoms and signs, a purpuric rash suggests septicaemia/meningitis. The patient should receive cefotaxime preceded by a blood culture.
- In a child with respiratory or circulatory difficulty, the presence of an urticarial rash or angio-oedema suggests anaphylaxis. Give epinephrine (10 μg/kg) IM.

Gastrointestinal

Gastrointestinal emergencies usually present with shock from fluid loss. This will become apparent during the primary assessment of the circulation or the secondary assessment of the cardiovascular system. The symptoms and signs shown in the box below may be useful in that they may suggest the need for surgical involvement.

Symptoms	Signs
Vomiting	Abdominal tenderness
Blood PR	Abdominal mass
Abdominal pain	

Further history

Developmental and social history

Particularly in a small child or infant, knowledge of the child's developmental progress and immunisation status may be useful. The family circumstances may also be helpful, sometimes prompting parents to remember other details of the family's medical history.

Drugs and allergies

Any medication that the child is currently on or has been on should be recorded and in addition any medication in the home that the child might have had access to if poisoning is a possibility.

SUMMARY

The structured approach to the seriously ill child outlined here allows the practitioner to focus on the appropriate level of diagnosis and treatment during the first hour of care. Primary assessment and resuscitation are concerned with the maintenance of vital functions, while secondary assessment and emergency treatment allow more specific urgent therapies to be started. This latter phase of care requires a system-by-system approach and this minimises the chances of significant conditions being missed.

In the following chapters the recognition, resuscitation and emergency management of children with:

- breathing difficulties
- shock
- abnormalities of pulse rate or rhythm
- decreased conscious level
- convulsions and
- poisoning

are discussed in more detail.

CHAPTER
9

The child with breathing difficulties

INTRODUCTION

Most children with breathing difficulties will have an upper or lower respiratory tract illness. These are the commonest causes of acute benign conditions in children but are also the most likely causes of life-threatening illness, especially in the very young. However, cardiac disease and also unintentional injury such as choking and poisoning can present as breathing difficulties. This chapter will provide the student with an approach to the assessment, resuscitation and emergency management of such children.

While parents are usually alert to breathing difficulties in toddlers and older children, abnormal respiration may be more difficult for them to detect in infants. Infants with breathing difficulties may present as acute feeding problems. Feeding is one of an infant's most strenuous activities and parents are accustomed to seeing feeding as a gauge of their infant's wellbeing.

SUSCEPTIBILITY OF CHILDREN TO SEVERE RESPIRATORY ILLNESS

Disorders of the respiratory tract are the commonest illnesses of childhood. They are the most frequent reason for children to be seen by their general practitioner and they account for 30–40% of acute medical admissions to hospital in children. Despite advances in the management of respiratory illnesses, they still result in almost 300 deaths in children between the ages of 4 weeks and 14 years in England and Wales each year: approximately half of these deaths are in children less than 12 months old (ONS 1998).

Most respiratory illnesses are self-limiting minor infections, but a few present as potentially life-threatening emergencies. In these, accurate diagnosis and prompt initiation of appropriate treatment are essential if unnecessary morbidity and mortality are to be avoided.

The pattern of severe respiratory illness in children is different from that in adults. These variations reflect important differences in the immune status, and the structure and function of the lungs and chest wall of children and adults.

- Children, and particularly infants, are susceptible to infection with many organisms to which adults have acquired immunity.
- The upper and the lower airways in children are smaller, and are more easily obstructed by mucosal swelling, secretions or a foreign body. Airway resistance is inversely proportional to the fourth power of the radius of the airway: a reduction in the radius by a half causes a 16-fold increase in airway resistance. Thus, 1 mm of mucosal oedema in an infant's trachea of 5 mm diameter results in a much greater increase in resistance than the same degree of oedema in the trachea of 10 mm diameter.
- The thoracic cage of young children is much more compliant than that of adults. When there is airways obstruction and increased inspiratory effort, this increased compliance results in marked chest wall recession and a reduction in the efficiency of breathing.
- The respiratory muscles of young children are relatively inefficient. In infancy, the diaphragm is the principal respiratory muscle, and the intercostal and accessory muscles make relatively little contribution. Respiratory muscle fatigue can develop rapidly and result in respiratory failure and apnoea.

APPROACH TO THE CHILD WITH BREATHING DIFFICULTIES

PRIMARY ASSESSMENT

Airway

Assess airway patency by the "look, listen, and feel" method.
Note the presence of inspiratory noises. *Stridor suggests an upper airway pathology.*

Breathing

Assess the adequacy of breathing.

- *Effort of breathing*
    Recession. *These signs are common to all conditions with breathing difficulty, but sternal recession is particularly associated with upper airway obstruction.*
    Respiratory rate. *Hypoventilation, i.e. a slow rate and/or shallow breaths in a child with serious breathing difficulty suggests exhaustion.*
    Grunting
    Accessory muscle use
    Flare of the alae nasi
- *Efficacy of breathing*
    Breath sounds
    Chest expansion/abdominal excursion
- *Effects of inadequate respiration*
    Heart rate
    Skin colour
    Mental status
    Check oxygen saturation on the pulse oximeter in air and in high flow oxygen

Note the presence of expiratory noises. *Wheeze suggests a lower airway pathology.*

Circulation

Assess the adequacy of circulation

- *Cardiovascular status*
   Heart rate and rhythm. *Tachycardia is expected; bradycardia is a sign of respiratory failure*
   Pulse volume
   Capillary refill
   Blood pressure
- *Effects of circulatory inadequacy on other organs*
   Acidotic sighing respirations
   Pale or cyanosed skin colour. *Central cyanosis that does not improve with high flow oxygen suggests a congenital heart disease with a right to left shunt*
   Mental status: agitation or depressed conscious level
   Urinary output
- Note the presence of signs of heart failure *which will suggest a cardiac cause for the breathlessness.*
   Tachycardia
   Raised jugular venous pressure (often absent in infants with heart failure)
   Lung crepitations on auscultation
   Gallop rhythm
   Enlarged liver

and listen for a heart murmur.

Disability

- Assess neurological function.
- A rapid measure of level of consciousness should be recorded using the AVPU scale.
- Note the child's posture. *Children in respiratory failure are usually hypotonic.*
- The presence of convulsive movements should be noted.

Exposure

- Take the child's core temperature. *A fever suggests an infectious cause (although the absence of a fever does not exclude infection).*
- Look for a rash. *An urticarial rash suggests anaphylaxis.*

RESUSCITATION

Airway

- A patent airway is the first requisite. If the airway is not patent an airway opening manoeuvre should be used. The airway should then be secured with a pharyngeal airway device or by intubation with experienced senior help.

Breathing

- All children with breathing difficulties should receive high flow oxygen through a face mask with oxygen as soon as the airway has been demonstrated to be adequate

- If the child is hypoventilating with a slow respiratory rate or weak effort, respiration should be supported with oxygen via a bag-valve-mask device and experienced senior help summoned

Key features

While the primary assessment and resuscitation are being carried out a focused history of the child's health and activity over the previous 24 hours and any significant previous illness should be gained.

All children with breathing difficulties will have varying degrees of respiratory distress and cough so these are not useful diagnostic discriminators.

Certain key features which will be identified clinically in the above assessment and from the focused history can point the clinician to the likeliest working diagnosis for emergency treatment.

- Inspiratory noises, i.e. *stridor* point to upper airway obstruction.
- Expiratory noises, i.e. *wheeze* point to lower airway obstruction.
- Fever without stridor points to *pneumonia*.
- Signs of heart failure point to congenital or acquired *heart disease*.
- Suspicion of ingestion and absence of cardio-respiratory pathology point to *poisoning*.

APPROACH TO THE CHILD WITH STRIDOR

Obstruction of the upper airway (larynx and trachea) is potentially life-threatening. The small cross-sectional area of the upper airway renders the young child particularly vulnerable to obstruction by oedema, secretions or an inhaled foreign body.

Table 9.1. Causes of stridor

Incidence (UK)	Diagnoses
Very common	Croup – viral laryngotracheitis
Common	Croup – recurrent or spasmodic croup
Uncommon	Laryngeal foreign body
Rare	Epiglottis
	Croup – bacterial tracheitis
	Trauma
	Infectious mononucleosis
	Angioneurotic oedema
	Retropharyngeal abscess
	Inhalation of hot gases
	Diphtheria

Reassess airway

Is the airway partially obstructed or narrowed and what is the likely cause?
Note the presence of inspiratory noises.

- If "bubbly" noises are heard, the airway is full of secretions requiring clearance. This also suggests that the child is either very *fatigued*, or has a *depressed conscious level* and cannot clear the secretions himself by coughing. The child with cerebral palsy may often demonstrate this sign as he may have permanently poor airway control.
- If stertorous (snoring) respiratory noises are heard, consider partial obstruction of the airway due to *depressed conscious level.*

- If there is a harsh stridor associated with a barking cough, upper airway obstruction due to *croup* should be suspected.
- If a quiet stridor in a sick looking child is present, consider *epiglottitis*.
- With a very sudden onset, no prodromal symptoms and a history suggestive of inhalation, consider a laryngeal *foreign body*.

Reassess the breathing: what degree of *effort* is needed for breathing and what is its *efficacy* and *effect*?

The answer to this question will inform the clinician as to the severity of the upper airway obstruction.

A pulse oximeter should be put in place and the oxygen saturation both on breathing air and high flow oxygen noted.

AIRWAY EMERGENCY TREATMENT

In the child with a compromised but functioning airway an important principle in all cases is to avoid worsening the situation by upsetting the child. Crying and struggling may quickly convert a partially obstructed airway into a completely obstructed one. Administration of oxygen, nebulised epinephrine or the performance of a radiograph may all require skill. Parents' help should be enlisted.

Partial obstruction from secretions/depressed conscious level

An airway partially obstructed by secretions should be cleared by suction as long as there is no stridor. The child with the stertorous breathing of partial obstruction due to a depressed conscious level or extreme fatigue is in danger of losing the airway completely. The airway must be supported by a chin lift or jaw thrust manoeuvre and an anaesthetist asked to attend urgently. Consideration should be given to maintaining the airway with an oro-pharyngeal or naso-pharyngeal airway and the child may require intubation.

Croup syndromes

Patients with severe respiratory distress in association with harsh stridor and barking cough should be given nebulised epinephrine (5 ml of 1:1 000) with oxygen through a face mask. This will produce a transient improvement for 30–60 minutes but rarely alters the long-term course of the illness. This treatment should be given only to children with signs of severe obstruction. Epinephrine reduces the clinical severity of obstruction, but does not improve arterial blood gases, reduce the duration of hospitalization or the need for intubation. Children who have received epinephrine will appear improved for a short while only and need to be observed very closely with continuous ECG and oxygen saturation monitoring. They may later require tracheal intubation. A marked tachycardia is usually produced by the epinephrine, but other side effects are uncommon. This treatment is best used to "buy time" in which to assemble an experienced team to treat a child with severe croup.

Many children admitted to hospital with croup have hypoxaemia as a result of alveolar hypoventilation secondary to airways obstruction and ventilation perfusion imbalance. The degree of hypoxaemia correlates poorly with clinical signs: the respiratory rate and the degree of sternal recession are the best clinical indicators. Humidified oxygen should be given through a face-mask, and, the oxygen saturation monitored. Oxygen saturation measurements are helpful in assessing severity and response to treatment but hypoventilation may be masked when the child is receiving high ambient oxygen. The oxygen saturation with the child breathing air should be checked intermittently.

Inhalation of warm moist air is widely used but is of unproven benefit.

Foreign body

Children with severe respiratory distress and a significant history of foreign body inhalation may require laryngoscopy if the "choking child" procedure has been unsuccessful. Do not jeopardise the airway by unpleasant or frightening interventions, but contact a senior anaesthetist/ENT surgeon urgently. However, in extreme cases of life threat immediate direct laryngoscopy with Magills forceps to remove a visible foreign body may be necessary.

Epiglottitis

Children with severe respiratory distress and a soft inspiratory stridor are candidates for epiglottitis. Intubation may be required. Contact a senior anaesthetist urgently. Do not jeopardise the airway by unpleasant or frightening interventions. The diagnosis of acute epiglottitis is made from the characteristic history and clinical findings. Lateral radiographs of the neck have been used to confirm the diagnosis, but these should be avoided as they disturb the child and have precipitated fatal total airway obstruction.

There is no evidence that nebulised epinephrine or steroids are beneficial. The child will need intubation after careful gaseous induction of anaesthesia. This must be done by an experienced anaesthetist unless there has been a respiratory arrest. When deeply anaesthetised the child can be laid on his back to allow laryngoscopy and intubation. Tracheal intubation may be difficult because of the intense swelling and inflammation of the epiglottis ("cherry red epiglottis"). A much smaller tube than the one usually required for the child's size will be necessary.

Anaphylaxis

In addition to oxygen, the specific treatment for anaphylaxis is intramuscular epinephrine (10 micrograms/kg). Nebulised adrenaline as described above in the treatment of croup may also be given (see also page 107).

Further treatment for upper airway conditions

Croup

There is now good evidence that steroids modify the natural history of croup. Children with mild, moderate or severe croup can benefit from steroid treatment. Current treatments are either systemic dexamethasone 0·15 mg/kg or inhaled nebulised budenoside 1 milligram. Dexamethasone can be continued once daily for two to three days if symptoms persist and budenoside may be repeated 30–60 minutes later if clinically indicated. Budenoside and dexamethasone are equally effective. The choice will depend on which route is most appropriate for the individual child but oral dexamethasone is the treatment of choice. The use of steroids in croup gives rise to some clinical improvement within hours and may lead to a reduction in hospital stay.

Fewer than 5% of children admitted to hospital with croup require tracheal intubation. The decision to intubate is a clinical one based on increasing tachycardia, tachypnoea and chest retraction, or the appearance of cyanosis, exhaustion or confusion. Ideally, the procedure should be performed under general anaesthetic by an experienced paediatric anaesthetist, unless there has been a respiratory arrest. A much smaller gauge tracheal tube than usual is often required. If there is doubt about the diagnosis, or difficulty in intubation is anticipated, an ENT surgeon capable of performing a tracheotomy should be present. The median duration of intubation in croup is 3 days: the younger the child, the longer intubation is usually required. Prednisolone (1 mg/kg every 12 hours) reduces the duration of intubation and the need for re-intubation in children with severe croup. All intubated children must have continuous CO_2 and SaO_2 monitoring.

Over 80% of children with the rarer bacterial tracheitis need intubation and ventilatory support to maintain an adequate airway, as well as intravenous antibiotics (combination of flucloxacillin and cefotaxime).

Epiglottitis

This is now a rare condition in countries where HiB immunisation has been introduced. However, it does still occur, in an older age group, in cases of vaccine failure and in unimmunised children. Once the airway has been secured, blood should be sent for culture and treatment with intravenous cefotaxime or ceftriaxone commenced. With appropriate treatment, most children can be extubated after 24–36 hours and have recovered fully within 3–5 days. Complications such as hypoxic cerebral damage, pulmonary oedema and other serious *Haemophilus* infections are rare but in the under two year old, immunity is not secure and there are cases of secondary HiB meningitis occurring after successful treatment of epiglottitis. In countries where the HiB vaccine is in use there should be an investigation into vaccine failure.

Foreign body

In the case of the stridulous child with a relatively stable airway and a strong suspicion of foreign body inhalation, careful gaseous induction of anaesthesia should be induced by an experienced anaesthetist, with the presence of an ENT surgeon to perform a tracheotomy in case of disaster. The foreign body can then be removed under controlled conditions. In some cases, prior to anaesthesia, it may be appropriate to perform a careful lateral neck radiograph in the emergency room (taking extreme care not to distress the child, thus provoking complete obstruction) to ascertain the position and nature of the object.

Anaphylaxis

If there has not been significant improvement with the initial dose of epinephrine, a further intramuscular dose can be given after five minutes. Chlorpheniramine and steroids are also given to patients with anaphylaxis but their onset of action (if any) is delayed (see page 109).

Background information on conditions causing acute upper airway obstruction

Most cases of upper airway obstruction in children are the result of infection, but inhalation of a foreign body or hot gases (house fires), angioneurotic oedema and trauma can all result in obstruction and the normal airway will become obstructed in the unconscious, supine patient.

Croup

Croup is defined as an acute clinical syndrome with inspiratory stridor, a barking cough, hoarseness and variable degrees of respiratory distress. This definition embraces several distinct disorders. Acute viral laryngotracheobronchitis (viral croup) is the commonest form of croup and accounts for over 95% of laryngotracheal infections. Parainfluenza viruses are the commonest pathogens but other respiratory viruses, such as respiratory syncytial virus and adenoviruses produce a similar clinical picture. The peak incidence of viral croup is in the second year of life and most hospital admissions are in children aged between 6 months and five years.

The typical features of a barking cough, harsh stridor and hoarseness are usually preceded by fever and coryza for 1–3 days. The symptoms often start, and are worse, at night. Many children have stridor and a mild fever (<38·5°C), with little or no respiratory difficulty. If tracheal narrowing is minor, stridor will be present only when the child hyperventilates or is upset. As the narrowing progresses, the stridor becomes both inspiratory and expiratory and is present even when the child is at rest. Some children, and particularly those below the age of three, develop the features of increasing obstruction and hypoxaemia with marked sternal and subcostal recession, tachycardia, tachypnoea and agitation. If the infection extends distally to the bronchi, wheeze may also be audible.

Some children have repeated episodes of croup without preceding fever and coryza. The symptoms are often of sudden onset at night, and usually persist for only a few hours. This recurrent or spasmodic croup is often associated with atopic disease (asthma, eczema, hay-fever). The episodes can be severe, but are more commonly self-limiting. They are difficult to distinguish clinically from infectious croup and appear to respond identically to treatment.

Bacterial tracheitis, or pseudomembranous croup, is an uncommon but life-threatening form of croup. Infection of the tracheal mucosa with *Staphyloccocus aureus*, streptococci or *Haemophilus influenzae* B (HiB) results in copious, purulent secretions and mucosal necrosis. The child appears toxic with a high fever and the signs of progressive upper airway obstruction. The croupy cough and the absence of drooling helps distinguish this condition from epiglottitis. Over 80% of children with this illness need intubation and ventilatory support to maintain an adequate airway, as well as intravenous antibiotics (combination of flucloxacillin and cefotaxime).

Acute epiglottitis

Acute epiglottitis shares many clinical features with croup but it is a quite distinct entity. Although much less common than croup, its importance is that unless the diagnosis is made rapidly and appropriate treatment commenced, total obstruction and death are likely to ensue. In countries where routine immunisation of infants with the conjugate vaccine against HiB has been introduced, there has been a dramatic reduction in the incidence of epiglottitis.

Infection with *Haemophilus influenzae* B causes intense swelling of the epiglottis and the surrounding tissues and obstruction of the larynx. Epiglottitis is most common in children aged 1–6 years, but it can occur in infants and in adults.

The onset of the illness is usually acute with high fever, lethargy, a soft inspiratory stridor and rapidly increasing respiratory difficulty over 3–6 hours. In contrast to croup, cough is minimal or absent. Typically the child sits immobile, with the chin slightly raised and the mouth open, drooling saliva. He looks very toxic, pale and has poor peripheral circulation (most are septicaemic). There is usually a high fever ($>39°C$). Because the throat is so painful, the child is reluctant to speak and unable to swallow drinks or saliva. Disturbance of the child, and particularly attempts to lie the child down, to examine the throat with a spatula, or to insert an intravenous cannula, can precipitate total obstruction and death, and must be avoided.

Other causes of upper airways obstruction

Although croup accounts for the large majority of cases of acute upper airways obstruction, several other uncommon conditions need to be considered in the differential diagnosis. *Diphtheria* is seen only in children who have not been immunised against the disease. Always ask about immunisations in any child with fever and the signs of upper airways obstruction, particularly if they have been to endemic areas recently.

Marked tonsillar swelling in *infectious mononucleosis or acute tonsillitis* can rarely compromise the upper airway. The passage of a nasopharyngeal tube may give instant relief. *Retropharyngeal abscess* is uncommon nowadays, but can present with fever and the features of upper airway obstruction together with feeding difficulties. Treatment is by surgical drainage and intravenous antibiotics.

Anaphylaxis is a potentially life-threatening immunologically mediated syndrome in which laryngeal oedema can develop over minutes often with swelling (angioneurotic oedema) of the face, mouth and tongue. Food allergies, especially nuts and drug reactions, especially contrast media and anaesthetic drugs are usual causes of this.

Prodromal symptoms of flushing, itching, facial swelling and urticaria usually precede stridor. Abdominal pain, diarrhoea, wheeze and shock may be additional or alternative manifestations of anaphylaxis (page 108).

A severe episode of anaphylaxis can be predicted in patients with a previous severe episode or a history of increasingly severe reaction, a history of asthma or treatment with beta blockers.

The inquisitive and fearless toddler and the infant with toddler siblings is at risk of inhaling a *foreign body*. If an inhaled foreign body lodges in the larynx or trachea, the outcome is often fatal at home, unless measures such as those discussed in Chapter 4 are performed. Should a child present to hospital, especially during waking hours, with very sudden onset of stridor and other signs of acute upper airway obstruction, and particularly if there is no fever or preceding illness, then a laryngeal foreign body is the likely diagnosis. A history of eating or of playing with small objects immediately prior to the onset of symptoms is strong supportive evidence. Foodstuffs (nuts, sweets, meat) are the commonest offending items. In 1998 16 children in England and Wales died from choking. In all but one food was the cause of obstruction. In some instances, objects may compress the trachea from their position of lodgement in the upper oesophagus producing a similar but less severe picture of airway obstruction.

The object may pass through the larynx into the bronchial tree, where it produces a persistent cough of very acute onset, and unilateral wheezing. Examination of the chest may reveal decreased air entry on one side or evidence of a collapsed lung. Inspiratory and expiratory chest radiographs may show mediastinal shift on expiration due to gas-trapping distal to the bronchial foreign body. Removal through a bronchoscope under general anaesthetic should be performed as soon as possible as there is a risk of coughing moving the object into the trachea and causing life-threatening obstruction.

APPROACH TO THE CHILD WITH WHEEZE

Asthma and bronchiolitis are the two common causes of lower respiratory obstruction. Almost without exception, bronchiolitis is confined to the under one year olds and asthma is much more commonly diagnosed in the over ones.

It is often difficult to assess the *severity* of an acute exacerbation of asthma. Important points in the history include the duration of symptoms, what treatment has already been given in this episode and the response to that treatment, and the course of previous attacks. Children who have previously required intravenous therapy, and particularly those who have required admission to an intensive care unit are at high risk of life-threatening episodes.

Physical signs such as wheeze and respiratory rate are poor indicators of severity. Use of accessory muscles, recession and pulse rate are better guides. Pulsus paradoxus (the difference between systolic pressure on inspiration and expiration) is no longer considered a reliable sign to assess the severity of asthma although its presence is usually associated with moderate to severe asthma. Cyanosis, fatigue and drowsiness are a late signs indicating life-threatening asthma and are usually accompanied by a silent chest on auscultation, indicating that virtually no air is being exchanged.

The peak expiratory flow rate (PEFR) is a valuable measure of severity and should be a routine part of the assessment. Children below the age of five and those who are very dyspnoeic, are usually unable to produce reliable readings. Arterial oxygen saturation as measured non-invasively by a pulse oximeter (SaO_2) is useful in assessing severity, monitoring progress and predicting outcome in acute asthma. All children with a PEFR < 33% of their predicted value, or those with a saturation of less than 85% in air have life-threatening asthma (see box). Other concerns include a poor response to repeated doses of bronchodilator at home, or increasing exhaustion. A chest radiograph is indicated only if there is severe dyspnoea, uncertainty about the diagnosis, asymmetry of chest signs or signs of severe infection.

Some physical signs have been quantified to assist the clinician in assessing severity and thereby urgency. Two characteristic levels are described to indicate the appearance of asthmatic children at the most severe end of the spectrum. These are *severe* and *life-threatening* asthma.

<table>
<tr><td>

Features of severe asthma

- Too breathless to feed or talk
- Recession/use of accessory muscles
- Respiratory rate > 50 breaths/min
- Pulse rate >140 beats/min
- Peak flow < 50% expected/best

</td><td>

Features of life-threatening asthma

- Conscious level depressed/agitated
- Exhaustion
- Poor respiratory effort
- Oxygen saturation < 85% in air/cyanosis
- Silent chest
- Peak flow < 33% expected/best

</td></tr>
</table>

Young children with severe asthma are especially difficult to assess.

Table 9.2. Predicted values of peak expiratory flow rate in children

Height (cm)	Peak flow (litres/min)
110	150
120	200
130	250
140	300
150	350
160	400
170	450

Reassess ABC

Asthma emergency treatment

- Give high flow oxygen via a face mask with reservoir bag. Attach pulse oximeter.
- Attempt peak expiratory flow measurement (may not be possible in child with severe respiratory distress and in the under fives).
- Give salbutamol (2·5 mg/5 mg for <5 years/>5 years) and ipratropium bromide (250 micrograms/500 micrograms for <5 years/>5 years) nebulised with oxygen to any child with respiratory distress known to have asthma, or if this is their first wheeze episode, over the age of nine months.
- If an infant or child is clearly in respiratory failure with poor respiratory effort, depressed conscious level and poor saturation despite maximum oxygen therapy, attempt to support ventilation with bag-valve-mask: give an intravenous salbutamol infusion (give a loading dose of 5 micrograms/kg) to any in whom a diagnosis of asthma is suspected and summon experienced support.

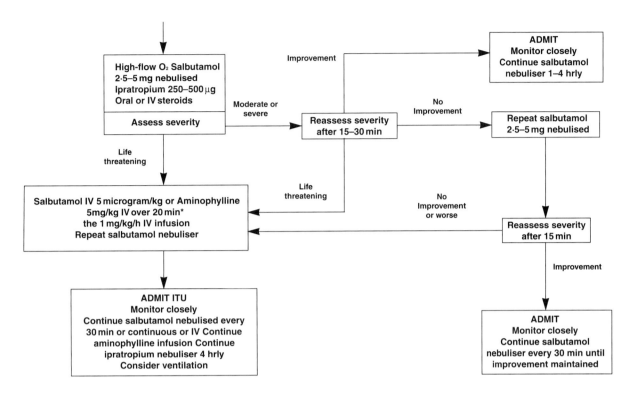

Figure 9.1. Algorithm for the management of acute asthma
*Omit if on oral theophylline

Asthma further treatment

High dose nebulised ß₂-bronchodilators (usually salbutamol but terbutaline is also used), steroids, and oxygen form the foundation of the therapy of acute asthma. There is now evidence that adding nebulised ipratropium bromide to maximal doses of ß₂-bronchodilators is beneficial in severe acute asthma in children. As soon as the diagnosis has been made, the child should be given nebulised ß₂-bronchodilator and ipratropium. The nebuliser should be driven by oxygen (4–6 l/min) in all but the mildest of cases. This can be repeated every one to two hours until there is improvement. As an alternative to nebulised treatment 10–20 puffs of a bronchodilator from a metered dose inhaler can by given (one puff at a time) through a spacer but this cannot be supplemented with oxygen. In severe or life-threatening asthma half-hourly or even continuous nebulised bronchodilator may be needed until the child's condition stabilises.

Corticosteroids expedite recovery from acute asthma. Although a oral single dose of prednisolone is effective, many paediatricians use a 3–5 day course. There is no need to taper off the dose, unless the child is on maintenance treatment with oral or high dose inhaled steroids. Unless the child is vomiting, there is no advantage in giving steroids parenterally.

Intravenous salbutamol has been shown to offer an advantage over nebulised delivery. Although nebulised drugs should be given first as they are accessible and more acceptable to the child, intravenous salbutamol has a place in severe or life-threatening episodes that do not respond promptly to nebulised therapy. Important side-effects include sinus tachycardia and hypokalaemia: serum potassium levels should be checked 12 hourly and supplementation may be needed.

The increased use of nebulised bronchodilators and oral steroids has been associated with a reduction in the use of intravenous aminophyllline. It still has a role in the child who fails to respond adequately to nebulised therapy. A loading dose is given over 15 minutes, followed by a continuous infusion. The pulse should be regularly checked for irregularities with continuous ECG monitoring during infusion of the loading dose. If the child has received a slow-release theophylline in the previous 12 hours, the loading dose should be omitted. Seizures, severe vomiting, and fatal cardiac arrhythmias may follow rapid infusion. There is no place for rectal administration of these drugs, as absorption is unpredictable.

If the child responds poorly to the above measures, a paediatric intensive care team should contacted for further advice and discussion of intensive care transfer. The child must continue under constant observation, and ECG and oxygen saturation monitoring. The frequency of nebulised ß$_2$-bronchodilator should be increased to half-hourly, or be administered continuously or given intravenously.

Intravenous fluids should normally be restricted to approximately two-thirds of the normal daily requirements as there is increased secretion of antidiuretic hormone in severe asthma. Antibiotics should only be given if there are clear signs of infection.

Several studies have shown that intravenous magnesium sulphate infusion can be effective in critically ill children with severe acute asthma where other therapies have failed but there is as yet little clinical experience with this treatment.

Mechanical ventilation is rarely required. There are no absolute criteria for ventilation, but it should be considered if there is a P_{CO_2} of > 8 kPa, persistent hypoxaemia (P_{CO_2} < 8 kPa in an inspired oxygen of 60%), or increasing exhaustion, despite intensive drug therapy. In skilled hands, the prognosis is good but complications such as air-leak, and lobar collapse are common. Children with acute asthma who require mechanical ventilation should be transferred to a paediatric intensive care unit. All intubated children must have continuous CO_2 monitoring

Table 9.3. Drug treatment of severe acute asthma

Oxygen	High flow
Nebulised beta-2-bronchodilator	Salbutamol 2·5–5 mg 30 min–4 hourly
	Terbutaline 2–10 mg 30 min–4 hourly
Prednisolone	2mg/kg/day in 2 doses, for 3–5 days (max dose/day 60 mg)
	OR
	Intravenous hydrocortisone succinate loading dose 4 mg/kg continuous infusion 1 mg/kg/hour
Aminophylline	Loading dose 5 mg/kg iv over 15 minutes*
	Continuous infusion 1mg/kg/h
Intravenous salbutamol	Loading dose 4–6 µg/kg over 10 min
	Continuous infusion 0·5-1·0 µg/kg/min
Nebulised ipratropium	125–250 µg 6-hourly

* Omit if child has received oral theophyllline in previous 12 hours

Whatever treatment is needed, it is important to monitor the response to treatment carefully. Assessment is based on physical signs and oxygen saturation measurements performed immediately before and 15–30 minutes after nebulised treatment. An improved peak flow measurement is expected. When there has been considerable improvement (Sao_2>92% in air, minimal recession, PEFR >50% normal value) intravenous treatment can be discontinued and the frequency of nebulised therapy reduced. The child's maintenance treatment should be reviewed and altered if inadequate. Inhaler technique should be checked.

Bronchiolitis emergency treatment

As there is no specific treatment for bronchiolitis, management is supportive. Humidified oxygen is delivered into a headbox at a rate that will maintain Sao_2 above 92%, and intravenous or nasogastric fluids are commenced if required. Pulse oximetry is helpful in assessing the severity of hypoxemia. Because of the risk of apnoea, small infants and those with severe disease should be attached to oxygen saturation and respiratory monitors. Antibiotics, bronchodilators and steroids are of no value. The precise role of the nebulised antiviral agent ribavirin is unclear and its use should be reserved for children with pre-existing lung disease, those with impaired immunity and infants with congenital heart disease. Mechanical ventilation is required in 2% of infants admitted to hospital, either because of recurrent apnoea, exhaustion, or hypercapnia and hypoxaemia secondary to severe small airways obstruction. All intubated infants must have continuous Sao_2 and CO_2 monitoring. Naso-pharyngeal CPAP may be sufficient ventilatory support for some infants.

Most children recover from the acute infection within two weeks. However, as many as half will have recurrent episodes of cough and wheeze over the next 3–5 years. Rarely, there is severe permanent damage to the airways (bronchiolitis obliterans).

Background information on asthma and bronchiolitis

Acute exacerbation of *asthma* is the commonest reason for a child to be admitted to hospital in this country. Admissions for acute asthma in children aged 0–4 years increased seven-fold between 1970 and 1986 and admissions for children in the 5-14 age group tripled. In the early 1990s asthma represented 10–20% of all acute medical admissions in children but rates have fallen over the last 3–5 years. There were 24 deaths from asthma in children in England and Wales in 1998 (ONS). Consultations with General Practitioners for asthma have doubled in the last 15 years. These increases reflect a real increase in the prevalence of asthma in children.

Except in the young infant, there is rarely any problem in making a diagnosis of acute asthma. An inhaled foreign body, bronchiolitis, croup and acute epiglottitis should be considered as alternative diagnoses. The classic features of acute asthma are cough, wheeze and breathlessness. An increase in these symptoms and difficulty in walking, talking or sleeping, all indicate worsening asthma. Decreasing relief from increasing doses of a bronchodilator always indicates worsening asthma.

Upper respiratory tract infections are the commonest precipitant of symptoms of asthma in the preschool child. Ninety per cent of these infections are caused by viruses. Exercise-induced symptoms are more frequent in the older child. Heat and water loss from the respiratory mucosa appears to be the mechanism by which exercise induces bronchoconstriction. Acute exacerbations may also be precipitated by emotional upset, laughing or excitement. It is hard to assess the importance of allergen exposure to the onset of acute symptoms in an individual asthmatic, partly because of the ubiquitous nature of the common allergens (house dust mite, grass pollens, moulds) and partly because delay in the allergic response makes a cause and effect relationship difficult to recognise. A rapid fall in air temperature, exposure to a smoky atmosphere and other chemical irritants such as paints, and domestic aerosols may trigger an acute attack.

Bronchiolitis is the most common serious respiratory infection of childhood: it occurs in 10% of all infants and 2–3% are admitted to hospital with the disease each year. Ninety per cent of patients are aged 1–9 months: it is rare after one year of age. There is an annual winter epidemic. Respiratory syncytial virus is the pathogen in 75% cases, the remainder of cases being caused by other respiratory viruses, such as parainfluenza,

influenza and adenoviruses. Acute bronchiolitis is never a primary bacterial infection, and it is likely that secondary bacterial involvement is uncommon.

Fever and a clear nasal discharge precede a dry cough and increasing breathlessness. Wheezing is often, but not always, present. Feeding difficulties associated with increasing dyspnoea are often the reason for admission to hospital. Recurrent apnoea is a serious and potentially fatal complication and is seen particularly in infants born prematurely. Children with pre-existing chronic lung disease (e.g. cystic fibrosis, bronchopulmonary dysplasia in premature infants), and children with congenital heart disease or immune deficiency syndromes are at particularly high risk of developing severe respiratory failure with bronchiolitis.

The findings on examination are characteristic.

Table 9.4. Bronchiolitis – characteristic findings on examination

Tachypnoea	50-100 breaths/minute
Recession	Subcostal and intercostal
Cough	Sharp, dry
Hyperinflation of the chest	Sternum prominent, liver depressed
Tachycardia	140-200 beats per minute
Crackles	Fine end-inspiratory
Wheezes	High-pitched expiratory > inspiratory
Colour	Cyanosis or pallor
Breathing pattern	Irregular breathing/recurrent apnoea

Risk factors for severity in bronchiolitis

- Age under 6 weeks
- Premature birth
- Chronic lung disease
- Congenital heart disease
- Immunodeficiency

The chest radiograph shows hyperinflation with downward displacement and flattening of the diaphragm due to small airways obstruction and gas-trapping. In one third of infants there is also evidence of collapse or consolidation, particularly in the upper lobes. Respiratory syncytial virus can be cultured or identified with a fluorescent antibody technique on nasopharyngeal secretions. Blood gas analysis, which is required in only the most severe cases, shows lowered oxygen and raised carbon dioxide levels.

APPROACH TO THE CHILD WITH FEVER

Although many causes of breathing difficulties are associated with infection, a high fever is usually associated only with pneumonia, epiglottitis and bacterial tracheitis. Although many cases of asthma are precipitated by an URTI, the asthmatic child is rarely febrile and a low grade fever is characteristic of bronchiolitis. Therefore in the absence of stridor and wheeze, breathing difficulties in association with a significant fever are likely to be due to pneumonia.

Reassess ABC

Airway and breathing support may be especially needed in children with neurological handicap who may have poor airway control and weak respiratory muscles even when well.

Caution should be exercised in fluid administration to children with pneumonia. Some have inappropriate ADH secretion which can contribute to fluid overload and worsening breathlessness.

Pneumonia emergency treatment

- As it is not possible to differentiate reliably between bacterial or viral infection on clinical or radiological grounds, all children diagnosed as having pneumonia should receive antibiotics. Cefotaxime will be effective against most bacteria but flucloxacillin should be added if *Staphylococcus aureus* is suspected and erythromycin added if *Chlamydia* or *Mycobacteria pneumoniae* thought to be responsible.
- Clinical examination and the chest radiograph may reveal a pleural effusion. If this is large, it should be tapped to relieve breathlessness. Details of the procedure can be found on page 235.

Background to pneumonia

Pneumonia in childhood is still responsible for over 130 deaths each year in England and Wales. Infants, and children with congenital abnormalities or chronic illnesses are at particular risk. In adults, two-thirds of cases of pneumonia are caused by either *Streptococcus pneumoniae* or *Haemophilus influenzae*. A much wider spectrum of pathogens causes pneumonia in childhood, and different organisms are important in different age groups.

In the newborn, organisms from the mother's genital tract, such as *Escherichia coli* and other Gram-negative bacilli, group B beta-haemolytic *Streptococcus* and increasingly, *Chlamydia trachomatis*, are the most common pathogens. In infancy respiratory viruses, particularly respiratory syncytial virus, are the most frequent cause, but *Pneumococcus*, *Haemophilus* and, less commonly, *Staphylococcus aureus* are also important. In older children, viruses become less frequent pathogens and bacterial infection is more important. *Mycoplasma pneumonia* is a common cause of pneumonia in the school-age child. *Bordatella pertussis* can present with pneumonia as well as with classical whooping cough, even in children who have been fully immunised.

Fever, cough, breathlessness, and lethargy following an upper respiratory infection are the usual presenting symptoms. The cough is often dry initially but then becomes loose. Older children may produce purulent sputum but in those below the age of 5 years it is usually swallowed. Pleuritic chest pain, neck stiffness and abdominal pain may be present if there is pleural inflammation. Classical signs of consolidation such as impaired percussion, decreased breath sounds and bronchial breathing are often absent, particularly in infants, and a chest radiograph is needed. This may show lobar consolidation, widespread bronchopneumonia or less commonly, cavitation of the lung. Pleural effusions are quite common, particularly in bacterial pneumonia. An ultrasound of the chest will delineate a pleural effusion and be helpful in the placing of a chest drain. Blood cultures, swabs for viral isolation, and a full blood count should also be performed.

As it is not possible to differentiate reliably between bacterial or viral infection on clinical or radiological grounds, all children diagnosed as having pneumonia should receive antibiotics. The initial choice of antibiotics depends on the age of the child. Antibiotics should be given for 7–10 days, except in staphylococcal pneumonia, where a flucloxacillin course of 4–6 weeks duration is needed. Many older children have no respiratory difficulty and can be treated at home with penicillin, a cephalosporin or erythromycin. Infants, and children who look toxic or have definite dyspnoea should be admitted and usually require intravenous treatment initially. Local antibiotic policies should be followed. Physiotherapy, an adequate fluid intake and oxygen (in severe pneumonia), are also required. Mechanical ventilation is rarely required unless there is serious underlying condition. If a child has recurrent or persistent pneumonia, investigations to exclude underlying conditions such as cystic fibrosis or immunodeficiency should be performed.

APPROACH TO THE CHILD IN HEART FAILURE

Infants and children with serious cardiac pathology may present with breathlessness, cyanosis or cardiogenic shock. The immediate management of the latter is described in Chapter 10.

Table 9.5. Causes of heart failure which may present as breathing difficulties

Left ventricular volume overload or excessive pulmonary blood flow
Ventricular septal defect
Atrioventricular septal defect
Persistent arterial duct
Common arterial trunk

Left heart obstruction
Hypertrophic cardiomyopathy
Critical aortic stenosis
Aortic coarctation
Hypoplastic left heart syndrome

Primary "pump" failure
Myocarditis
Cardiomyopathy

Reassess ABC

HEART FAILURE EMERGENCY TREATMENT

- If there are signs of shock — poor pulse volume or low blood pressure with extreme pallor and depressed conscious level, treat the child for *Cardiogenic Shock* (page 109).
- If circulation is adequate and oxygen saturation is normal or improves significantly with oxygen by face mask but there are signs of heart failure, then the breathing difficulty is due to pulmonary congestion secondary to a large left to right shunt. The shunt may be through a VSD, AVSD, PDA or more rarely a truncus arteriosus. In many cases a heart murmur will be heard. A chest radiograph will also give confirmatory evidence with a large, usually globular heart and radiological signs of pulmonary congestion. Give high flow oxygen by face mask with a reservoir and diuretics such as frusemide (1 mg/kg IV followed by initial maintenance dose of 1–2 mg/kg/day in 1–3 divided doses). If there is no diuresis within 2 hours, the intravenous bolus can be repeated.
- Babies in the first few days of life who present with breathlessness and increasing cyanosis largely unresponsive to oxygen supplementation are likely to have a duct-

dependent congenital heart disease such as tricuspid or pulmonary atresia. An infusion of alprostadil at an initial dose of 0·05 micrograms/kg/min will maintain or increase the patent ductus arteriosus size temporarily until the patient can be transferred to a neonatal cardiology unit. Patients should be intubated and ventilated for transfer both because of the seriousness of their condition and also because the alprostadil may cause apnoea. As oxygen tends to promote ductal closure, oxygen concentration for ventilation should be individually adjusted using pulse oximetry to monitor the most effective concentration for each infant.

- Children of all ages who present with breathlessness from heart failure may have myocarditis. This is characterised by a marked sinus tachycardia and the absence of signs of structural abnormality. The patients should be treated with oxygen and diuretics.

Full blood count, serum urea and electrolytes, calcium, glucose and arterial blood gases should be performed on all patients in heart failure. A routine infection screen including blood cultures is recommended especially in infants. A full 12-lead electrocardiogram and chest radiograph are essential. All patients suspected of having heart disease should be discussed with a paediatric cardiologist, echocardiography will establish the diagnosis in almost all cases.

Background to heart failure in infancy and childhood

In infancy heart failure is usually secondary to structural heart disease and medical treatment is directed to improving the clinical condition prior to definitive surgery. With modern obstetric management many babies are now discharged from the maternity unit only hours after birth. Therefore babies with serious congenital neonatal heart disease may present to paediatric or Accident and Emergency departments.

Infants with common congenital heart diseases are usually diagnosed in utero or at the post-natal examination but a few will present acutely after discharge from medical care as the lowering pulmonary vascular resistance over the first hours to days of life allows increasing pulmonary flow in infants with left to right shunts such as VSD, persistent PDA, truncus arteriosus. The increasing left to right shunt causes increasing pulmonary congestion and heart failure and the infant presents with poor feeding, sweating and breathlessness. In addition, some may present at a few months of age when heart failure is precipitated by a respiratory infection, usually bronchiolitis.

Duct-dependent congenital heart disease

There are also several rarer and more complex congenital heart defects in which the presence of a patent ductus arteriosus is essential to maintain pulmonary or systemic flow. The normal patent ductus arteriosus closes functionally in the first 24 hours of life. This may be delayed in the presence of congenital cardiac anomalies.

The pulmonary obstructive lesions include pulmonary atresia, critical pulmonary valve stenosis, tricuspid atresia, severe Fallot's tetralogy and some cases of transposition of the great vessels. In all of these lesions there is no effective route for blood to take from the right ventricle into the pulmonary circulation and therefore pulmonary blood flow and oxygenation of blood are dependent on flow from the aorta via a patent ductus.

Babies with critical pulmonary obstructive lesions present in the first few days of life with increasing cyanosis, breathlessness or cardiogenic shock. On examination there may be a characteristic murmur but more frequently there is no murmur audible. An enlarged liver is a common finding. The clinical situation has arisen from the gradual closure of the ductus arteriosus. Complete closure will result in the death of the infant from hypoxia.

Additionally, there are some congenital heart malformations where systemic blood flow is dependent on the ductus arteriosus delivering blood to the aorta from the pulmonary circulation. This is characteristic of severe coarctation, critical aortic stenosis and hypoplastic left heart syndrome.

In these congenital heart lesions the baby ceases to be able to feed and becomes breathless, grey and collapsed with a poor peripheral circulation. On examination the babies are in heart failure and in more severe cases in cardiogenic shock. In this situation even in coarctation of the aorta all pulses are difficult to feel.

In the older child myocarditis and cardiomyopathy are the most common causes of the acute onset of heart failure and remains rare (see Table 9.1.).

How to differentiate the infant with heart failure from the infant with bronchiolitis

The common features of heart failure in infancy are:

- Breathlessness
- Feeding difficulty with growth failure
- Restlessness
- Sweating
- Tachycardia
- Tachypnoea
- Sternal and sub-costal recession
- The extremities are cool and pale with cardiomegaly and hepatomegaly
- Auscultation reveals a gallop rhythm and occasionally basal crackles

In babies and children peripheral oedema is less commonly seen than in adults. It can therefore be difficult to differentiate the infant with heart failure from the infant with bronchiolitis but the cardinal additional features in the infant in heart failure is the greater degree of hepatomegaly, the enlarged heart with displaced apex beat and the presence of a gallop rhythm and/or a murmur. A chest radiograph will often be helpful in showing cardiomegaly and pulmonary congestion rather than the over-inflation of bronchiolitis.

Older children presenting in heart failure will almost certainly have myocarditis or cardiomyopathy and present with fatigue, effort intolerance, anorexia, abdominal pain and cough. On examination a marked sinus tachycardia, hepatomegaly and raised JVP is found.

METABOLIC AND POISONING

Diabetes

As hyperventilation is a feature of the severe acidosis produced by diabetes, occasionally a child may be presented as a primary breathing difficulty. The correct diagnosis is usually easy to establish and management is described in Appendix B.

Poisoning

There may be apparent breathing difficulties following the ingestion of a number of poisons.

The repiratory rate may be increased by poisoning with:
- Salicylates

- Ethylene glycol (anti-freeze)
- Methanol
- Cyanide.

But usually only poisoning with salicylates causes any diagnostic dilemma.

Poisoning with drugs that cause a depression of ventilation will present as a diminished conscious level

The management of the poisoned child is dealt with in Chapter 14.

10

The child in shock

INTRODUCTION

Shock results from an acute failure of circulatory function. Inadequate amounts of nutrients, especially oxygen, are delivered to body tissues and there is inadequate removal of tissue waste products. These functions involve several body systems which means that there are several causes of shock and therefore the clinician must consider which of several alternative emergency treatments will be effective for an individual patient. This chapter will provide the student with an approach to the assessment, resuscitation and emergency management of children in shock.

Maintenance of adequate tissue perfusion depends on a pump (the heart) delivering the correct type and volume of fluid (blood) through controlled vessels (arteries, veins, and capillaries) without abnormal obstruction to flow. Inadequate tissue perfusion resulting in impaired cellular respiration (i.e. shock) may result from defects of the pump (cardiogenic), loss of fluid (hypovolaemic), abnormalities of vessels (distributive), flow restriction (obstructive), or inadequate oxygen releasing capacity (dissociative).

From the box it can be seen that the most common causes of shock in the paediatric patient are hypovolaemia from any cause, septicaemia, and the effects of trauma.

**Classification of causes of shock
(common causes are emboldened)**

Cardiogenic
    Arrhythmias
    Cardiomyopathy
    Heart failure
    Valvular disease
    Myocardial contusion
    Myocardial infarction
Hypovolaemic
    Haemorrhage
    Gastroenteritis
    Volvulus

Burns
Peritonitis
Distributive
Septicaemia
Anaphylaxis
Vasodilating drugs
Anaesthesia
Spinal cord injury
Obstructive
Tension pneumothorax
Haemopneumothorax
Flail chest
Cardiac tamponade
Pulmonary embolism
Hypertension
Dissociative
Profound anaemia
Carbon monoxide poisoning
Methaemoglobinaemia

Children in shock are usually presented by parents who are aware that their child is worryingly ill or seriously injured even though they may not be able to express their concerns clearly. The child may be presented primarily with a fever, a rash, with pallor, poor feeding or drowsiness or with a history of trauma or poisoning. The initial assessment will identify which patients are in shock

APPROACH TO THE CHILD IN SHOCK

PRIMARY ASSESSMENT

Airway

Assess airway patency by the "look, listen, and feel" method.

If the child can speak or cry, this indicates that the airway is patent, that breathing is occurring and there is adequate circulation.

If there is no evidence of air movement then chin lift or jaw thrust manoeuvres should be carried out and the airway reassessed. If there continues to be no evidence of air movement then airway patency can be assessed by performing an opening manoeuvre and giving rescue breaths (see Basic life support, Chapter 4).

Breathing

Assess the adequacy of breathing
Monitor oxygen saturation with a pulse oximeter.

- Effort of breathing
  Recession
  Respiratory rate
  Grunting
  Accessory muscle use
  Flare of the alae nasi

- Efficacy of breathing
   Breath sounds
   Chest expansion/abdominal excursion
- Effects of breathing
   Heart rate
   Skin colour
   Mental status

Circulation

Assess the adequacy of circulation.

Cardiovascular status

Heart rate

A raised heart rate is a common response to many types of stress (fever, anxiety, hypoxia, hypovolaemia). In shock, tachycardia is caused by catecholamine release, and is an attempt to maintain cardiac output by increasing heart rate in the face of falling stroke volume. *Bradycardia in a shocked child is caused by hypoxia and acidosis and is a preterminal sign.*

Pulse volume

Examination of central and peripheral pulses may reveal a poor pulse volume peripherally or, more worryingly, centrally. In early septic shock there is sometimes a high output state which will produce bounding pulses.

Capillary refill

Poor skin perfusion can be a useful early sign of shock. Slow capillary refill (>2 seconds) after blanching pressure for 5 seconds is evidence of reduced skin perfusion. When testing for capillary refill press on the skin of the sternum or a digit held at the level of the heart. Mottling, pallor, and peripheral cyanosis also indicate poor skin perfusion. All these signs may be difficult to interpret in patients who have just been exposed to cold.

In early shock, there may be a hyperdynamic circulation due to vasodilataion in which peripheries are warm but the capillary refill is delayed.

Blood pressure

Blood pressure is a difficult measure to obtain and interpret especially in young infants. A formula for calculating normal systolic blood pressure is:

$$80 + (2 \times \text{Age in years})$$

Children's cardiovascular systems compensate well initially in shock. *Hypotension is a late and often sudden sign of decompensation and, if not reversed, will be rapidly followed by death.* Serial measurements of blood pressure should be performed frequently.

Effects of circulatory inadequacy on other organs

Acidotic sighing respirations

The acidosis produced by poor tissue perfusion in shock leads to rapid deep breathing.

Pale, cyanosed or cold skin

A core/toe temperature difference of more than 2°C is a sign of poor skin perfusion.

Mental status

Agitation or depressed conscious level. Early signs of brain hypoperfusion are agitation and confusion, often alternating with drowsiness. Infants may be irritable but drowsy with a weak cry and hypotonia. They may not focus on the parent's face. These are important early cerebral signs of shock. Later the child becomes progressively drowsier until consciousness is lost.

Urinary output

Urine flow is decreased or absent in shock. Hourly measurement is helpful in monitoring progress. A minimum flow of 1 ml/kg/h in children and 2 ml/kg/h in infants indicates adequate renal perfusion.

NOTE: Poor capillary refill, core/toe temperature difference and differential pulse volumes are neither sensitive nor specific indicators of shock when used in isolation. There are helpful when used in conjunction with the other signs described.

Look for the presence of signs of heart failure

- Tachycardia
- Raised jugular venous pressure (often not seen in infants in heart failure)
- Lung crepitations on auscultation
- Gallop rhythm
- Enlarged liver

And listen for a heart murmur.

Monitor heart rate/rhythm, blood pressure and core/toe temperature difference. If heart rate is above 200 in an infant or above 150 in a child or if the rhythm is abnormal perform a standard ECG.

Disability

Assess neurological function.

- A rapid measure of level of consciousness should be recorded using the AVPU scale.
- A **ALERT**
- V responds to **VOICE**
- P responds to **PAIN**
- U **UNRESPONSIVE**
- Pupillary size and reaction should be noted.
- Note the child's posture: *children in shock are usually hypotonic.*
- The presence of convulsive movements should be noted.

Exposure

- Take the child's core and toe temperatures.
- Look for a rash: *if one is present, ascertain if it is purpuric.*
- Look for evidence of poisoning.

RESUSCITATION

Airway

- A patent airway is the first requisite. If the airway is not patent an airway opening manoeuvre should be used. The airway should then be secured with a pharyngeal airway device or by intubation with experienced senior help.

Breathing

- All children in shock should receive high flow oxygen through a face mask with a reservoir as soon as the airway has been demonstrated to be adequate.
- If the child is hypoventilating, respiration should be supported with oxygen via a bag-valve-mask device and experienced senior help summoned.

Circulation

Gain intravenous or intraosseous access.

- Take blood for FBC, U&Es, blood culture, cross-match, glucose stick test and laboratory test
- Give 20 ml/kg rapid bolus of crystalloid to all patients except for those with signs that heart failure is their primary pathology.
- The initial bolus should be colloid and an antibiotic such as cefotaxime 100 mg/kg should be used for those in whom a diagnosis of septicaemia is made obvious by the presence of a purpuric rash.
- If a tachyarrhythmia is identified as the cause of shock, up to three synchronous electrical shocks at 0·5, 1·0, 2·0 Joules should be given.
If the arrhythmia is broad complex and the synchronous shocks are not activated by the defibrillator then attempt an asynchronous shock.
A conscious child should be anaesthetised first if this can be done in a timely manner.
If the shocked child's tachyarrhythmia is SVT then he can be treated with intravenous/intraosseous adenosine if this can be administered more quickly than a synchronous electrical shock.

Circulatory access

A short, wide-bore peripheral venous or intraosseous cannula should be used. Upper central venous lines are unsuitable for the resuscitation of hypovolaemic children because of the risk of iatrogenic pneumothorax, or exacerbation of an unsuspected neck injury; both these complications can be fatal. Femoral vein access is safer, if peripheral or intraosseous access is impossible. It is wise to obtain two separate intravenous and/or intraosseous lines both to give large volumes of fluid quickly and also in case one line is lost.

Techniques for vascular access are described in Chapter 23.

Antibiotics

In paediatric practice, septicaemia is the commonest cause of a child presenting in shock. Therefore, unless an alternative diagnosis is very clear (such as trauma, anaphylaxis or poisoning) an antibiotic, usually a third-generation cephalosporin such as cefotaxime or ceftriaxone, is given as soon as a blood culture has been taken. An anti-staphyloccocal antibiotic (flucloxacillin or vancomycin) should be considered in possible toxic shock syndrome i.e. post burns/cellulitis.

Hypoglycaemia
Hypoglycaemia may give a similar clinical picture to that of compensated shock. This must always be excluded by urgent glucose stick test and blood glucose estimation. Shock and hypoglycaemia may coexist as the sick infant or small child has poor glucose-producing reserves.

Key features

While the primary assessment and resuscitation are being carried out a focused history of the child's health and activity over the previous 24 hours and any significant previous illness should be gained.

Certain key features which will be identified clinically in the above assessment, from the focused history and from the initial blood test results can point the clinician to the likeliest working diagnosis for emergency treatment.

- A history of vomiting and/or diarrhoea points to *fluid loss* either externally (e.g. gastroenteritis) or into the abdomen (e.g. volvulus, intussusception).
- The presence of fever and/or a rash points to *septicaemia*.
- The presence of urticaria, angio-neurotic oedema and a history of allergen exposure points to *anaphylaxis*.
- The presence of cyanosis unresponsive to oxygen or a grey colour with signs of heart failure in a baby under 4 weeks points to *duct-dependent congenital heart disease*.
- The presence of heart failure in an older infant or child points to *cardiomyopathy*.
- A history of sickle cell disease or a recent diarrhoeal illness and a very low haemoglobin points to *acute haemolysis*.
- An immediate history of major trauma points to blood loss, and more rarely, *tension pneumothorax, haemothorax, cardiac tamponade or spinal cord transection* (see Part IV The Seriously Injured Child for management).
- The presence of severe tachycardia and an abnormal rhythm on the ECG points to an *arrhythmia* (see Chapter 11).
- A history of polyuria and the presence of acidotic breathing and a very high blood glucose points to *diabetes* (see Appendix B for management).
- A history of drug ingestion points to *poisoning* (see Chapter 14 for management).

APPROACH TO THE CHILD WITH FLUID LOSS

Infants are more likely than older children to present with shock due to sudden fluid loss in gastroenteritis or with concealed fluid loss secondary to a "surgical abdomen" such as a volvulus. This is due both to the infant's low physiological reserve and increased susceptibility to these conditions.

In infants gastroenteritis may occasionally present as a circulatory collapse with little or no significant preceding history of vomiting or diarrhoea. The infecting organism can be any of the usual diarrhoeal pathogens, of which the most common is rotavirus. The mechanism leading to this presentation is that there is a sudden massive loss of fluid from the bowel wall into the gut lumen, causing depletion of the intravascular volume and the appearance of shock in the infant. This occurs before the stool is passed so that the diagnosis may be unsuspected. Usually during resuscitation of these infants, copious watery diarrhoea is evacuated.

Having completed the primary assessment and resuscitation and identified by means of the key features that fluid loss is the most likely diagnosis, the child is reassessed to identify the response to the first fluid bolus.

REASSESS ABC

Fluid loss – emergency treatment

If the child still shows clinical signs of shock after the first bolus of fluid, give a second 20 ml/kg bolus of crystalloid. If there is clinical suspicion of a surgical abdominal problem, such as bile-stained vomiting or abdominal guarding, seek an urgent surgical opinion. An abdominal radiograph and an ultrasound scan may be helpful in showing distended bowel, intra-abdominal air or fluid.

In the case of infants with gastroenteritis, two boluses of crystalloid is usually sufficient to restore the circulating volume. If after this amount of fluid, the child is still in shock when assessed clinically, give the third bolus as colloid (human albumen is the most widely used in paediatric practice) and consider whether there is an additional or alternative diagnosis, such as an intra-abdominal surgical problem (e.g. volvulus, peritonitis) in the patient originally thought to have gastro-enteritis or co-existent septicaemia in the patient with the "surgical abdomen".

Obtain surgical and anaesthetic advice if not already obtained and give antibiotics intravenously if more than two boluses of fluid have been required

The child should be catheterised in order to assess accurately the urinary output.

Intubation and ventilation should be strongly considered in a patient who has failed to respond adequately to two boluses of fluid (i.e. half the estimated intravascular volume). Acid–base status should be checked by means of an arterial blood gas.

In the patient with gastroenteritis who has stabilised after treatment for shock there will still be a need to treat dehydration and electrolyte imbalance. See Appendix B for further management

APPROACH TO THE CHILD WITH SEPTICAEMIA

The cardinal sign of meningococcal septicaemia is a purpuric rash in an ill child. At the onset, however, the rash is not florid and a careful search should be made for purpura in any unwell child. In about 13% of patients with meningococcal septicaemia, a blanching erythematous rash replaces a purpuric one, and in 7% of cases no rash occurs. In the much rarer toxic shock syndrome, the initial clinical picture includes a high fever, headache, confusion, conjunctival and mucosal hyperaemia, scarlatiniform rash with secondary desquamation, subcutaneous oedema, vomiting and watery diarrhoea. Early administration of antibiotics, concurrent with initial resuscitation is vital.

In countries where the vaccine against *Meningococcus* C has been introduced a fall in the number of cases of infection is occurring.

Having completed the primary assessment and resuscitation and identified by means of the key features that septicaemia is the most likely dignosis, the child is reassessed.

REASSESS ABC

Septicaemia emergency management

If the child is still in shock after the first bolus of fluid a second 20 ml/kg fluid bolus should be given over five to ten minutes. In septicaemia it remains usual practice to give fluid as 4·5% human albumin. (A discussion of the relative merits of fluids can be found on page 114)

Children in septic shock often require several boluses of fluid to achieve relative stability. Once the third bolus of fluid has been commenced, the patient should be intubated by rapid sequence induction of anaesthesia and ventilated. This is done both to support a seriously ill patient by maximising oxygenation and to anticipate the development of pulmonary oedema caused by fluid leak in the lungs. All intubated children must have continuous SaO_2 and CO_2 monitoring. The child should be catheterised in order to assess accurately the urinary output.

In septic shock, myocardial depression is a co-existent feature. Therefore, at the same time as the third bolus of fluid is commenced an infusion of dobutamine should be started at an initial rate of 10 micrograms/kg/min. This can be given through a peripheral vein as it is unlikely that central venous access will yet have been obtained. The rate of infusion should be adjusted to the patient's response. Do not hesitate to increase the infusion rapidly in the face of a poor response. Consider the use of epinephrine if maximal does of dobutamine and/or dopamine are unsuccessful. Epinephrine should be preferably given through a central vein but do not delay if this is not available.

Further investigations

In addition to the blood tests taken during resuscitation, the following blood tests are needed in the septic child: calcium, magnesium, phosphate, coagulation screen and arterial blood gas. Electrolyte and acid–base derangements can have a deleterious effect on myocardial function. They should be sought and corrected.

Table 10.1. Corrective measures for electrolyte and acid–base derangements

Result	Treat if less than	Correct with
Glucose	3 mmol/l	3 ml/kg 10% dextrose
Acid–base	7·15	1 mmol/kg $NaHCO_3$: ventilate
Potassium	3·5 mmol/l	0·25 mmol/kg KCl over 30 min: ECG
Calcium	2 mmol/l	0·3 ml/kg 10% Ca gluconate over 30 min
Magnesium	0·75 mmol/l	0·2 ml/kg 50% $MgSO_4$ over 30 min
Phosphate	0·7 mmol/l	0·2 mmol/kg over 30 min

It is difficult to manage a patient so seriously ill as to require ventilation and inotropic support without intensive care facilities and invasive monitoring. If these treatments are required, a paediatric intensive care unit must be involved early to give advice and to retrieve the patient

Reassess disability

This is an assessment of the neurological status of the septicaemic child.

• Both hypoxia and shock produce neurological effects on their own account and the conscious level is part of the assessment of the severity of these conditions. In addition, in children with meningococcal septicaemia, many have both *septicaemia* and *meningitis*. Of these some, generally in the school age group have clinically significant raised intracranial pressure (RICP). These children must be identified as the clinician may need to prevent or treat this problem.
• The level of consciousness should be assessed using the Glasgow Coma Scale.
• Pupillary size and reaction should be noted.
• The presence of abnormal posturing should be noted. This may require a painful stimulus to demonstrate its presence.

Disability emergency treatment

• If, despite effective treatment of shock, the child has a decreasing conscious level and/or abnormal posturing, possibly also with focal neurological signs, he may have raised intracranial pressure. He should be intubated using rapid sequence induction if this has not already been done and capnography used to monitor CO_2 levels which should be kept in the range 4–4·5 kPa. A diuretic such as mannitol (0·5–1·0 g/kg) or frusemide (1 mg/kg) can be given intravenously. The child should be catheterised in order to assess accurately the resulting urinary output. This will temporarily relieve the intracranial pressure. The presence of relative bradycardia and hypertension is a pre-terminal sign of imminent brain stem coning and death. This should be treated vigorously with diuretics and hyperventilation.

• If the shocked state has been effectively treated, only maintenance fluids should be continued although close monitoring is required as continued capillary fluid leak will lead to a return of shock. If the patient is still shocked then treatment of the shocked state takes priority. An adequate blood pressure is necessary to perfuse a swollen brain.

• Lumbar puncture must be avoided as its performance may cause death through coning of the brain through the foramen magnum.

Paediatric intensive care skills and monitoring is paramount in these patients. Seek advice early.

APPROACH TO THE CHILD WITH ANAPHYLAXIS

Anaphylaxis is a potentially life-threatening syndrome which may progress to shock, although in most cases a rash is the only symptom. It is immunologically mediated. The most common causes are allergy to penicillin, to radiographic contrast media, and to certain foods, especially nuts.

Prodromal symptoms of flushing, itching, facial swelling, urticaria, abdominal pain, diarrhoea, wheeze, and stridor may precede shock or may be the only manifestations of anaphylaxis. The presence of these additional symptoms confirms anaphylaxis as the cause of shock in a child. Most patients will have a history of previous attacks and some may have a "medic-alert" bracelet.

Anaphylaxis can be life-threatening because of the rapid onset of airway compromise due to laryngeal oedema, breathing difficulties due to sudden severe broncho-constriction and/or the development of shock due to acute vasodilatation and fluid loss from the intravascular space caused by increased capillary permeability.

Key points in the history may point to a severe reaction. These are shown in the box.

Symptoms and signs vary according to the body's response to the allergen. These are shown in Table 10.2.

> Previous severe reaction
> History of increasingly severe reaction
> History of asthma
> Treatment with ß-blockers

Table 10.2. Symptoms and signs in allergic reaction

	Symptoms	Signs
Mild	Burning sensation in mouth	Urticarial rash
	Itching of lips, mouth, throat	Angio-oedema
	Feeling of warmth	Conjunctivitis
	Nausea	
	Abdominal pain	
Moderate (Mild +)	Coughing/wheezing	Bronchospasm
	Loose bowel motions	Tachycardia
	Sweating	Pallor
	Irritability	
Severe (Moderate +)	Difficulty breathing	Severe bronchospasm
	Collapse	Laryngeal oedema
	Vomiting	Shock
	Uncontrolled defaecation	Respiratory arrest
		Cardiac arrest

The management of anaphylactic shock requires good airway management, administration of epinephrine (adrenaline), and aggressive fluid resuscitation.

Note that the intramuscular route is the preferred route for the delivery of epinephrine. Intravenous epinephrine should be reserved for children with life-threatening shock for whom intramuscular injection has been ineffective. The patient must be carefully monitored.

Having completed the primary assessment and resuscitation and identified by means of the key features that anaphylaxis is the most likely diagnosis, the child is reassessed

Remove allergen if possible.

Reassess airway

If there is stridor then the child has laryngeal oedema.

Airway emergency management

- If the child has airway obstruction with stridor call for urgent anaesthetic and ENT help.
- Give epinephrine 10 micrograms/kg IM and also nebulised epinephrine 5 ml 1:1000.
- Consider the need for intubation or a surgical airway.

Reassess breathing
- Assess *effort, efficiency* and *effect*
- Check oxygen saturation on the pulse oximeter
- If there is wheeze then the child has bronchoconstriction

Breathing emergency treatment

If the child has bronchoconstriction give nebulised salbutamol 2·5–5 mg. If no parenteral epinephrine has been given then give epinephrine 10 micrograms/kg IM.

Reassess circulation
- Look for signs of shock.
- Check pulse rate and rhythm on the ECG.

Circulation emergency treatment

If the child is in shock give colloid 20 ml/kg IV/IO. If no parenteral epinephrine has been given yet then give epinephrine 10 micrograms/kg IM.

Further emergency management

Depending whether upper airway obstruction, bronchoconstriction or shock predominate in the clinical picture of anaphylaxis, the clinician should

1. secure the airway by intubation
2. follow the protocol for asthma
3. continue to treat for shock with boluses of colloid and ventilatory support
4. give further doses of epinephrine intramuscularly every five minutes if the symptoms are not reversed.

Additional inotropes will not be needed as the epinephrine used for the treatment of anaphylaxis is a powerful inotrope. However, in the face of shock resistant to intramuscular epinephrine and one or two boluses of fluid, an infusion of intravenous epinephrine may be life-saving. The dose is 0·1–5·0 micrograms/kg/min and the patient should be closely monitored for pulse and blood pressure.

In addition to the above treatment it is also customary to give patients with anaphylaxis an antihistamine and steroids. There is no evidence of the part these drugs play in management and their onset of action is too delayed to be of much benefit in the first hour.

Drug doses in anaphylaxis	
Epinephrine 10 micrograms/kg	
Chlorpheniramine	
>12 years	10–20 milligrams
6–12 years	5–10 milligrams
1–5 years	2·5–5 milligrams
1 month–1 year	250 micrograms/kg
Do not use in neonates	
Hydrocortisone	4 milligrams/kg

APPROACH TO THE INFANT WITH A DUCT-DEPENDENT CONGENITAL HEART DISEASE

Babies with critical pulmonary obstructive lesions present in the first few days of life with increasing cyanosis, breathlessness or cardiogenic shock. On examination there may be a characteristic murmur but in fact more frequently there is no murmur audible. An enlarged liver is a common finding.

Babies with critical systemic obstructive lesions also present in the first few days of life with inability to feed, breathlessness, a grey appearance and collapse with poor peripheral circulation. On examination the babies are in heart failure and in more severe cases in cardiogenic shock. In this situation, even in coarctation of the aorta, all pulses are difficult to feel.

The clinical situation has arisen from the gradual closure of the ductus arteriosus on which, in these congenital heart anomalies, a functioning circulation depends. Complete closure will result in the death of the infant.

Having completed the primary assessment and resuscitation and identified by means of the key features that duct-dependent congenital heart disease is the most likely diagnosis, the child is reassessed.

Reassess ABC

DUCT-DEPENDENT CONGENITAL HEART DISEASE EMERGENCY TREATMENT

Babies in the first few days of life who present with breathlessness and increasing cyanosis or a grey appearance largely unresponsive to oxygen supplementation are likely to have a duct-dependent congenital heart disease such as tricuspid or pulmonary atresia, critical aortic stenosis or hypoplastic left heart syndrome. An infusion of alprostadil at an initial dose of 0·05 micrograms/kg/min will maintain or increase the patent arteriosus ductus size temporarily until the patient can be transferred to a neonatal cardiology unit. Patients should be intubated and ventilated for transfer both because of the seriousness of their condition and also because the prostaglandin may cause apnoea.

Full blood count, serum urea and electrolytes, calcium, glucose and arterial blood gases should be performed on all sick infants with congenital heart disease. A routine infection screen including blood cultures is also recommended. A full 12-lead electrocardiogram and chest radiograph are essential. All patients suspected of having heart disease should be discussed with a paediatric cardiologist, echocardiography will establish the diagnosis in almost all cases.

APPROACH TO THE CHILD WITH CARDIOMYOPATHY

Cardiomyopathy/myocarditis is most uncommon but may rarely be found in an infant or child presenting in shock and with signs of heart failure but with no history of congenital heart disease.

If such a patient were in the first few weeks of life, a trial of alprostadil would be appropriate and harmless.

Having completed the primary assessment and resuscitation and identified by means of the key features that cardiomyopathy/myocarditis is the most likely diagnosis, the child is reassessed.

Reassess ABC

Cardiomyopathy emergency treatment

- As the circulation is already overloaded with fluid, a diuretic, such as frusemide, should be given and the failing heart supported with an infusion of dobutamine which has some vasodilatory as well as inotropic effects.
- Urgent cardiology advice should be sought. Echocardiography should establish the diagnosis in almost all cases.

Full blood count, serum urea and electrolytes, calcium, glucose and arterial blood gases should be performed on all children with heart disease. A routine infection screen including blood cultures is also recommended. A full 12-lead electrocardiogram and chest radiograph are essential.

APPROACH TO THE CHILD WITH PROFOUND ANAEMIA

The most usual situation in which a child develops sudden severe haemolysis is in the case of septicaemia associated with sickle cell disease

In this situation, the child should be treated as for sepsis with volume support, intubation and inotropes. However, the volume infused should be fresh blood as soon as it can be obtained. These children may have an already damaged myocardium causing them to be candidates for cardiogenic as well as septic and dissociative shock.

An exchange transfusion may be life-saving in selected cases. These children will all need early paediatric intensive care advice and transfer.

BACKGROUND TO SHOCK

Shock results from an acute failure of circulatory function. Inadequate amounts of nutrients, especially oxygen, are delivered to body tissues and there is inadequate removal of tissue waste products. Shock is a complex clinical syndrome that is the body's response to cellular metabolic deficiency.

In hypovolaemic or distributory shock the initial haemodynamic abnormality of fluid loss or fluid shift is followed by compensatory mechanisms under neuroendocrine control. Later, shock is worsened by the production of vasoactive mediators and the products of cellular breakdown. The identity and relative importance of these chemicals are as yet poorly understood.

Shock is a progressive syndrome but it can be divided into three phases: compensated, uncompensated, and irreversible. Although artificial, this division is useful because each phase has characteristic clinicopathological manifestations and outcome.

Phase 1 (compensated) shock

In this phase vital organ function (brain and heart) is conserved by sympathetic reflexes which increase systemic arterial resistance, divert blood away from non-essential tissues, constrict the venous reservoir and increase the heart rate to maintain cardiac output. The systolic blood pressure remains normal whereas the diastolic pressure may be elevated due to increased systemic arterial resistance. Increased secretion of angiotensin and vasopressin allows the kidneys to conserve water and salt, and intestinal fluid is reabsorbed from the digestive tract. Clinical signs at this stage include mild agitation or confusion, skin pallor, increased heart rate, and cold peripheral skin with decreased capillary return.

Phase 2 (uncompensated) shock

In uncompensated shock, the compensatory mechanisms start to fail and the circulatory system is no longer efficient. Areas that have poor perfusion can no longer metabolise aerobically, and anaerobic metabolism becomes their major source of energy production. Anaerobic metabolism is comparatively inefficient. Only 2 moles of adenosine triphosphate (ATP) are produced for each mole of glucose metabolised compared to 38 moles of ATP per mole of glucose metabolised aerobically.

Anaerobic pathways produce excess lactate leading to systemic acidosis. The acidosis is compounded by intracellular carbonic acid formed because of the inability of the circulation to remove CO_2. Acidosis reduces myocardial contractility and impairs the response to catecholamines.

A further result of anaerobic metabolism is the failure of the energy dependent sodium–potassium pump, which maintains the normal homoeostatic environment in which the cell functions.

Lysosomal, mitochondrial, and membrane functions deteriorate without this homoeostasis. Sluggish flow of blood and chemical changes in small vessels lead to platelet adhesion, and may produce damaging chain reactions in the kinin and coagulation systems leading to a bleeding tendency.

Numerous chemical mediators have been identified in shocked patients, but the roles of each have not been clearly identified. They include histamine, serotonin, cytokines (especially tumour necrosis factor and interleukin 1), xanthine oxidase (which generates oxygen radicals), platelet-aggregating factor, and bacterial toxins. They are largely produced by cells of the immune system, especially monocytic macrophages. It has been suggested that these mediators, which developed as initial adaptive responses to severe injury and illness, may have deleterious consequences in the "unnatural" setting of the resuscitated patient. When the role of these chemical mediators is more fully understood, blocking agents may be produced which will improve the treatment in phase 2 shock.

The result of these cascading metabolic changes is to reduce tissue perfusion and oxidation further. Blood pools in some areas because arterioles can no longer control flow in the capillary system. Furthermore, abnormal capillary permeability allows further fluid loss from the circulation into the interstitium.

Clinically, the patient in phase 2 shock has a falling blood pressure, very slow capillary return, tachycardia, cold peripheries, acidotic breathing, depressed cerebral state, and absent urine output.

Phase 3 (irreversible) shock

The diagnosis of irreversible shock is a retrospective one. The damage to key organs such as the heart and brain is of such magnitude that death occurs despite adequate restoration of the circulation. Pathophysiologically, the high energy phosphate reserves in cells (especially those of the liver and heart) are greatly diminished. The ATP has been degraded via adenosine to uric acid. New ATP is synthesised at only 2% an hour and the body can be said to have run out of energy. This underlies the clinical observation that during the progression of shock a point is reached at which death of the patient is inevitable, despite therapeutic intervention. *Hence early recognition and effective treatment of shock are vital.*

A closer study of septic shock illustrates many of these points.

Septic shock

In sepsis the cardiac output may be normal or raised but may still be too low to deliver sufficient oxygen to the tissues. This is because abnormal distribution of blood in the microcirculation leads to decreased tissue perfusion.

The release of bacterial toxins triggers complex interacting haemodynamic and metabolic changes. Mediators and activators are released and react to produce the "septic syndrome". These activators may be vasodilators or vasoconstrictors; some promote and activate the coagulation cascade; others are cardiac depressants.

In septic shock cardiac function may be depressed Oxygen delivery to the heart from the coronary arteries occurs mainly in diastole, and the tachycardia and increased oxygen demand of the myocardium in septic shock may jeopardise cardiac oxygenation. Metabolic acidosis also damages myocardial cells at mitochondrial level. The function of the left ventricle is affected more than the right ventricle. This may be due to myocardial oedema, adrenogenic receptor dysfunction, or impaired sarcolemmal calcium influx. The right ventricle is less important in maintaining cardiac output than the left, but increased

112

pulmonary vascular resistance can limit the hyperdynamic state and oxygen delivery.

In septic shock cells do not use oxygen properly   There appears to be a block at the mitochondrial level in the mechanism of oxygen uptake, and in progressive shock the difference between arterial and venous saturation levels of oxygen is inappropriately narrow. This progressive deterioration in cell oxygen consumption heralds multiple organ failure.

Early (compensated) septic shock

This is characterised by a raised cardiac output, decreased systemic resistance, warm extremities, and a wide pulse pressure. This pattern is seen more typically in adults and may never be seen in infants in whom cold peripheries are much more common. The hyperdynamic state is recognised by hyperpyrexia, hyperventilation, tachycardia, and mental confusion. All of these signs may be minimal: mental confusion in particular needs to be looked for carefully, if septic shock is not to be overlooked at this stage. Decreased capillary return is a useful sign in these circumstances.

Late (uncompensated) septic shock

If no effective therapy is given, the cardiovascular performance deteriorates and cardiac output diminishes. Even with a normal or raised cardiac output, shock develops. The normal relationship between cardiac output and systemic vascular resistance breaks down and hypotension may persist as a result of decreased vascular resistance.

The cardiac output may fall gradually over several hours, or precipitously in minutes. As tissue hypoxia develops, plasma lactic acid levels increase.

Infants, who have little cardiac reserve, often present with hypotension and a hypodynamic picture. These sick babies are a diagnostic challenge but sepsis must be assumed and treated as quickly as possible.

Survival in septic shock depends on the maintenance of a hyperdynamic state. Several factors mitigate against this by encouraging hypovolaemia:

1. Increased microvascular permeability.
2. Arteriolar and venous dilatation with peripheral pooling of blood.
3. Inadequate fluid intake.
4. Fluid loss secondary to fever, diarrhoea, and vomiting.
5. Inappropriate polyuria.

AFTER RESUSCITATION AND EMERGENCY TREATMENT

Following successful restoration of adequate circulation, varying degrees of organ damage may remain, and should be actively sought and managed after the initial resuscitation and emergency treatment has stabilised the patient. The problems are similar but of less degree than those expected following resuscitation from cardiac arrest.

Kidneys

Prerenal failure, acute tubular necrosis, and the more severe cortical necrosis may be sequelae of phase 2 shock. Once haemodynamic parameters are improving, fluid administration should be reviewed and serum electrolytes, urea, and creatinine analysed.

Lung

"Shock lung" appears to be a more common sequel in adults than in children. Patients with this complication develop respiratory failure because of increased lung water. Ventilation with high inspired oxygen is necessary, and positive end-expiratory pressure (PEEP) may be required.

Heart

Despite adequate volume restoration, and even if shock was not primarily cardiogenic, poor myocardial perfusion often leads to decreased contractility. Inotropic agents need to be continued and vasodilators may be required.

Coagulation abnormalities

As described above, sludging of blood and the production of chemical mediators may initiate microvascular clotting which leads to a consumption coagulopathy. Clotting times and a platelet count should be estimated and fresh frozen plasma given if clinically indicated.

Other organs

The liver and bowel may be damaged in shock, leading to gastrointestinal bleeding. Endocrine organs may be variously affected and patients must be monitored for glucose and mineral homoeostasis.

FLUID RESUSCITATION

Underlying considerations

Crystalloid or colloid fluids or blood are available for volume replacement.

The distribution of different fluids through the main compartments within the body (in decreasing volume: intracellular, interstitial and intravascular) is determined by constituents of the fluid. In general, the large molecules in colloids ensure that a greater proportion of the volume given as colloid will be retained in the intravascular space, the compartment where fluid resuscitation is directed. Blood is retained best in the intravascular space. The ability of the osmotically active particles of colloid to remain intravascular, and retain intravascular fluid volume, is varied. The complex starches used in heta- or pentastarch remain in the vascular space for a prolonged period. The gelatin derivatives of Gelofusine or Haemaccel of other colloids do so for only a few hours. Albumin will exchange readily with the albumin in the interstitial fluid, but remains in the intravascular space for more than 24 hours in health. Albumin loss to the tissue fluid will be enhanced where the endothelial barrier function is degraded by endothelial inflammation.

Again with crystalloids, distribution is determined by the constituents. The sodium and chloride of normal saline will ensure that it is localised more to the whole extracellular compartment (where sodium is the main osmotically active particle), and so when given intravenously, only a minor part will remain in the intravascular compartment as the majority of extracellular fluid is tissue fluid. This is in contrast to the distribution of 5% glucose, which after the metabolism of the glucose is effectively free water, which then disperses through all the fluid compartments of the body and so even less is retained intravascularly.

Those who support colloid resuscitation emphasis the importance of oncotic pressure in maintaining intravascular volume and tissue perfusion. Those who favour crystalloids respond that as the endothelium becomes leakier in ill patients, the colloid will also leak and serve to retain fluid in the tissues. To equal the increase of intravascular volume produced by a colloid, approximately three to five times as much crystalloid must be given.

Colloids are in general more expensive than crystalloids, and of the colloids, human albumin solution (HAS) is the most expensive and most restricted in availability. Anaphylactic reactions are commoner with the colloids and more so with the gelatine-based colloids. Transmission of viral infections is a concern with the use of HAS.

Most of the fluids used in resuscitation are (close to) isotonic. Hypertonic solutions, particularly hypertonic saline has been used to resuscitate patients usually following blood loss. Experience in paediatrics is not extensive, but certainly some reports are favourable. An underlying concept is that smaller volumes of hypertonic solutions may adequately resuscitate the intravascular volume, without excess tissue oedema.

Further details on the composition of fluids can be found in Appendix B.

If blood is needed, it may be given after full cross-match which takes about 1 hour to perform. In more urgent situations type-specific non-cross-matched blood (which is ABO rhesus compatible but has a higher incidence of transfusion reactions) should be requested. It takes about 15 minutes to prepare. In dire emergencies O-negative blood must be given.

Fluids should be warmed if this can be done without delay. Isotonic electrolyte solution should be kept available in a warmed cabinet. Further details on the management of shock in trauma, burns and diabetes can be found in Chapters 15, 20 and Appendix B.

Clinical considerations

Many trials contrasting fluid resuscitation regimens have been carried out, though few have been in paediatrics. None have produced a definitive answer. A recent Cochrane analysis suggesting that use of albumin increased mortality provoked considerable debate in the literature but there were few paediatric trials included and many of the studies were not done in the emergency situation. A further Cochrane review found no evidence that any colloid solution was more effective than any other, though neither was there a demonstrable benefit to albumin resuscitation

Furthermore, although all forms of shock are often treated as one, there is no reason to expect all forms of shock to respond to treatment in the same way, as their underlying biology differs.

Although the debate is often described as "crystalloid versus colloid", within each group there are important differences between individual crystalloids and individual colloids.

Where the electrolytes or tonicity are disturbed, the immediate concern is to reverse shock or disturbances of perfusion. Chronic disturbances of electrolytes or tonicity should be corrected more slowly (over 24–48 hours) as compensatory mechanisms will have developed. Over rapid correction is likely to contribute to morbidity. The fluid used will depend on the disturbance of electrolytes.

Clinical decisions

The clinical decisions which must be made are essentially: When should we give fluid; how much fluid should we give, and which fluid should we give?

When should we give fluid?

Fluids should be given where perfusion is compromised. Assessment of perfusion is difficult, and relies on assessment of organ function – urine output, mentation, peripheral perfusion. In a retrospective review of children with septic shock, early administration of large volumes of fluid (>40 ml/kg in the first hour) was associated with better outcome than smaller volume resuscitation encouraging a vigorous approach in septicaemia. In contrast, where shock is caused by penetrating trauma requiring definitive surgical management, maximal fluid resuscitation may be best delayed until operation as improving perfusion without improving oxygen-carrying capacity as well results in a worse outcome.

How much fluid should we give?

Administration of fluid should be guided by the response. Smaller volumes may be judged by their effect on the feature (for example peripheral perfusion) which provoked the administration of the fluid bearing in mind the caveats in Chapter 3 on the interpretation of these signs. If large volumes are needed, resuscitation is best guided by measurement of cardiac filling pressures and therefore patients requiring large volume resuscitation need prompt paediatric intensive care advice and timely transfer.

Which fluid should we give?

No definitive answer can be given. Where small volumes of fluid are used it may not matter. When larger volumes of fluid are used it must be more important.

In acute collapse, a smaller volume of colloid is needed than crystalloid to produce a given increase in intravascular volume, and so more rapid correction of haemodynamic derangement may be possible with colloid if it is readily available.

When larger volumes of fluid are used, the choice of fluid becomes more important. As the circulating volume of a child is approximately 80 ml/kg, if more than 40 ml/kg of fluid is used over a short time, one half of the child's circulating volume will have been given. If much more fluid transfusion is needed, significant haemodilution may result, and consideration should be given to using blood for fluid resuscitation with measurements of the central venous pressure (effectively cardiac preload) to guide fluid resuscitation. Where large volumes are used human albumin solution is generally preferred in paediatric practice although most adult patients are resuscitated with synthetic colloids, crystalloid, or hypertonic solutions.

IN CONCLUSION

There is no definitive evidence demonstrating which fluid is best for resuscitation. Other important questions – how much and when should fluids be used also remain to be answered. Clinical trials will be needed to answer these questions, though they are likely to be difficult to perform. Whilst awaiting more clinical trials, fluid resuscitation guided by a knowledge of the pathophysiology underlying the disease, and of the different roles of the different fluids will remain optimal management.

11

The child with an abnormal pulse rate or rhythm

INTRODUCTION

Most tachyarrhythmias in children are caused by a re-entrant congenital conduction pathway abnormality but some are secondary to poisoning or metabolic disturbance, follow cardiac surgery or occur in the course of cardiomyopathy. In tachyarrhythmias the rate is fast but the rhythm largely regular.

Most bradyarrhythmias are secondary to hypoxia and shock and are pre-terminal events although a few follow conduction pathway damage during cardiac surgery. The rate is slow and the rhythm usually irregular.

Children with congenital conduction pathway abnormalities will present in one of two ways. If they are able to communicate effectively, i.e the older child, they will present early, usually in good condition, with a perception of palpitations. If they are unable to communicate, i.e the younger child and infants, they will present later with poor feeding or even shock if their parent has not noticed the abnormal heart rate.

Those with other causes of tachyarrhythmias, such as poisoning, may present with additional symptoms, depending on the cause and progress of the underlying problem.

Children with bradyarrhythmias will almost always be in severe and pre-terminal respiratory failure or shock on presentation.

This chapter will provide the student with an approach to the assessment, resuscitation and emergency management of children with abnormal pulse rate or rhythm.

APPROACH TO THE CHILD IN WITH AN ABNORMAL PULSE RATE OR RHYTHM

PRIMARY ASSESSMENT

Airway

Assess airway patency by the "look, listen, and feel" method.
If the child can speak or cry, this indicates that the airway is patent, that breathing is

occurring and there is adequate circulation.

If there is no evidence of air movement then chin lift or jaw thrust manoeuvres should be carried out and the airway reassessed. If there continues to be no evidence of air movement then airway patency can be assessed by performing an opening manoeuvre and giving rescue breaths (see Basic Life Support, Chapter 4).

Breathing

Assess the adequacy of breathing.

- Effort of breathing
  Recession
  Respiratory rate
  Grunting
  Accessory muscle use
  Flare of the alae nasi
- Efficacy of breathing
  Breath sounds
  Chest expansion/abdominal excursion

Monitor oxygen saturation with a pulse oximeter.

Circulation

Assess the adequacy of circulation
Cardiovascular status

Heart rate and rhythm

This is the defining observation for this presentation. An abnormal pulse rate is defined as one falling outside the normal range given in Chapter 3. In practice, most serious disease or injury states are associated with a sinus tachycardia. In infants this may be as high as up to 220 bpm and in children up to 180 bpm. Rates over these figures are highly likely to be tachyarrhythmias, but in any case of significant tachycardia, i.e 200 in an infant and 150 in a child, an ECG rhythm strip should be examined and, if in doubt, a full 12-lead ECG performed. Very high rates may be impossible to count manually and the pulse oximeter is often unreliable in this regard. Again a rhythm strip is advised.

An abnormally slow pulse rate is defined as less than 60 beats per minute or a rapidly dropping heart rate associated with poor systemic perfusion. If a bradyarrhythmia is found it will almost always be in a child who clearly requires major resuscitation.

Pulse volume

Examination of central and peripheral pulses may show a poor volume peripherally or, more worryingly, also centrally.

Capillary refill

If there is poor skin perfusion with a rhythm abnormality there may be shock. Slow capillary refill (>2 seconds) after blanching pressure for 5 seconds is evidence of reduced skin perfusion. When testing for capillary refill press on the skin of the sternum or a digit held at the level of the heart. Mottling, pallor, and peripheral cyanosis also indicate poor skin perfusion. All these signs may be difficult to interpret in patients who have just been exposed to cold.

Blood pressure

Children's cardiovascular systems compensate well initially in tachyarrhythmias. *Hypotension is a late and often sudden sign of decompensation and, if not reversed, will be rapidly followed by death.*

Serial measurements of blood pressure should be performed frequently.

Effects of circulatory inadequacy on other organs

Acidotic sighing respirations

The acidosis produced by poor tissue perfusion leads to rapid deep breathing.

Pale, cyanosed or cold skin

A core/toe temperature difference of more than 2°C is a sign of poor skin perfusion.

Mental status: agitation or depressed conscious level

Early signs of brain hypoperfusion are agitation and confusion, often alternating with drowsiness. Infants may be irritable but drowsy with a weak cry and hypotonia. They may not focus on the parent's face. These are important early cerebral signs of shock. Later the child becomes progressively drowsier until consciousness is lost.

Urinary output

Urine flow is decreased or absent in shock. It is not a useful initial assessment but hourly measurement is helpful in monitoring progress. A minimum flow of 1 ml/kg/h in children and 2 ml/kg/h in infants indicates adequate renal perfusion.

NOTE Poor capillary refill, core/toe temperature difference and differential pulse volumes are neither sensitive nor specific indicators of shock when used in isolation. There are helpful when used in conjunction with the other signs described.

Look for the presence of signs of heart failure

- Tachycardia
- Raised jugular venous pressure
- Lung crepitations on auscultation
- Gallop rhythm
- Enlarged liver

And listen for a heart murmur.

Monitor heart rate/rhythm, blood pressure and core/toe temperature difference.

If heart rate is above 200 in an infant or above 150 in a child or if the rhythm is abnormal perform a standard ECG.

Disability

Assess neurological function.
- A rapid measure of level of consciousness should be recorded using the AVPU scale.
- Pupillary size and reaction should be noted.
- Note the child's posture: children in shock are usually hypotonic.
- The presence of convulsive movements should be noted.

Exposure

- Take the child's core and toe temperatures.
- Look for evidence of poisoning.

RESUSCITATION

Airway

If the airway is not open, an airway opening manoeuvre should be performed and an airway adjunct placed. Seek urgent anaesthetic help to secure the airway.

Breathing

- All children in shock with an abnormal rhythm should receive high flow oxygen through a face mask with a reservoir as soon as the airway has been demonstrated to be adequate.
- If the child is hypoventilating or has bradycardia, respiration should be supported with oxygen via a bag-valve-mask device and experienced senior help summoned.

Circulation

- If the heart rate is below 60 in a patient with shock, chest compressions should be commenced.
- If a child in shock has a narrow complex tachyarrhythmia up to three synchronous electrical shocks at 0·5, 1 and 2J should be given. If the arrhythmia is broad complex give asynchronous shocks. A conscious child should be anaesthetised or sedated first if this can be done in a timely manner. Synchronisation relies on the ability of the defibrillator to recognise the QRST complex, and is designed to avoid shock delivery at a point in the cardiac cycle likely to precipitate ventricular fibrillation. Ventricular tachycardia in children is usually fast and has no recognisable QRST complexes; in such circumstances it will prove impossible to deliver a shock to the child in synchronous mode, as the defibrillator will fail to "spot" a favourable time for shock delivery. In order to overcome the problem and ensure prompt delivery of effective treatment, non-synchronous shocks are recommended.
The reason this approach is not advocated in stable ventricular tachycardia is that there is more time available to deliver the synchronous shock, because if it takes 30–40 seconds it does not matter.
- If the shocked child's tachyarrhythmia is SVT then he can be treated with intravenous/intraosseous adenosine if this can be administered more quickly than a synchronous electrical shock
Gain intravenous or intraosseous access.

- Take blood for FBC and U&Es, glucose stick test and laboratory test.
- Give a bolus of crystalloid to a patient with bradycardia who is in shock.

While the primary assessment and resuscitation are being carried out a focused history of the child's health and activity over the previous 24 hours should be gained.

Certain key features which will be identified clinically in the primary assessment, from the focused history, from the initial blood tests and from the rhythm strip and 12-lead ECG can point the clinician to the likeliest working diagnosis for emergency treatment.

From the ECG the arrhythmia can be categorised by the following simple questions:

1. Is the *rate*:
    too fast?
    too slow?
2. Is the *rhythm*:
    regular?
    irregular?
3. Are the QRS *complexes*:
    narrow?
    broad?

- *Bradycardia* is most usually a preterminal rhythm. It is usually seen as the final response to profound *hypoxia and ischaemia* and its presence is ominous. It can also be precipitated by *vagal stimulation* as occurs in tracheal intubation and suctioning and may be found in post-operative cardiac patients. The rhythm is usually irregular.
- In addition bradycardia may be seen in patients with *raised intracranial pressure*. These patients will have presented with coma and their management can be found in Chapters 12 and 18.
- *Bradycardia* can be a side effect of *poisoning* with *digoxin* or *beta-blockers* and the management can be found in Chapter 14.
- A rapid heart rate with a narrow QRS complex on the ECG is *supra-ventricular tachycardia*. The rhythm is usually regular.
- A rapid heart rate with a wide QRS complex on the ECG is *ventricular tachycardia*.
- *Ventricular tachycardia* can be provoked by *hyperkalaemia* and by poisoning with *tricyclic antidepressant*s, with a combination of *cisapride and macrolide antibiotics* and by *terfenadine taken with grapefruit juice*. Additional details on the management of the poisoned child with ventricular tachycardia can be found in Chapter 14.

APPROACH TO THE CHILD WITH BRADYCARDIA

In paediatric practice bradycardia is almost always a preterminal finding in patients with respiratory or circulatory insufficiency. Airway, breathing, and circulation should always be assessed and treated if neeeded before pharmacological management of bradycardia.

Reassess ABC

BRADYCARDIA EMERGENCY TREATMENT

Continue to treat hypoxia and shock vigorously with intubation, ventilation, and volume expansion. If these measures do not lead to rapid improvement, consider a bolus of epinephrine 10 µg/kg IV followed by an epinephrine infusion. The starting dose of epinephrine for infusion is 0·05 micrograms/kg/min.

In the patient who has developed bradycardia from vagal stimulation during suctioning or tracheal intubation, volume expansion is unlikely to be needed but good ventilation should be ensured prior to giving atropine 0·02 mg/kg IV (minimum dose 0·1 mg, maximum 2·0 mg/dose). The drug counteracts excess vagal tone.

Small doses of atropine may produce paradoxical bradycardia therefore, the recommended dose is 0·02 mg/kg, with a minimum dose of 0·1 mg and a maximum single dose of 0·5 mg in a child and 1·0 mg in an adolescent. The dose may be repeated in 5 minutes, to a maximum total dose of 1·0 mg in a child and 2·0 mg in an adolescent. If intravenous/intraosseous access is not readily available, atropine (0·04 mg/kg) may be administered tracheally, although absorption into the circulation may be unreliable.

Seek expert toxicology help for the management of bradycardia caused by poisoning.

APPROACH TO THE CHILD WITH SUPRAVENTRICULAR TACHYCARDIA

Supraventricular tachycardia (SVT) is the most common non-arrest arrhythmia during childhood and is the most common arrhythmia that produces cardiovascular instability during infancy. SVT in infants generally produces a heart rate > 220 bpm, and sometimes as high 300 bpm. Lower heart rates occur in children during SVT. The QRS complex is narrow making differentiation between marked sinus tachycardia due to shock and SVT difficult, particularly because SVT may also be associated with poor systemic perfusion.

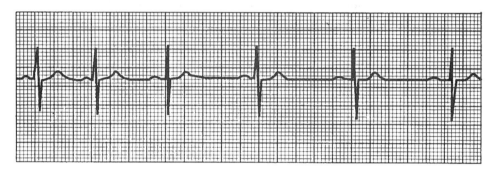

Figure 11.1. Sinus bradycardia during suctioning

The following characteristics may help to distiguish between sinus tachycardia and SVT:

1. Sinus tachycardia is typically characterised by a heart rate less than 200 per minute in infants and children whereas infants with SVT typically have a heart rate greater than 220 beats per minute.
2. P-waves may be difficult to identify in both sinus tachycardia and SVT once the ventricular rate exceeds 200 beats per minute. If P-waves are identifiable, they are usually upright in leads I and AVF in sinus tachycardia while they are negative in leads II, III and AVF in SVT.
3. In sinus tachycardia, the heart rate varies from beat to beat and is often responsive to stimulation, but there is no beat-to-beat variability in SVT.
4. Termination of SVT is abrupt whereas the heart rate slows gradually in sinus tachycardia in response to treatment.
5. A history consistent with shock (e.g., gastroenteritis or septicaemia) is usually present with sinus tachycardia.

Cardiopulmonary stability during episodes of SVT is affected by the child's age, duration of SVT, prior ventricular function and ventricular rate. Older children usually complain of lightheadedness, dizziness, chest discomfort or note the fast heart rate, but very rapid rates may be undetected for long periods in young infants until they develop a low cardiac output state and shock. This deterioration in cardiac function occurs

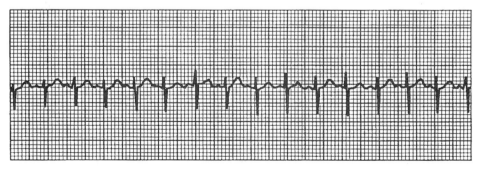

Figure 11.2. Sinus tachycardia

122

because of increased myocardial oxygen demand and limitation in myocardial oxygen delivery during the short diastolic phase associated with very rapid heart rates. If baseline myocardial function is impaired (e.g., in a child with a cardiomyopathy), SVT can produce signs of shock in a relatively short time.

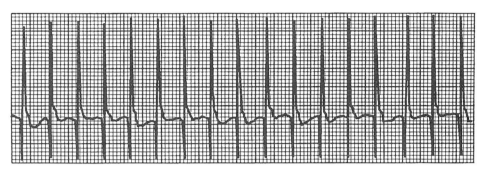

Figure 11.3. Supraventricular tachycardia

Reassess ABC

SUPRAVENTRICULAR TACHYCARDIA EMERGENCY TREATMENT

Try vagal stimulation while continuing ECG monitoring. The following techniques can be used:

1. Elicit the "diving reflex" which produces an increase in vagal tone, slows atrioventricular conduction and interrupts the tachycardia. In the case of a baby, the infant should be wrapped in a towel and his whole face immersed in iced water for about five seconds. There is no need to obstruct the mouth or nostrils as the baby will be temporarily apnoeic. For an older child an ice-water soaked cloth is placed on the nose and mouth.
2. One-sided carotid body massage.
3. Older children can try a Valsalva manoeuvre. Some children know that a certain position or action will usually effect a return to sinus rhythm. Blowing hard through a straw may be effective for some children.

Do not use ocular pressure in an infant or child as ocular damage may result.

If these manoeuvres are unsuccessful, give:

Intravenous adenosine Start with a bolus dose of 50 micrograms/kg intravenously and increase the dose to 100 micrograms/kg after 2 minutes if success is not achieved. The next dose should be 250 micrograms/kg. The maximum total dose that should be given is 500 micrograms/kg (300 micrograms/kg under one month). Adenosine is a very rapidly acting drug with a half-life of less than 10 seconds. This means that side effects (flushing, nausea, dyspnoea, chest tightness) are short-lived. It also means, however, that the effect may be short-lasting and the supraventricular tachycardia may recur.

For the same reason if the drug is given through a small peripheral vein, an insufficiently high concentration may reach the heart and therefore a larger dose may need to be given. Preferably, the drug should be given into a large peripheral vein and rapidly followed by a saline flush. Adenosine is the drug of choice for supraventricular tachycardia because of its efficacy and safety record.

If a child with stable supraventricular tachycardia has not been converted to a normal rhythm with intravenous adenosine it is essential to seek the advice of a paediatric cardiologist before further treatment. The use of one of the following may be suggested.

Flecainide 2 mg/kg over 20 minutes This drug is particularly useful in refractory Wolff–Parkinson–White type tachycardia. It is a membrane stabiliser but can be pro-arrhythmic and has a negative inotropic effect.

Digoxin Dosage schedules vary with age and underlying condition. Seek advice.

Verapamil This drug has been associated with irreversible hypotension and asystole when given to infants. It therefore should *not be used in children under 1 year of age*. The dose for 1–5 years is 50 micrograms/kg intravenously slowly, from 5 to 10 years 100 micrograms/kg, from 10 to 15 years 150 micrograms/kg. The drug should be terminated when sinus rhythm is seen even though the calculated dose has not been given. *Do not use if a patient has received β-blockers, flecainide or amiodarone.*

Amiodarone This drug can be used in refractory atrial tachycardia. The dose is 5 mg/kg over 20–30 min diluted in approximately 4 ml/kg of 5% dextrose.

Propranolol 50 micrograms/kg slowly intravenously. Only if pacing is available as asystole may occur. *Do not give propranolol if the patient has been given verapamil.*

It is unsafe to give verapamil and propranolol to the same patient as they both have negative inotropic actions. It is, however, safe to give propranolol and digoxin.

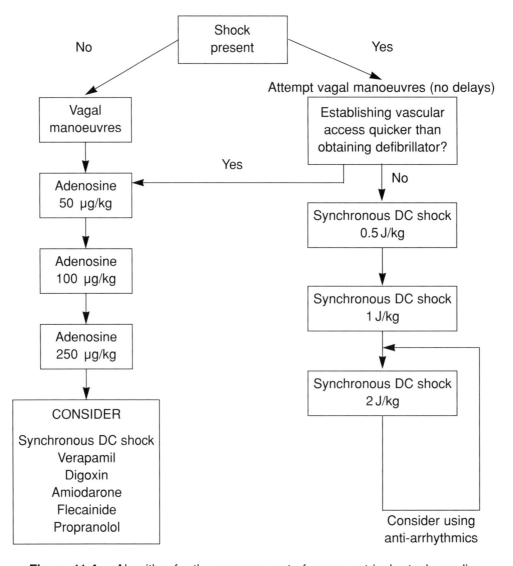

Figure 11.4. Algorithm for the management of supraventricular tachycardia

APPROACH TO THE CHILD WITH VENTRICULAR TACHYCARDIA

Reassess ABC

VENTRICULAR TACHYCARDIA EMERGENCY TREATMENT

In the haemodynamically stable child with ventricular tachycardia a history should be carefully obtained to identify an underlying cause for the tachycardia as this will often determine ancillary therapy.

Ask about:

- Congenital heart disease and surgery.
- Possibility of poisoning with tricyclic antidepressants, procainamide, quinidine, cisapride and macrolide antibiotics and terfenadine with grapefruit juice: the mere presence of such drugs in the home in association with a previously well child is presumptive evidence of causation.
- A history of renal disease suggesting hyperkalaemia.

Look for:

- Characteristics of the ECG suggestive of torsades-de-pointes.
- Serum K, Mg, Ca.

Analysis of the ECG should be done in consultation with a paediatric cardiologist to whom it should faxed.

The treatment of the haemodynamically stable child with ventricular tachycardia should always include early consultation with a pediatric cardiologist. They may suggest amiodarone (5 mg/kg over 60 minutes) or intravenous procainamide (15 mg/kg over 30–60 minutes) but especially in cases where the ventricular arrhythmia has been caused by drug toxicity sedation/anaesthesia and DC shock may be the safest approach.

It is important not to delay a safe therapeutic intervention for longer than necessary in VT as the rhythm often deteriorates quite quickly into pulseless VT or VF.

Both amiodarone and procainamide can cause hypotension which should be treated with volume expansion.

Torsades-de pointes ventricular tachycardia

This is a polymorphic ventricular tachycardia characterised by an ECG appearance of QRS complexes which change in amplitude and polarity so that they appear to rotate around an isoelectric line. It is seen in conditions characterised by a long QT interval. Quinidine, disopyramide, amiodarone, tricyclic antidepressants and digoxin are all reported causes. In addition, pharmacokinetic interactions may cause torsades de pointes with the interaction between cisapride and erythromycin being a recently recognised problem. The treatment is magnesium sulphate in a rapid IV infusion (several minutes) of 25–50 mg/kg (up to 2 g).

Wide-QRS SVT (i.e., SVT with aberrant conduction) is uncommon in infants and children. Correct diagnosis and differentiation from ventricular tachycardia depends on careful analysis of at least a 12-lead ECG that may be supplemented by information from an oesophageal lead. The patient and family history should be evaluated to help identify the presence of an underlying condition predisposing to stable ventricular tachycardia. Since either SVT or VT can cause haemodynamic instability, assumptions about the mechanism (i.e., ventricular versus supraventricular) should not be based

125

solely on the haemodynamic status of the patient.

A dose of adenosine may help identify the underlying aetiology of the arrhythmia, but should be used with extreme caution in haemodynamically stable children with wide-complex tachycardia as acceleration of the tachycardia and significant hypotension are known risks.

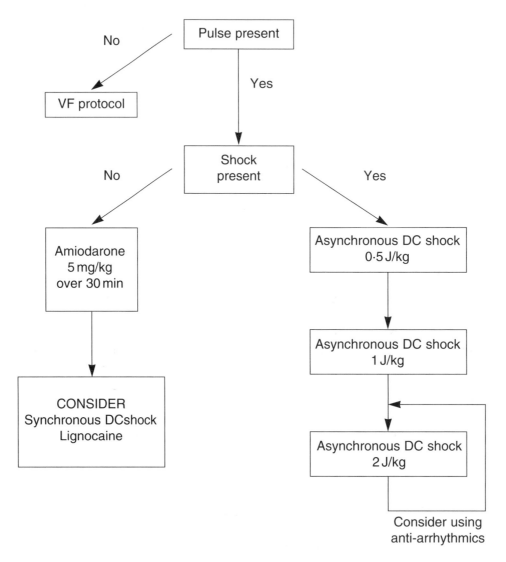

Figure 11.5. Algorithm for the management of ventricular tachycardia

12

The child with a decreased conscious level

INTRODUCTION

The conscious level may be altered by disease, injury, or intoxication. The level of awareness decreases as a child passes through stages from drowsiness (mild reduction in alertness and increase in hours of sleep) to unconsciousness (unrousable unresponsiveness). Because of variability in the definition of words describing the degree of coma, the Glasgow and the Children's Coma Scales have been developed as semi-quantitative measures and, more importantly, as an aid to communication between carers. The Glasgow Coma Scale was developed and validated for use in the head injured patient but has come to be used as an unvalidated tool for the description of conscious states from all pathologies.

In children, coma is caused by a diffuse metabolic insult (including cerebral hypoxia and ischaemia) in 95% of cases, and by structural lesions in the remaining 5%. Metabolic disturbances can produce diffuse, incomplete, and asymmetrical neurological signs falsely suggestive of a localised lesion. Early signs of metabolic encephalopathy may be subtle with reduced attention and blunted affect. The conscious level in metabolic encephalopathies is often quite variable from minute to minute. The most common causes of coma are summarised in the box.

Disorders causing coma in children

Hypoxic ischaemic brain injury
   Following respiratory or circulatory failure
Epileptic seizures
Trauma
   Intracranial haemorrhage, brain swelling
Infections
   Meningitis
   Encephalitis
Poisoning
Metabolic
   Renal, hepatic failure, Reye's syndrome, hypoglycaemia, diabetes, hypothermia, hypercapnia
Vascular lesions
   Bleeding, arteriovenous malformations, arterial or venous thrombosis
Hypertension

Table 12.1. Glasgow Coma Scale and Children's Coma Scale

Glasgow Coma Scale (4–15 years)		Child's Glasgow Coma Scale (<4 years)	
Response	Score	Response	Score
Eye opening		*Eye opening*	
Spontaneously	4	Spontaneously	4
To verbal stimuli	3	To verbal stimuli	3
To pain	2	To pain	2
No response to pain	1	No response to pain	1
Best motor response		*Best motor response*	
Obeys verbal command	6	Spontaneous or obeys verbal command	6
Localises to pain	5	Localises to pain or withdraws to touch	5
Withdraws from pain	4	Withdraws from pain	4
Abnormal flexion to pain (decorticate)	3	Abnormal flexion to pain (decorticate)	3
Abnormal extension to pain (decerebrate)	2	Abnormal extension to pain (decerebrate)	2
No response to pain	1	No response to pain	1
Best verbal response		*Best verbal response*	
Orientated and converses	5	Alert, babbles, coos, words to usual ability	5
Disorientated and converses	4	Less than usual words spontaneous irritable cry	4
Inappropriate words	3	Cries only to pain	3
Incomprehensible sounds	2	Moans to pain	2
No response to pain	1	No response to pain	1

Children with a decreased conscious level are usually presented by parents who are very aware of the seriousness of the symptom. They may also have noted other features such as fever, headache, exposure to poisoning which may aid the clinician to make a presumptive diagnosis

APPROACH TO THE CHILD WITH A DECREASED CONSCIOUS LEVEL

Primary assessment

The first steps in the management of the patient with a decreased conscious level are to assess and if necessary support airway, breathing and circulation. This will ensure that the diminished conscious level is not secondary to hypoxia and/or ischaemia and that whatever the cerebral pathology it will not be worsened by lack of oxygenated blood supply to the brain.

Airway

Assess airway patency by the "look, listen, and feel" method.

If the child can speak or cry in response to a stimulus, this indicates that the airway is patent, that breathing is occurring and that there is adequate circulation. If the child responds only with withdrawal to a painful stimulus (AVPU score "P".) his airway is at risk.

If there is no evidence of air movement then chin lift or jaw thrust manoeuvres should be carried out and the airway reassessed. If there continues to be no evidence of air movement then perform an opening manoeuvre and give rescue breaths (see Basic Life Support, Chapter 4).

Breathing

Assess the adequacy of breathing.

- *Effort of breathing*
  Recession
  Respiratory rate
  Grunting
  Accessory muscle use
  Flare of the alae nasi
  Breath sounds
  Chest expansion/abdominal excursion
- *Effects of breathing*
  Heart rate
  Skin colour
  Mental status

Monitor oxygen saturation with a pulse oximeter.

Circulation

Assess the adequacy of circulation.

- *Cardiovascular status*
  Heart rate. *The presence of an inappropriate bradycardia will suggest raised intracranial pressure*
  Pulse volume
  Capillary refill
  Blood pressure
  Significant hypertension may indicate a possible aetiology for the coma or be a result of it
- *Effects of circulatory inadequacy on other organs*
  Acidotic sighing respirations. *This may suggest metabolic acidosis from diabetes or salicylate or ethylene glycol poisoning as a cause for the coma.*
  Pale, cyanosed or cold skin.

Monitor heart rate/rhythm, blood pressure and core/toe temperature difference.
If heart rate is above 200 in an infant or above 150 in a child or if the rhythm is abnormal perform a standard ECG.

Disability

- Assess neurological function.
- A rapid measure of level of consciousness should be recorded using the AVPU scale.
- A **ALERT**
- V responds to **VOICE**
- P responds to **PAIN**
- U **UNRESPONSIVE**

Pupillary size and reaction should be noted. *Very small pupils suggest opiate poisoning, large pupils amphetamines, atropine, tricyclic antidepressants and others (see page 156).*

Note the child's posture. *Decorticate or decerebrate posturing in a previously normal child should suggest raised intracranial pressure.*

Look for neck stiffness in a child and a full fontanelle in an infant which suggest *meningitis.*

The presence of convulsive movements should be sought: these may be subtle.

Exposure

Take the child's core and toe temperatures. *A fever is suggestive evidence of an infectious cause (but its absence does not the suggest the opposite) or poisoning with ecstasy, cocaine or salicylates. Hypothermia suggests poisoning with barbiturates or ethanol.*

Look for a rash. *If one is present, ascertain if it is purpuric as an indicator of meningococcal disease or non-accidental injury*

Look for evidence of poisoning.

RESUSCITATION

Airway

- A patent airway is the first requisite. If the airway is not patent it should be opened and maintained with an airway manouvre and the child ventilated by bag-valve-mask oxygenation. An airway adjunct can be used. The airway should then be secured by intubation by experienced senior help.
- If the child has an AVPU score of "P", his airway is at risk. It should be maintained by an airway manoeuvre or adjunct and senior help requested to secure it.

Breathing

- All children with a decreased conscious level should receive high flow oxygen through a face mask with a reservoir as soon as the airway has been demonstrated to be adequate.
- If the child is hypoventilating, respiration should be supported with oxygen via a bag-valve-mask device and experienced senior help summoned.

Circulation

Gain intravenous or intraosseous access.

- Take blood for FBC, U&Es, blood culture, cross-match, glucose stick test and laboratory glucose. Give 5 ml/kg of 10% dextrose to any hypoglycaemic patient (glucose stick test < 3 mmol/l) if possible, take 10 ml of clotted blood before giving the dextrose for later investigation of the hypoglycaemic state.
- Give 20 ml/kg rapid bolus of crystalloid to any patient with signs of shock. Colloid and an antibiotic such as cefotaxime should be used for those in whom a diagnosis of septicaemia is made obvious by the presence of a purpuric rash.
- Give an antibiotic such as cefotaxime to any child in whom a diagnosis of meningitis is made obvious by a stiff neck or bulging fontanelle.

KEY FEATURES

While the primary assessment and resuscitation are being carried out a focused history of the child's health and activity over the previous 24 hours and any significant previous illness should be gained.

Specific points for history taking include:

- Recent trauma
- Pre-existing neurological disability
- History of epilepsy
- Poison ingestion
- Known chronic condition (e.g. renal disease, cardiac abnormality, diabetes)
- Last meal
- Recent trips abroad.

In a patient in coma, it is often impossible to be certain of the diagnosis in the first hour. The main immediate aims are therefore to maintain homoeostasis and "treat the treatable".

If the situation remains unstable or is deteriorating, further urgent primary assessment and resuscitation must be initiated.

If the patient is stable, a further and more detailed neurological examination will reassess the earlier findings, help localise the site of neurological dysfunction, and provide a reference for further examinations.

1. Eye examination:
   - Pupil size and reactivity (see box)
   - Fundal changes – haemorrhage and papilloedema
   - Ophthalmoplegia – lateral or vertical deviation
2. Reassess Coma Score.
3. Reassess posture and tone – look for lateralisation.
4. Assess deep tendon reflexes and plantar responses – look for lateralisation.

Lateralisation suggests a localised rather than a generalised lesion but this is often a false indicator in childhood. The child will almost certainly need a CT scan.

Summary of pupillary changes	
Pupil size and reactivity	*Cause*
Small reactive pupils	Metabolic disorders
	Medullary lesion
Pin-point pupils	Metabolic disorders
	Narcotic/organophosphate ingestions
Fixed midsize pupils	Midbrain lesion
Fixed dilated pupils	Hypothermia
	Severe hypoxia
	Barbiturates (late sign)
	During and postseizure
	Anticholinergic drugs
Unilateral dilated pupil	Rapidly expanding ipsilateral lesion
	Tentorial herniation
	Third nerve lesion
	Epileptic seizures

General physical examination

The physical examination may add clues to point to a working diagnosis. Specific points to include are the following:

1. Skin: rash, haemorrhage, trauma, evidence of neurocutaneous syndromes.
2. Scalp: evidence of trauma.
3. Ears and nose:
    (a) Bloody or clear discharge. *Base of skull fracture (page 185)*
    (b) Evidence of otitis media. *May accompany meningitis*
4. Neck: tenderness or rigidity. *Meningitis, cerebrovascular accident.*
5. Odour. *Metabolic disorders and poisoning.*
6. Abdomen: enlarged liver. *(In conjunction with hypoglycaemia: Reye's syndrome.)*

The *key features* which will be identified clinically, from the focused history and from the initial blood test results can point the clinician to the likeliest working diagnosis for emergency treatment.

Additionally, unless meningitis can be excluded by the clear identification of another cause for coma, it should be assumed present as the consequence of missed diagnosis is catastrophic and the risk of unnecessary treatment with antibiotics small. Acyclovir should also be *considered* as herpes encephalitis has a worse prognosis when treatment is *seriously* delayed. Senior advice should be sought.

Lumbar puncture should not be performed in a child in coma. It can be performed some days later when the child's condition allows, to confirm or refute the diagnosis of meningitis/*encephalitis* if antibiotic treatment/*acyclovir* has been started (see page 134).

- Coma that develops over several hours, associated with irritability and/or fever and a rash points to *meningitis/encephalitis* (but this should also be a default working diagnosis in the absence of a clear alternative one).
- A history of opiate ingestion and/or pin-point pupils points to *poisoning with opiates.*
- A history of onset of coma over an hour or so in an otherwise well child is suggestive of *poisoning* (see Chapter 14 for management of poisoning in general).
- Hyperglycaemia points to *diabetes* (see Appendix B).
- A vague and inconsistent history and/or suspicious bruising in an infant is suggestive of *intracerebral bleeding from child abuse:* the presence of retinal haemorrhage is strong presumptive evidence of the same (see management of head injury in Chapter 18).
- A history of very sudden onset of coma often with a preceding headache points to a *cerebrovascular accident* (rare in childhood).
- Coma associated with significant hypertension points to *hypertensive encephalopathy.*

APPROACH TO THE CHILD WITH MENINGITIS/ENCEPHALITIS

After the neonatal period, the commonest cause of bacterial meningitis is *Neisseria meningitidis (Meningococcus)*. There is still a mortality rate of more than 5% and a similar rate of permanent serious sequelae. Widespread Hib vaccination has reduced the incidence of *Haemophilus influenzae* infection. Infection with *Streptococcus pneumoniae* remains uncommon and should prompt a search for an abnormal immune state or a cerebral sinus.

Diagnosis of bacterial meningitis

In the under 3-year-old child

Bacterial meningitis is difficult to diagnose in its early stages in this age group. The classic signs of neck rigidity, photophobia, headache, and vomiting are often absent. A bulging fontanelle is a sign of advanced meningitis in an infant, but even this serious and late sign will be masked if the baby is dehydrated from fever and vomiting. Almost all children with meningitis have some degree of raised intracranial pressure, so that, in fact, the signs and symptoms of meningitis are primarily those of raised intracranial pressure. The following are signs of possible meningitis in infants and young children:

* Coma.
* Drowsiness (often shown by lack of eye contact with parents or doctor).
* Irritability that cannot be easily soothed by parent.
* Poor feeding.
* Unexplained pyrexia.
* Convulsions with or without fever.
* Apnoeic or cyanotic attacks.
* Purpuric rash.

Older children of 4 years and over

These children are more likely to have the classic signs of headache, vomiting, pyrexia, neck stiffness, and photophobia. Some present with coma or convulsions. In all unwell children, and children with an unexplained pyrexia, a careful search should be made for neck stiffness and for a purpuric rash. The finding of such a rash in an ill child is almost pathognomic of meningococcal infection for which immediate treatment is required (see Chapter 10).

Reassess ABCD

* If there is an abnormal breathing pattern this may suggest raised intracranial pressure.
* Decorticate or decerebrate posturing in a previously normal child should suggest raised intracranial pressure.

MENINGITIS EMERGENCY TREATMENT

After the above assessment, any child in whom meningitis is suspected and who has not yet received intravenous cefotaxime or other suitable antibiotic should now receive this.

There is evidence that dexamethasone (0·15 mg/kg) given intravenously before or at the same time as the initial antibiotic improves outcome in cases of *Haemophilus influenzae* meningitis. There is no evidence of benefit in meningitis caused by other organisms.

As many of the clinical signs of meningitis are actually caused by raised intracranial pressure, a specific assessment should be made of its severity.

Raised intracranial pressure

There are very few absolute signs of raised ICP, these being papilloedema, a bulging fontanelle, and absence of venous pulsation in retinal vessels. All three signs are often absent in acutely raised ICP.

In a previously well, unconscious child (Glasgow Coma Scale <9) who is not in a postictal state, the signs in the box are suggestive of raised intracranial pressure:

Signs of raised intracranial pressure

1. Abnormal oculocephalic reflexes; avoid in patients with neck injuries:
   (a) when the head is turned to the left or right a normal response is for the eyes to move away from the head movement; an abnormal response is no (or random) movement;
   (b) when the head is flexed, a normal response is deviation of the eyes upward, a loss of his conjugate upward gaze is a sign suggestive of raised ICP.
2. Abnormal posture:
   (a) decorticate (flexed arms, extended legs)
   (b) decerebrate (extended arms, extended legs).
   Posturing may need to be elicited by a painful stimulus.
3. Abnormal pupillary responses unilateral or bilateral dilation suggests raised ICP.
4. Abnormal breathing patterns. There are several recognisable breathing pattern abnormalities in raised ICP. However, they are often changeable and may vary from hyperventilation to Cheyne–Stokes breathing to apnoea.
5. Cushing's triad: slow pulse, raised blood pressure, and breathing pattern abnormalities are a late sign of raised ICP.

Raised ICP emergency treatment

- If there is evidence of raised intracranial pressure, seek advice from a paediatric neurologist or intensivist.
- The patient should be intubated and CO_2 monitored by capnography. The PCO_2 should kept in the range 28–32 mmHg.
- Mannitol 0·5–1·0 g/kg should be infused if there is evidence of impending coning as shown by Cushing's triad.

Lumbar puncture

The purpose of a lumbar puncture is to confirm the diagnosis of meningitis and to identify the organism and its antibiotic sensitivity. There is a risk of coning and death if a lumbar puncture is performed in a child with significantly raised intracranial pressure. Normal fundi are quite consistent with acutely, severely raised intracranial pressure. It is now usual practice to treat a child with obvious meningitis with antibiotics immediately and perform a diagnostic lumbar puncture if necessary some days later when the child is clearly no longer suffering from raised intracranial presssure. The relative contraindications to a lumbar puncture are shown in the box.

Relative contraindications to lumbar puncture

- Prolonged or focal seizures.
- Focal neurological signs, e.g. asymmetry of limb movement and reflexes, ocular palsies.
- A widespread purpuric rash in an ill child. In this case intravenous cefotaxime should be given immediately after a blood culture.
- Glasgow Coma Scale – score of less than 13.
- Pupillary dilatation.
- Impaired oculocephalic reflexes (doll's eye reflexes).
- Abnormal posture or movement decerebrate or decorticate posturing or cycling movements of the limbs.
- Inappropriately low pulse, elevated blood pressure, and irregular respirations (i.e. signs of impending brain herniation).
- Coagulation disorder.
- Papilloedema.
- Hypertension.

APPROACH TO THE CHILD POISONED WITH OPIATES

These children are usually toddlers who have drunk the green liquid form of methadone.

Reassess ABC

- The sedative effect of the drug may reduce the conscious level sufficiently to put the airway at risk.
- These patients will usually hypoventilate.
- Support ventilation with bag-valve-mask before giving naloxone (see Chapter 5).

Opiate poisoning emergency treatment

Following stabilisation of airway, breathing and circulation, the specific antidote is naloxone. An initial bolus dose of 10 micrograms/kg is used but some children need doses as high as 100 micrograms/kg up to a maximum of 2 mg. Naloxone has a short half-life, relapse ofter occurring after 20 minutes. Further boluses, or an infusion of 10–20 micrograms/kg/min may be required.

It is important to normalise CO_2 before the naloxone is given as adverse events such as ventricular arrhythmias, acute pulmonary oedema, asystole or seizures may otherwise occur. This is because the opioid system and adrenergic system are interrelated. Opioid antagonists and hypercapnia stimulate sympathetic nervous system activity. Therefore if ventilation is not provided to normalise carbon dioxide prior to naloxone administration, the sudden rise in epinephrine (adrenaline) concentration can cause arrhythmias.

Transfer

After the child has been stabilised and conditions such as hypoglcaemia, meningitis and opiate poisoning treated as indicated some children will remain a puzzle.

These children and those in whom there is any suggestion of lateralisation or intra-cranial bleeding should have an urgent CT scan: get senior advice

Children who remain very ill and those in whom the cause of coma is as yet unidentified will require referral to a paediatric neurologist and may need transfer to a paediatric intensive care unit.

Patients may need paralysis, intubation, and ventilation for safe transfer (see Chapter 25). In such patients neurological assessment cannot be continued, and there should therefore be clear documentation of neurological signs before paralysis is commenced.

Raised intracranial pressure

The initial priority in the management of the unconscious child is the maintenance of adequate respiration, circulation, and metabolic homoeostasis. Once this has been done, the possibility of raised intracranial pressure should be considered.

In very young children, before the cranial sutures are closed, considerable intracranial volume expansion may occur if the process is slow. However, if the process is rapid and in children with a fixed volume cranium, increase in volume due to brain swelling, haematoma, or cerebral spinal fluid (CSF) blockage will cause raised intracranial pressure (ICP). Initially cerebrospinal fluid and venous blood within the cranium decrease in volume. Soon, this compensating mechanism fails and as the intracranial

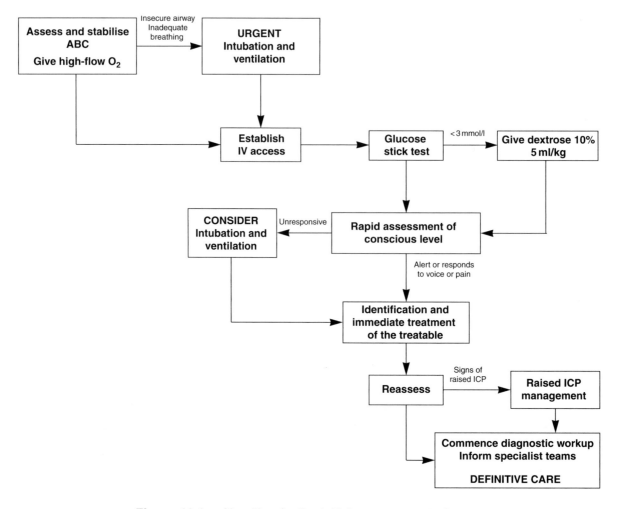

Figure 12.1. Algorithm for the initial management of coma

pressure continues to rise the cerebral perfusion pressure (CPP) falls and arterial blood flow is reduced.

$$CPP = MAP - ICP$$

where MAP is mean arterial pressure. Reduced CPP reduces cerebral blood flow (CBF). Normal CBF is over 50 ml/100 g brain tissue/min. If the CBF falls below 20 ml/100 g brain tissue/min, the brain suffers ischaemia.

Increasing intracranial pressure will push brain tissue against more rigid intracranial structures. Two clinical syndromes are recognisable by the site of localised brain compression.

Central syndrome

The whole brain is pressed down towards the foramen magnum and the cerebellar tonsils herniate through it ("coning"). Neck stiffness may be noted. A slow pulse, raised blood pressure, and irregular respiration leading to apnoea are seen terminally.

Uncal syndrome

The intracranial volume increase is mainly in the supratentorial part of the intracranial space. The uncus, which is part of the hippocampal gyrus, is forced through the tentorial opening and compressed against the fixed free edge of the tentorium. If the pressure is unilateral (for example, from a subdural or extradural haematoma), this

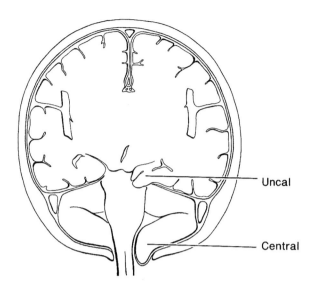

Uncal

Central

Figure 12.2. Herniations of the brain

leads to third nerve compression and an ipsilateral dilated pupil. Next, an external oculomotor palsy appears, so the eye cannot move laterally. Hemiplegia may then develop on either or both sides of the body, depending on the progression of the herniation.

CHAPTER

13

The convulsing child

INTRODUCTION

Generalised convulsive (tonic-clonic) status epilepticus (CSE) is currently defined as a generalised convulsion lasting 30 minutes or longer or when successive convulsions occur so frequently that the patient does not recover consciousness between them. Although the outcome of CSE is mainly determined by its cause, the duration of the convulsion is also relevant. In addition, the longer the duration of the episode, the more difficult it is to terminate it. In general, convulsions that persist beyond five minutes may not stop spontaneously so it is usual practice to institute treatment when the episode has lasted between five and ten minutes.

Tonic-clonic status occurs in approximately 1–5% of patients with epilepsy. Up to 5% of children with febrile seizures will present in status epilepticus.

Status epilepticus can be fatal, but mortality is lower in children than in adults at about 4%. Death may be due to complications of the convulsion, such as obstruction of the airway or aspiration of vomit, to overmedication, or to the underlying disease process.

Neurological sequelae (persistent epilepsy, motor deficits, learning and behavioural difficulties) are age dependent, occurring in 6% of those over three years but 29% of those under one year.

A generalised convulsion increases the cerebral metabolic rate at least threefold. Initially, there is an increased sympathetic activity with release of catecholamines which lead to peripheral vasoconstriction and increased systemic blood pressure. There is also loss of cerebral arterial regulation and, following the increase in systemic blood pressure, there is a resulting increase in cerebral blood flow to provide the necessary oxygen and energy. If convulsions continue, the systemic blood pressure falls and this is followed by a fall in cerebral blood flow. Lactic acid accumulates and there is subsequently cell death, oedema, and raised intracerebral pressure resulting in further worsening of cerebral perfusion. Cellular metabolism of calcium and sodium is also impaired, with further cell death.

PRIMARY ASSESSMENT

The first steps in the management of the patient who is convulsing are to assess and if necessary support airway, breathing and circulation. This will ensure that the convulsion is not secondary to hypoxia and/or ischaemia and that whatever the cerebral pathology it will not be worsened by lack of oxygenated blood supply to the brain.

Airway

Assess airway patency by the "look, listen, and feel" method.

If there is no evidence of air movement then chin lift or jaw thrust manoeuvres should be carried out and the airway reassessed. If there continues to be no evidence of air movement then airway patency can be assessed by performing an opening manoeuvre and giving rescue breaths (see Basic Life Support, Chapter 4).

Breathing

Assess the adequacy of breathing

- Effort of breathing
  Recession
  Respiratory rate
  Grunting. *This may be caused by the convulsion and not be a sign of respiratory distress in this instance*
- Efficacy of breathing
  Breath sounds
  Chest expansion/abdominal excursion
- Effects of breathing
  Heart rate
  Skin colour

Monitor oxygen saturation with a pulse oximeter.

Circulation

Assess the adequacy of circulation

Cardiovascular status
  Heart rate. The presence of an inappropriate bradycardia will suggest raised intracranial pressure
  Pulse volume
  Capillary refill
  Blood pressure. *Significant (>97th percentile for age) hypertension indicates a possible aetiology for the convulsion*
Effects of circulatory inadequacy on other organs
  Pale, cyanosed or cold skin

Monitor heart rate/rhythm, blood pressure and core/toe temperature difference.

If heart rate is above 200 in an infant or above 150 in a child or if the rhythm is abnormal perform a standard ECG.

Disability

Assess neurological function.

- The AVPU score cannot be measured meaningfully as the convulsing patient has an abnormal conscious level by virtue of the convulsion.
- Pupillary size and reaction should be noted. *Very small pupils suggest opiate poisoning, large pupils amphetamines, atropine, tricyclic antidepressants and others (see page 156).*

Note the child's posture. Decorticate or decerebrate posturing in a previously normal child should suggest raised intracranial pressure. These postures can sometimes be mistaken for the tonic phase of a convulsion. Consider also the possibility of a drug-induced dystonic reaction or a psychogenic, pseudo-epileptic attack. All these movement disorders are distinguishable from tonic-clonic status epilepticus as long as they are considered.

Look for neck stiffness in a child and a full fontanelle in an infant which suggest *meningitis.*

Exposure

- Take the child's core and toe temperatures. *A fever is suggestive evidence of an infectious cause (but its absence does not the suggest the opposite) or poisoning with ecstasy, cocaine or salicylates. Hypothermia suggests poisoning with barbiturates or ethanol.*
- Look for a rash. *If one is present, ascertain if it is purpuric as an indicator of meningococcal disease or non-accidental injury.*
- Look for evidence of poisoning.

RESUSCITATION

Airway

- A patent airway is the first requisite. If the airway is not patent it should be opened and maintained with an airway manoeuvre and the child ventilated by bag-valve-mask oxygenation. An airway adjunct can be used. The airway should later be secured by intubation by experienced senior help.
- Even if the airway is open the oropharynx may need secretion clearance by gentle suction.

Breathing

- All convulsing children should receive high flow oxygen through a face mask with a reservoir as soon as the airway has been demonstrated to be adequate.
- If the child is hypoventilating, respiration should be supported with oxygen via a bag-valve-mask device and experienced senior help summoned.

Circulation

Gain intravenous or intraosseous access.

- Take blood for glucose stick test and laboratory test. Give 5 ml/kg of 10% dextrose to any hypoglycaemic patient. If possible, take 10 mls of clotted blood before giving the dextrose for later investigation of the hypoglycaemic state.

- Give 20 ml/kg rapid bolus of crystalloid to any patient with signs of shock. Colloid and an antibiotic such as cefotaxime should be used for those in whom a diagnosis of septicaemia is made obvious by the presence of a purpuric rash after blood has been taken for culture.
- Give an antibiotic such as cefotaxime to any child in whom a diagnosis of meningitis is made obvious by a stiff neck or bulging fontanelle after blood has been taken for culture.

Key features

While the primary assessment and resuscitation are being carried out a focused history of the child's health and activity over the previous 24 hours and any significant previous illness should be gained.

Specific points for history taking include:

- Current febrile illness
- Recent trauma
- History of epilepsy
- Poison ingestion
- Last meal

The immediate emergency treatment requirement, after ABC stabilisation and exclusion or treatment of hypoglycaemia is to stop the convulsion.

Reassess ABC

CONVULSION EMERGENCY TREATMENT

This evidence-based consensus guideline is not intended to cover all circumstances. There are patients with chronic epilepsy whose physicians recognise that they respond to certain drugs and not to others and for these children an individual protocol is more appropriate. In addition, seizures in neonates are managed differently to those of infants and children.

The protocol is for the majority of children in CSE who present acutely on wards or in an Accident and Emergency department.

Step 1

- For those patients in whom intravenous access is already established or can be established quickly, *lorazepam 0·1 mg/kg* is used in the first instance.
- In children in whom intravenous access is unsuccessful, *rectal diazepam 0·5 mg/kg* should be given.

Step 2

- If, after 10 minutes the convulsion continues, a second dose of *lorazepam* is given (0·1 mg/kg).
- If the child has received rectal diazepam, now has intravenous access and is still convulsing, he should be given a dose of intravenous *lorazepam* (0·1 mg/kg).
- If intravenous access still has not been achieved, then a dose of *rectal paraldehyde* (0·4 ml/kg) can be given mixed with an equal volume of olive oil.

In the majority of children, treatment in steps 1 to 2 will be effective.

Step 3

At this stage senior help is needed to reassess the child and advise on management. It is also wise to seek anaesthetic or intensive care advice as the child will need anaesthetising and intubating if this step is unsuccessful.

- While the phenytoin (18 mg/kg over 20 minutes) is being prepared, *paraldehyde* should be given to any child who has not yet received it.
- If the convulsion stops before phenytoin is started, the infusion should not be commenced without specialist advice.
- If the convulsion stops after phenytoin has been started, the complete dose should still be given as this will have an anticonvulsive effect for up to 24 hours.
- In the case of children already receiving phenytoin as maintenance treatment for their epilepsy, *phenobarbitone* (20 mg/kg over 20 minutes) should be used in place of phenytoin.

Step 4

If 20 minutes after Step 3 has started, the child remains in CSE an anaesthetist must be present. Check airway, breathing, and circulation. Take blood for glucose, arterial blood gas, urea, electrolytes, and calcium. Treat any vital function problem and correct metabolic abnormalities slowly. Treat pyrexia with paracetamol or diclofenac rectally. Consider mannitol (0·5 g/kg intravenously over 30–60 minutes).

- Rapid sequence induction of anaesthesia is performed with *thiopentone* and a short-acting paralysing agent.
- Further advice on management should be sought from a paediatric neurologist.

In children under three years with a history of chronic, active epilepsy, a trial of *pyridoxine* should be insituted.

Drugs

Lorazepam

Lorazepam is equally or more effective than diazepam and possibly produces less respiratory depression. It has a longer duration of action (12–24 hours) than diazepam (less than one hour). It appears to be poorly absorbed from the rectal route.

Lorazepam is not available in every country. If this is the case, diazepam can be substituted at a dose of 0·25 mg/kg IV/IO.

Diazepam

This is an effective, quick-acting anticonvulsant, which takes effect within minutes but whose action is short-lasting (about 40 minutes to 1 hour). It has a depressant effect on respiration and this is enhanced by the addition of other anticonvulsants such as phenobarbitone. Also, repeated doses make side effects more marked. The rectal dose is well absorbed.

Paraldehyde

Dose: 0·4 ml/kg per rectum (0·3 ml/kg under 6 months of age), made up as a 50:50 solution in olive oil or physiological saline. Arachis oil should be avoided as children with peanut allergy may react to it. Paraldehyde can cause rectal irritation, but intramuscular paraldehyde causes severe pain and may lead to sterile abscess formation. Paraldehyde causes little respiratory depression. It should not be used in liver disease.

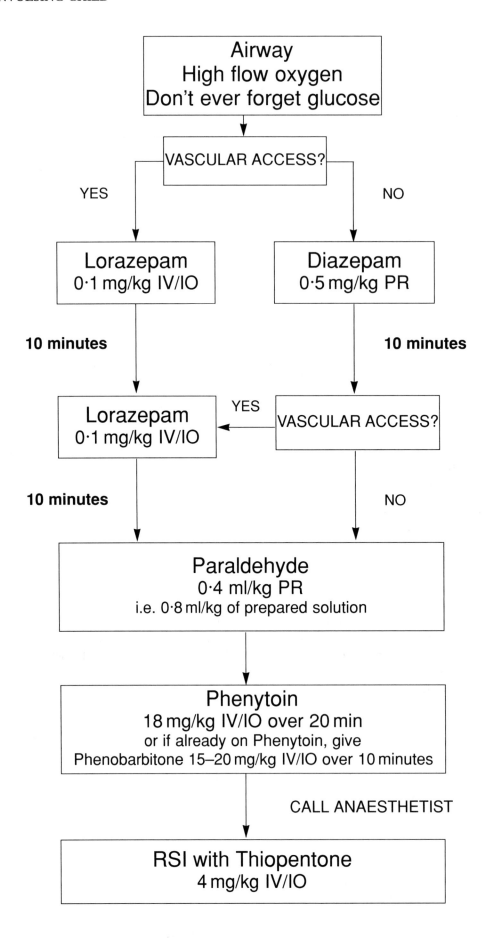

Figure 13.1. Status epilepticus algorithm

Paraldehyde takes 10–15 minutes to act and its action is sustained for 2–4 hours.
Do not leave paraldehyde standing in a plastic syringe for longer than a few minutes.

Phenytoin

Dose: 18 mg/kg intravenously. Rate of infusion no greater than 1 mg/kg/min. Infusion to be made up in 0·9% sodium chloride solution to a maximum concentration of 10 mg in 1 ml.

Measure plasma phenytoin levels 90–120 minutes after the completion of the infusion.

Phenytoin can cause dysrhythmias and hypotension, and therefore an ECG monitor should be used and the BP monitored. It has little depressant effect on respiration.

Do not use this if the child is known to be on oral phenytoin until the blood level of phenytoin is known. Then only give it if the phenytoin level is less than 2·5 micrograms/ml. Phenytoin has a peak action within 1 hour but a long half-life that is dose-dependent. Its action therefore is more sustained than diazepam.

Fosphenytoin

This is a recently produced pro-drug of phenytoin. It is not itself anticonvulsant but is rapidly converted into phenytoin once administered. Because it does not need propylene glycol as a solvent, it can be administered more rapidly than phenytoin over 7–10 minutes and is said to cause fewer cardiac side effects. It can be given intramuscularly At present there are no paediatric efficacy data on use in CSE in children. If used it is prescribed in "phenytoin equivalents" which could cause confusion. 75 mg fosphenytoin is equivalent to 50 mg phenytoin.

Thiopentone sodium

Induction dose 4–8 mg/kg intravenously.

This is an alkaline solution which will cause irritation if the solution leaks into subcutaneous tissues.

It has no analgesic effect and is a general anaesthetic agent. Repeated doses have a cumulative effect. It is a potent drug with marked cardiorespiratory effects and should be used only by experienced staff who can intubate a child.

It is not an effective long-term anticonvulsant and its principal use in status epilepticus is to facilitate ventilation and the subsequent management of cerebral oedema due to the prolonged seizure activity. Other antiepileptic medication must be continued.

The child should not remain paralysed as continued seizure activity cannot universally be adequately monitored by cerebral function analysis monitoring. When the child is stable he or she will need transfer to a paediatric intensive care unit. A paediatric neurologist should continue to give clinical advice and support. There are several regimes for continued drug control of the convulsions but they are outside the scope of this text.

General measures

Fluid input should be kept to 50–60% normal requirements, using 0·45% saline and 5% dextrose. Monitoring includes pulse, blood pressure, respiratory rate, oxygen saturation, urine output, blood levels of glucose, urea, creatinine and electrolytes. The role of cerebral function analysis monitoring is still unclear. At the current time clinical features and standard EEG are the preferred method of assessing seizure activity.

Additional treatments will depend on the clinical situation.

Frequent reassessment of ABC is mandatory as therapy may cause depression of ventilation or hypotension.

Further management

Following cessation of the fit, all children will need continuous monitoring for vital functions and to observe for further convulsions. It is particularly important to ensure that breathing is adequate since the benzodiazepines used to control the fit may cause respiratory depression.

After the fit has been controlled the clinician must consider the underlying cause of the convulsion. In many cases there will be an infectious cause, either a benign, self-limiting infection causing 'febrile status' or possibly meningitis. See Chapter 12.

SYSTEMIC HYPERTENSIVE CRISIS

Hypertension is uncommon in children. Blood pressure is rarely measured routinely in otherwise healthy children and therefore hypertension usually presents with symptoms which may be diverse in nature. Neurological symptoms are more common in children than in adults. There may be a history of severe headaches, with or without vomiting, suggestive of raised intracranial pressure. Children may also present acutely with convulsions or in coma. Some children will present with a facial palsy or hemiplegia and small babies may even present with apnoea.

Blood pressure measurement

This may be difficult in small children and misleading if not done correctly. The following guidelines should be observed.

- Always use the biggest cuff that will fit comfortably on the upper arm. A small cuff will give erroneously high readings.
- The systolic blood pressure may give a more reliable reading than the diastolic because the fourth Korotkoff sound is frequently either not heard or is audible down to zero.
- If using an electronic device and the result is unexpected, recheck it manually before acting on it.
- Raised blood pressure in a child who is fitting, in pain or screaming must be rechecked when the child is calm.
- If the child is very small or uncooperative, using a Doppler device may be helpful. Approximate systolic blood pressures may be obtained by the palpation method.

Blood pressure increases with age – the reading should be checked against normal ranges for the child's age. Any blood pressure over the 95th centile should be repeated and if persistently raised will need treatment. Blood pressures leading to symptomatology will be grossly elevated for the child's age and the diagnosis should not be difficult.

Reassess ABC

HYPERTENSION EMERGENCY TREATMENT

Initial treatment will be that of the presentation. Airway, breathing, and circulation should be assessed and managed in the usual way and neurological status assessed and monitored. Convulsions usually respond to lorazepam or diazepam and patients with clinical signs of raised intracranial pressure should be managed as in Chapter 12.

Once the patient has been resuscitated, management of the hypertension is urgent, but should only be commenced after discussion with a paediatric nephrologist or paediatric cardiologist because of the dangers of too rapid reduction.

Monitoring of visual acuity and pupils is crucial during this time as lowering the blood pressure may lead to infarction of the optic nerve heads. Any deterioration must be treated by urgently raising the blood pressure using intravenous saline or colloid. Some children may be anuric – renal function (serum creatinine, urea, and electrolytes) should be analysed promptly.

Some drugs commonly used to achieve blood pressure reduction in children are shown in Table 13.1.

Table 13.1. Drug therapy of severe hypertension

Drug	Dose	Comments
Labetalol	16–50 µg/kg/min	α- and ß-blocker. Titratable infusion. DO NOT USE in patients with fluid overload
Sodium nitroprusside	0·2–1 µg/kg/min	Vasodilator. Very easy to adjust dose. Protect from light. Monitor cyanide levels
Hydralazine	0·2–1 µg/kg/min	Vasodilator. Titratable infusion. Adjust as required
Nifedipine	0·25 mg/kg	Vasodilator. Fluid can be drawn up from capsules and squirted into mouth sublingually. Better to bite the capsule and swallow. May be difficult to control BP drop because it is given as a bolus

Some specialists may recommend the use of nifedipine as a temporary measure before transfer; if any drug is used, the child should have the blood pressure monitored as above and an intravenous infusion in place.

These children should be cared for in a unit experienced in paediatric hypertension. This will usually be the regional paediatric nephrology (or paediatric cardiology) centre. It is essential that adequate consultation takes place before transfer.

14

The poisoned child

INTRODUCTION

Suspected poisoning in children results in about 40,000 attendences at Emergency departments each year in England and Wales. Around half of these children are admitted to hospital for treatment or observation. Precise data on hospital admissions for poisonings are altered by the fact that many Emergency departments and paediatric wards have special areas where children who have taken a substance of low toxicity can be observed for a few hours without being formally admitted.

Deaths from ingested poisons are uncommon, and are due to drugs (especially tricyclic antidepressants), household products and, rarely, plants. As can be seen from Table 14.1, more children die each year from inhalation of carbon monoxide and other gases in household fires, than die from accidental poisoning by drugs although fire deaths are decreasing while poisoning deaths are not.

Table 14.1. Deaths in children (ages 1–14) from poisons in England and Wales

Cause of death	1988	1998
From poisoning by drugs, medicaments and biological substances	16	18
From toxic effects of carbon monoxide	36	15
From toxic effect of other gases, fumes or vapours	56	24

Office of National Statistics 1998

There has been a steady decline in the number of childhood deaths from poisonings. The selective introduction of child-resistant containers (CRCs) in 1976, together with other measures, has reduced the number of poisonings and hospital attendances. In the case of salicylate poisoning the introduction of CRCs saw an 85% fall in hospital admissions from 1975 to 1978. It should be remembered, however, that 20% of children under the age of five years are capable of opening CRCs!

Accidental poisoning

This is usually a problem of the young child or toddler, with a mean age of presentation of two and a half years. Accidental poisoning usually occurs when the child is unsupervised, and there is an increased incidence in poisoning following recent disruption in households, such as a new baby, moving house or where there is maternal depression.

Intentional overdose

Suicide or parasuicide attempts are usually made by young people in their teens although sometimes they may be as young as eight or nine years. These children or adolescents should undergo psychiatric and social assessment.

Drug abuse

Alcohol and solvent abuse are the commonest forms of drug abuse in children in the UK.

Iatrogenic

The commonest offender is diphenoxylate with atropine (Lomotil). This combination is toxic to some children at therapeutic doses. The most frequently fatal drug is digoxin.

Deliberate poisoning

Rarely, symptoms are induced in children by adults via the administration of drugs. A history of poisoning will often not be given at presentation.

Most poisoning episodes in childhood and adolescence are of low lethality and little or no treatment is required. This chapter will not address the milder cases but will enable the student to develop an approach to the seriously ill poisoned child with additional advice on the management of specific poisons.

PRIMARY ASSESSMENT

Airway

Assess airway patency by the "look, listen, and feel" method.

If the child can speak or cry in response to a stimulus, this indicates that the airway is patent, that breathing is occurring and that there is adequate circulation. If the child responds only with withdrawal to a painful stimulus (AVPU score "P") his airway is at risk.

If there is no evidence of air movement then chin lift or jaw thrust manoeuvres should be carried out and the airway reassessed. If there continues to be no evidence of air movement then airway patency can be assessed by performing an opening manoeuvre and giving rescue breaths (see Basic Life Support, Chapter 4).

Breathing

Assess the adequacy of breathing.

- Effort of breathing
    Recession
    Respiratory rate. The rate may be increased in poisoning from amphetamines, ecstasy, salicylates, ethylene glycol, methanol.
- Efficacy of breathing
    Breath sounds
    Chest expansion/abdominal excursion

Monitor oxygen saturation with a pulse oximeter.

Circulation

Assess the adequacy of circulation

- Cardiovascular status
    Heart rate. Tachycardia is caused by amphetamines, ecstasy, ß-agonists, phenothiazines, theophylline and tricyclic antidepressants. Bradycardia is caused by beta-blockers, digoxin, organophosphates.
    Pulse volume
    Capillary refill
    Blood pressure. Hypotension is commonly seen in serious poisoning hypertension is caused by ecstasy and monoamine oxidase inhibitors
- Effects of circulatory inadequacy on other organs
    Acidotic sighing respirations. This may suggest metabolic acidosis from salicylate or ethylene glycol poisoning as a cause for the coma.
    Pale, cyanosed or cold skin

Monitor heart rate/rhythm, blood pressure and core/toe temperature difference.
If heart rate is above 200 in an infant or above 150 in a child or if the rhythm is abnormal perform a standard ECG. QRS prolongation and ventricular tachycardia is seen in tricyclic antidepressant poisoning.

Disability

Assess neurological function:

- A rapid measure of level of consciousness should be recorded using the AVPU scale.
- *Depression of conscious level suggests poisoning with opiates, sedatives (such as benzodiazapines) antihistamines, hypoglycaemic agents.*
- Pupillary size and reaction should be noted *Very small pupils suggest opiate or organophosphate poisoning, large pupils amphetamines, atropine, tricyclic antidepressants.*
- Note the child's posture. *Hypertonia is seen in amphetamine, ecstasy, theophylline and tricyclic antidepressant poisoning.*
- The presence of convulsive movements should be sought. *Convulsions are associated with any drug that causes hypoglycaemia (ethanol) and with tricyclic antidepressant poisoning.*

Exposure

Take the child's core and toe temperatures. *A fever suggests poisoning with ecstasy, cocaine or salicylates. Hypothermia suggests poisoning with barbiturates or ethanol.*

RESUSCITATION

Airway

- A patent airway is the first requisite. If the airway is not patent it should be opened and maintained with an airway manoeuvre and the child ventilated by bag-valve-mask oxygenation. An airway adjunct can be used. The airway should then be secured by intubation by experienced senior help.
- If the child has an AVPU score of "P", his airway is at risk. It should be maintained by an airway manoeuvre or adjunct and senior help requested to secure it.

Breathing

- All children with respiratory abnormalities, shock or a decreased conscious level should receive high flow oxygen through a face mask with a reservoir as soon as the airway has been demonstrated to be adequate.
- A number of agents taken in overdose (particularly narcotics) can produce respiratory depression. Oxygen should be given, but it is important to remember that these patients may have an increasing carbon dioxide level despite a normal oxygen saturation whilst breathing oxygen. Inadequate breathing should be supported using a bag-valve-mask device with oxygen or by intermittent positive pressure ventilation in the intubated patient.

Circulation

- A number of poisons can produce shock, by a number of different mechanisms. Hypovolaemia may be caused by gastrointestinal bleeding from iron poisoning or there may be vasodilatation from barbiturates. Shock should be treated with a fluid bolus, as usual. If possible, inotropes should be avoided in poisoning cases as the combination of toxic substance producing shock and an inotrope may be pro-arrhythmogenic.
- Cardiac dysrhythmias can be expected in tricyclic antidepressant (TCA), digoxin, quinine and anti-arrhythmic drug poisoning. Some anti-arrhythmic treatments are contraindicated with certain poisons. See below for advice on TCA poisoning and contact a Poison Centre urgently for other advice.

Gain intravenous or intraosseous access

- Take blood for FBC, U&Es, toxicology, paracetamol and salicylate levels (in patients who have taken an unknown drug) glucose stick test and laboratory test. Give 5 ml/kg of 10% dextrose to any hypoglycaemic patient.
- Give 20 ml/kg rapid bolus of crystalloid to any patient with signs of shock.
- If a child has a tachyarrhythmia and is shocked, up to three synchronous electrical shocks at 0·5, 0·5 and 1 joule should be given. If the arrhythmia is broad complex and the synchronous shocks are not activated by the defibrillator then attempt an asynchronous shock. A conscious child should be anaesthetised first if this can be done in a timely manner. DC shock may be dangerous in digoxin poisoning. Use lignocaine, amiodarone or phenytoin.

Disability

- Treat convulsions with diazepam or lorazepam.
- Give a trial of naloxone established in cases where depressed conscious level and small pupils suggest opiate poisoning.

In all cases of serious poisoning early consultation with a Poisons Centre is mandatory. Such centres have a wealth of expertise in the management of poisoning and will advise on the individual patients needs.

Monitoring

- ECG.
- Blood pressure (use appropriate size cuff).
- Pulse oximetry.
- Core temperature.
- Blood glucose.
- Urea and electrolytes.
- Blood gases (where indicated).

Lethality assessment

At the end of the primary assessment, it is important to assess the potential lethality of the overdose. This requires knowledge of the substance that has been taken, the time it was taken and the dosage. This information may be unattainable in the unwitnessed poisoning episode of a toddler or that of an unconscious or uncooperative adolescent. Some clues about the drug ingested may be available from physical signs noted during the primary assessment (Table 14.2).

Table 14.2. Diagnostic clues from the primary assessment

Signs	Drug
Tachypnoea	Aspirin, theophylline, carbon monoxide, cyanide
Bradypnoea	Ethanol, opiates, barbiturates, sedatives
Metabolic acidosis (sighing respirations)	Ethanol, carbon monoxide, ethylene glycol
Tachycardia	Antidepressants, sympathomimetics, amphetamines, cocaine
Bradycardia	ß-blockers, digoxin, clonidine
Hypotension	Barbiturates, benzodiazepines, ß-blockers, calcium channel blockers, opiates, iron, phenothiazines, phenytoin, tricyclic antidepressants
Hypertension	Amphetamines, cocaine, sympathomimetic agents
Small pupils	Opiates, organophosphate insecticides, phenothiazines
Large pupils	Amphetamines, atropine, cannabis, carbamazepine, cocaine, quinine, tricyclic antidepressants
Convulsions	Carbamazepine, lindane organophosphate insecticides, phenothiazines, tricyclic antidepressants
Hypothermia	Barbiturates, ethanol, phenothiazines
Hyperthermia	Amphetamines, cocaine, ecstasy, phenothiazines, salicylates

Some investigation results can add clues to the diagnosis of an unknown poison.

1. *Metabolic acidosis can be found in poisoning from:*
   - Carbon monoxide
   - Ecstasy
   - Ethylene glycol
   - Iron
   - Methanol
   - Salicylates
   - Tricyclic antidepressants.
2. *Enlarged anion gap (Na + K)-(HCO₃ − Cl)>18 can be found in poisoning from:*
   - Ethanol
   - Ethylene glycol
   - Iron
   - Methanol
   - Salicylates
3. *Hypokalaemia can be found in poisoning from:*
   - ß-agonists
   - Theophylline
4. *Hyperkalaemia can be found in poisoning from:*
   - Digoxin

The risks of a particular overdose can be assessed once all the information has been gathered. Complex or life-threatening cases should be discussed with a Poisons Centre. The Poisons Centre will require the following information:

- Age and weight of the patient.
- The time since exposure.
- The substance.
- The amount taken together with any description or labelling.
- The patient's condition.

If the nature of the overdose is unknown then a high potential lethality should be assumed. Many childhood poisoning incidents have zero lethality and no treatment is required.

POISONING EMERGENCY TREATMENT

Drug elimination

Many children have taken a trivial overdose or an overdose of a non-poisonous substance. If the overdose episode is assessed as having a low lethality, then no treatment is required.

If the drug overdose is assessed as having a potentially high lethality or its exact nature is unknown, then measures to minimise blood concentrations of the drug should be undertaken. In general this means stopping further absorption. Occasionally measures to increase excretion can be employed and in some circumstances specific antidotes may be available. Seek advice from a Poisons Centre.

Activated charcoal
Activated charcoal has a surface area of $1000 \, m^2/g$ and is capable of binding a number of poisonous substances without being systemically absorbed. It is now widely used in cases of poisoning. However, there are some substances which it will not absorb. These include alcohol and iron. Repeated doses of activated charcoal are useful in some types of poisoning because they promote drug reabsorption from the circulation back into the bowel and interrupt enterohepatic cycling. These types include aspirin, barbiturates, and theophylline.

154

It is often difficult to give charcoal to children as it is unpalatable. Flavouring may be necessary but can diminish the charcoal's activity. The charcoal can be given via a nasogastric tube or lavage tube after a gastric washout. The dose is at least 10 times the estimated dose of poison ingested. Children should usually be given 25–50 g.

Aspirated charcoal causes severe lung damage, so airway protection is especially important in the child who is not fully conscious.

Emesis

Emesis caused by ipecacuanha is now rarely used although for many years was routinely given for the management of poisoning incidents in children. The dose schedule is 15 ml with water (10 ml in children of 6 months to 2 years) repeated once after 20 minutes if necessary. It must not be used in the child with a depressed conscious level. Evidence now suggests that unless emesis occurs within 1 hour of ingestion of the poison little of the poison will be eliminated. Only about 30% is retrieved even up to 1 hour.

Emesis should only be used for poisons requiring removal which are not bound by charcoal or in children who are at risk from developing symptoms from the poison they have taken, present within one hour of ingestion and will not take the charcoal.

Gastric lavage

This is indicated in children who have ingested significant amounts of drugs at high lethality but is only likely to be effective if performed within an hour of ingestion. Intubation (under anaesthetic) will be necessary for children who cannot protect their airway. After evacuation the lavage tube can be used as a route for a specific antidote or activated charcoal. The lavage fluid can be water or isotonic saline and aliquots of 10–20 ml/kg used. In children the usual indication is iron poisoning

There are a number of active elimination techniques such as haemoperfusion and plasmapheresis: their use is infrequent and should be guided by Poisons Centre advice.

EMERGENCY TREATMENT OF SPECIFIC POISONS

Iron

The child with iron poisoning presents with shock, which may be due to gut haemorrhage. If over 20 mg/kg of elemental iron has been taken, toxicity is likely. Over 150 mg/kg may be fatal. Intubation, ventilation, and circulatory support are necessary in the severely affected child.

Initial symptoms of toxicity are vomiting, diarrhoea and abdominal pain. These may lead on to drowsiness, fits and circulatory collapse.

Gastric lavage should be performed once the airway is secured and circulatory access has been gained. Charcoal is not helpful. Desferrioxamine can be left in the stomach, but the main treatment is to infuse desferrioxamine at a dose of 15 mg/kg/h. This treatment should be given immediately to children with serious symptoms such as shock, coma or fits and to all with a serum iron level (4 hours or more after ingestion) of 3 mg/l and GI symptoms, leucocytosis or hyperglycaemia

Radiography of the abdomen can help to show how much iron remains within. Whole bowel irrigation with polyethylene glycol-electrolyte solutions may have a place in severe cases.

Tricyclic antidepressant (TCA) poisoning

The toxic effects of these agents results from their inhibition of fast sodium channels in the brain and myocardium. This action is known as "quinidine-like". With serious intoxication, the cardiac problems are due to intraventricular conduction delay. This results in QRS prolongation (a QRS of more than 4 little squares on the ECG paper is predictive of serious effects).

TCA poisoning causes anticholinergic effects (tachycardia, dilated pupils, convulsions) and cardiac effects (conduction delay, any arrhythmia). Convulsions should be treated as described in Chapter 13.

Additionally, alkalinisation up to an arterial pH of at least 7·45 and preferable 7·5 has been shown to reduce the toxic effects on the heart. This can be achieved by hyperventilation (P_{CO_2} no lower than 3·33 kPa (25 mmHg)) and by infusing sodium bicarbonate (1–2 mmol/kg). Hypotension should be treated with volume expansion and if an inotrope is necessary, norepinephrine (noradrenaline) is superior to dopamine, dobutamine and epinephrine (adrenaline). Glucagon has an inotropic effect and can be used in this circumstance.

The use of antiarrhythmics should be guided from a Poisons Centre. Lignocaine and phenytoin may be helpful. Quinidine, procainamide and disopyramide are contraindicated.

Opiates (including methadone)

Following stabilisation of airway, breathing and circulation, the specific antidote is naloxone. An initial bolus dose of 100 micrograms/kg up to a maximum of 2 mg should be given. Naloxone has a short half-life, relapse often occurring after 20 minutes. Further boluses, or an infusion of 10–20 micrograms/kg/min may be required.

It is important to normalise CO_2 before the naloxone is given as adverse events such as ventricular arrhythmias, acute pulmonary oedema, asystole or seizures may otherwise occur. This is because the opioid system and adrenergic system are interrelated. Opioid antagonists and hypercapnia stimulate sympathetic nervous system activity. Therefore if ventilation is not provided to normalise carbon dioxide prior to naloxone administration, the sudden rise in epinephrine concentration can cause arrhythmias.

Paracetamol

Significant paracetamol poisoning in childhood is almost always intentional: the accidental ingestion of paediatric paracetamol elixir preparations by the toddler very rarely achieves toxicity. Doses of less than 150 mg/kg will not cause toxicity except in a child with hepatic or renal disease. Current treatment of paracetamol poisoning includes oral charcoal and a paracetamol blood level to be taken at 4 hours or later. Figure 14.1 shows a nomogram indicating the level of blood paracetamol at which acetylcysteine should be given intravenously. A total dose of 300 mg/kg is given over approximately 24 hours. Contact a Poisons Centre for individual details.

Salicylates

Aspirin slows stomach emptying so gastric lavage can be undertaken up to 4 hours after ingestion. Repeated charcoal doses should be given for patients who have ingested sustained release preparations. The salicylate level can be measured initially at 2 hours. However, repeated measurements are necessary and no reliance should be placed on a single salicylate level. The levels will usually rise significantly over the first 6 hours (longer if an enteric coated preparation is used). Salicylate poisoning causes a respiratory alkalosis and metabolic acidosis. Arterial blood gas estimation is necessary to manage the patient. Alkalinisation of the patient improves excretion of salicylate: 1 mmol/kg of sodium bicarbonate should be infused over 4 hours. Forced diuresis is no longer used.

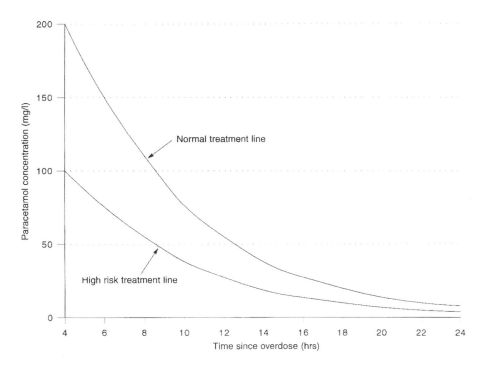

Figure 14.1. Nomogram showing level of blood paracetamol

Ethylene glycol

This sweet-tasting substance is available as an antifreeze and de-icer fluid for vehicles. It produces a clinical appearance of inebriation accompanied by metabolic acidosis and causes widespread cellular damage, especially to the kidneys. In unwitnessed ingestions the clue is in the metabolic acidosis with an inexplicable anion gap. Activated charcoal is ineffective. Ethanol is a competitive inhibitor of alcohol dehydrogenase and can block metabolism of the ethylene glycol to its poisonous metabolic byproducts. An oral loading dose of 2·5 ml/kg of 40% ethanol (the strength of most spirits) should be started. The aim is to have a blood ethanol concentration of 100 mg/dl. Haemodialysis may be necessary. Cofactors, thiamine, and pyridoxine are also recommended.

Cocaine

Cocaine poisoning leads to local accumulation of the neurotransmitters norepinephrine (noradrenaline), dopamine, epinephrine (adrenaline) and serotonin. Accumulation of norepinephrine and epinephrine leads to tachycardia which increases myocardial oxygen demand while reducing the time for diastolic coronary perfusion. Vasoconstriction causing hypertension results from the accumulation of neurotransmitter at peripheral ß-adrenergic receptors and peripheral 5-HT receptor stimulation causes coronary artery vasospasm. In addition, cocaine stimulates platelet aggregation. Together, these changes can produce what is effectively a coronary event in a child or adolescent.

Acute coronary syndrome producing chest pain and varying types of cardiac rhythm disturbances is the most frequent complication of cocaine use which leads to hospitalisation. Cocaine is also a sodium channel inhibitor, similar to a type I anti-arrhythmic agent so can prolong the QRS duration and impair myocardial contractility. Through the combination of adrenergic and sodium channel effects, cocaine use may cause various tachyarrhythmias including ventricular tachycardia and ventricular fibrillation. Treatment should be guided by a Poisons Centre.

157

Initial treatment of acute coronary syndrome consists of oxygen administration, continuous ECG monitoring, administration of a benzodiazepine (e.g., diazepam or lorazepam) aspirin and heparin. Hyperthermia should be treated with cooling. ß-adrenergic blockers are contraindicated in the setting of cocaine intoxication.

Ventricular tachycardia should be treated with DC shock as anti-arrhythmic drugs may cause further pro-arrhythmic effects

Since cocaine is a sodium channel blocker, administration of sodium bicarbonate in a dose of 1–2 meq/kg should be considered in the treatment of ventricular arrhythmias

Ecstasy

Most ecstasy tablets contain 30–150 mg of 3,4-methylenedioxymethamphetamine (MDMA). This drug, which has a half-life of around 8 hours, most probably stimulates both peripheral and central alpha- and beta-adrenergic receptors. Early deaths are usually due to cardiac dysrhythmias while deaths after 24 hours occur from a neuroleptic malignant-like syndrome.

Mild adverse effects occur at low doses and include increased muscle tone, agitation, anxiety and tachycardia. Mild elevation of temperature may also occur. At higher doses, hypertonia with hyperreflexia, tachycardia, tachypnoea and visual disturbance can be seen. In the worst affected children, coma, convulsions and cardiac dysrhythmias can occur. Hyperpyrexia with increased muscle tone can lead to rhabdomyolysis, metabolic acidosis with acute renal failure and disseminated intravascular coagulation.

Activated charcoal should be given to conscious patients. Blood pressure and temperature must be monitored. Diazepam can be used to control anxiety – major tranquilisers should not be used as they exacerbate symptoms. If core temperature exceeds 39°C then active cooling should be commenced and the use of dantrolene sodium (1 mg/kg over 10–15 min) should be considered. Some children may require ventilation.

TELEPHONE NUMBER OF POISONS CENTRES IN THE UK
THERE IS NOW A SINGLE NATIONAL ENQUIRY NUMBER 0870 600 6266

IV

THE SERIOUSLY INJURED CHILD

CHAPTER
15

The structured approach to the seriously injured child

Children and adults are affected quite differently by major injuries – physically, physiologically, and psychologically. A young child cannot describe pain, or even localise symptoms. The more frightened children become, the "younger" they behave, and the less they can contribute to management. All symptoms may be denied vehemently.

Although traumatised children have a number of unique problems, this in no way affects the validity of a structured approach. By following the principles outlined, problems will be identified and treated in order of priority. It should be emphasised from the start that, although assessment and management are discussed separately, this is purely to allow things to be shown clearly. When dealing with an injured child it is essential that appropriate resuscitative measures are taken as soon as a problem is found.

The form of the structured approach is shown in the box.

> **Structured approach**
>
> Primary survey
> Resuscitation
> Secondary survey
> Emergency treatment
> Definitive care

PRIMARY SURVEY

During the primary survey life-threatening conditions are identified. Assessment follows the familiar ABC pattern with significant additions:

A	**A**irway and cervical spine control
B	**B**reathing
C	**C**irculation and haemorrhage control
D	**D**isability
E	**E**xposure

Airway and cervical spine

Airway assessment following trauma should follow the

LOOK
LISTEN
FEEL

technique discussed in Chapters 4 and 5.

A cervical spine injury should be assumed to be present until adequate investigation and examination exclude it.

Breathing

Once the airway has been secured and the cervical spine controlled, breathing should be assessed. As discussed in earlier chapters the adequacy of breathing is gained from three sets of observations – the effort of breathing, the efficacy of breathing, and the effects of inadequate respiration on other organ systems. These are summarised in the box.

Assessment of the adequacy of breathing

Effort of breathing
  Recession
  Respiratory rate
  Inspiratory or expiratory noises
  Grunting
  Accessory muscle use
  Flare of the alae nasi
Efficacy of breathing
  Breath sounds
  Chest expansion
  Abdominal excursion
Effects of inadequate respiration
  Heart rate
  Skin colour
  Mental status

The normal resting respiratory rate changes with age. These changes are summarised in Table 15.2.

Circulation

Circulatory assessment in the primary survey consists of the rapid assessment of heart rate, systolic blood pressure, capillary refill time, skin colour and temperature, respiratory rate, and mental status. Using these measures an approximate estimate of the percentage of blood loss can be made as shown in Table 15.1. Remember the caveats on the clinical signs of differential pulse volume and capillary refill time in Chapter 3.

Table 15.1. Recognition of stages of shock

Sign	Assessment of percentage blood loss		
	<25	25–40	>40
Heart rate	Tachycardia+	Tachycardia++	Tachycardia/ bradycardia
Systolic BP	Normal	Normal or falling	Falling
Pulse volume	Normal/reduced	Reduced+	Reduced++
Capillary refill time (Normal <2s)	Normal/increased	Increased+	Increased++
Skin	Cool, pale	Cold, mottled	Cold Pale
Respiratory rate	Tachypnoea+	Tachypnoea++	Sighing respiration
Mental state	Mild agitation	Lethargic Uncooperative	Reacts only to pain

Resting heart rate, blood pressure, and respiratory rate vary with age, and circulatory assessment of a child must take this variation into account. The normal values are shown in Table 15.2. A recent study has shown that injured children have a relative systolic hypertension unrelated to age or trauma severity. The clinician should therefore view with suspicion a systolic pressure in the lower part of the normal range in an injured child.

Table 15.2. Vital signs: approximate range of normal

Age (years)	Respiratory rate (breaths/min)	Systolic BP (mmHg)	Pulse (beats/min)
<1	30–40	70–90	110–160
1–2	25–35	80–95	100–150
2–5	25–30	80–100	95–140
5–12	20–25	90–110	80–120
>12	15–20	100–120	60–100

Disability

The assessment of disability during the primary survey consists of a brief neurological examination to determine conscious level, and assessment of pupil size and reactivity. Conscious level determination is kept as simple as possible – and requires only that the child is put into one of the four following categories:

A   Alert
V   Responds to Voice
P   Responds to Pain
U   Unresponsive

Exposure

In order to assess a seriously injured child fully, it is necessary to take his or her clothes off. Children become cold very quickly, and may be acutely embarrassed when undressed in front of strangers. Although exposure is necessary the time taken for it should be minimised, and a blanket provided at all other times.

RESUSCITATION

Life-threatening problems should be treated as they are identified during the primary survey.

Airway and cervical spine

Airway

The airway may be compromised by extrinsic material (blood, vomit, or a foreign body), by the tongue, or by injury to the face, mouth, or upper airway. Whatever the cause, airway management should follow the sequence described in Chapters 4 and 5. This is summarised in the box.

> **Airway management sequence**
> - Jaw thrust
> - Suction/removal of foreign body
> - Oral/pharyngeal airways
> - Tracheal intubation
> - Surgical airway

Head tilt/chin lift is not recommended following trauma, because cervical spine injuries may be made worse.

Cervical spine

The cervical spine should be presumed to be damaged until proved intact, especially if there is obvious injury above the clavicle. Children can have significant spinal cord injury without radiographic abnormality (with devastating consequences if ignored). Even if normal radiographs are obtained the cervical spine must be protected in any patient where there is a high index of suspicion. If the child is unconscious or cooperative, his or her head and neck should be immobilised initially by in-line manual stabilisation, and then using a semi-rigid collar, sandbags, and tape. Uncooperative or combative patients should simply have a hard collar applied, because too rigid immobilisation of the head in such cases may increase neck movement as struggling occurs. Only when radiographs are normal, *and* the neurological examination has been demonstrated to be completely normal, should immobilising manoeuvres be discontinued. A full neurological assessment cannot be carried out if the child is paralysed and ventilated. Spinal immobilisation may need to be maintained for prolonged periods in such cases.

Breathing

If breathing is inadequate, ventilation must be commenced. Initially bag-mask ventilation should be performed. Generally speaking, a child who requires bag-mask ventilation initially following trauma will subsequently require intubation to control the airway. Following intubation, mechanical ventilation can be commenced.

The indications for intubation and mechanical ventilation are summarised in the box.

Indications for intubation and ventilation

- Inadequate oxygenation via bag-and-mask technique
- Prolonged ventilation required
- Controlled hyperventilation required
- Flail chest
- Inhalation burn injury

If breath sounds are unequal then pneumothorax, misplaced tracheal tube, or blocked main bronchus should be considered, and appropriate measures should be taken.

Circulation

All seriously injured children require vascular access to be established urgently. Two relatively large intravenous cannulae are mandatory. The percutaneous approach to peripheral veins is the preferred route, but, if this fails, other routes should be used. The external jugular veins and femoral veins can be cannulated, and a cut-down onto the cephalic vein at the elbow or long saphenous at the ankle should be considered. Intraosseous infusion may be used, and will usually prove quicker and easier than the more specialised techniques mentioned above. Vascular access techniques are discussed in detail in Chapter 23.

Central venous cannulation is particularly hazardous in children, and should not be attempted by the inexperienced. If a central venous line is inserted, its main use is for monitoring central venous pressure.

Fluid therapy should be commenced as a bolus using 20 ml/kg of crystalloid (e.g. normal (physiological) saline) or colloid (e.g. gelatin or starch compounds). The response should be assessed. If there is no change, a further bolus of fluid is given. If there is still no improvement, the next bolus should be of whole blood or packed cells, and a surgical opinion should be sought urgently – this is summarised in Figure 15.1.

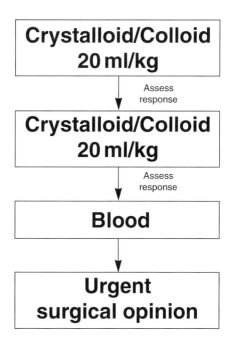

Figure 15.1. Fluids in hypovolaemic shock after trauma

Cross-matching of blood takes time, and clinical urgency may dictate that type-specific or O-negative blood must be given. The times necessary to obtain blood are shown in Table 15.3.

Table 15.3. Cross-match times

Blood type	Cross-match	Time (minutes)
O negative	Nil	0
Type specific	ABO	10–15
Full cross-match	Full	45–60

Other procedures carried out during resuscitation

History taking

History should be sought from the child, ambulance personnel, relatives, and witnesses of the accident. Ambulance staff should be able to provide a great deal of information, including details of the accident site and of pre-hospital care that was administered. Relatives should be able to give the child's past medical history and allergies, and provide details of the time of the last meal.

The mechanism of injury is useful in assessment. The information in Table 15.4 should be obtained if possible.

Table 15.4. Relevant history of injury mechanism

Road accident	Other
Car occupant/cyclist/pedestrian	Nature of accident
Position in vehicle	Objects involved
Restraints worn	Height of fall
Head protection	Landing surface
Thrown from vehicle	Environment
Speed of impact	Temperature
Damage to vehicle	Contamination
Other victim's injuries	

Blood tests

At the same time that intravenous access is obtained, blood should be taken for baseline haematology, baseline biochemistry, and cross-matching.

Radiographs

All seriously injured children must have radiographs of the *lateral cervical spine, chest* and *pelvis*. Other radiographs are taken later as dictated by clinical examination.

Urinary catheterisation

Catheterisation of a child should only be performed if the child cannot pass urine spontaneously, or if continuous accurate output measurement is required. The route (urethral or suprapubic) will depend on factors related to signs of urethral, bladder, intra-abdominal or pelvic injury (such as blood at the external meatus, or bruising in the scrotum or perineum). If a boy requires urethral catheterisation, urethral damage must be excluded first. The smallest possible silastic catheter should be used in order to reduce the risk of subsequent urethral stricture formation. If any doubt exists then the decision to catheterise the child can be left to the responsible surgeon. Urine should be sent for microscopy.

Nasogastric tube placement
Acute gastric dilatation is common in children and the stomach should be decompressed. If there is suspicion of base of skull fracture the tube should be passed orally.

Analgesia
Analgesia should be considered at this stage and administered unless there is very good reason for not doing so. Morphine is the drug of choice and should be given intravenously in a dose of 0·1–0·2 mg/kg. There is no place for the administration of intramuscular analgesia in trauma. Entonox (a 50/50 mix of O_2/N_2O) should be considered, but is contraindicated if there is a possibility of pneumothorax or base of skull fractures.

SECONDARY SURVEY

When the primary survey has been completed and resuscitation has stabilised the patient, the secondary survey can be started. If simple resuscitative measures do not stabilise the child, then operative intervention may be necessary before a formal secondary survey is undertaken. Whenever it is performed, it should identify all the injuries present in an anatomical and methodical way, and entails a thorough clinical examination, and relevant investigations.

Throughout this stage of management, the vital signs and neurological status should be continually reassessed, and any deterioration should lead to an immediate return to the primary survey.

Head

Clinical examination
- Inspect for bruising, haemorrhage, deformity, and CSF leak.
- Palpate for lacerations, bruising, and skull depressions.
- Perform otoscopy and ophthalmoscopy.
- Perform a mini-neurological examination:
    pupillary reflexes;
    Glasgow Coma Scale assessment (see Chapter 18);
    motor function – reflexes, tone, power.

Investigations (as indicated)
- Skull radiographs.
- CT brain scan.

Face

Clinical examination
- Inspect for bruising, lacerations, and deformity.
- Inspect the mouth inside and out.
- Palpate the bones for deformity.
- Palpate the teeth for looseness.

Investigations (as indicated)
Facial radiographs.

Neck

Clinical examination

Care should be taken not to move the cervical spine during this assessment. If the semi-rigid collar is removed, an assistant should maintain in-line cervical stabilisation throughout.

- Inspect the front and back of the neck for bruising and swelling.
- Palpate the cervical spine for tenderness, bruising, swelling, and deformity.
- Palpate for surgical emphysema.

Investigations (as indicated)
Further cervical spine images:
- Anteroposterior view.
- Odontoid view.
- Oblique view.
- MRI scan
- CT scan.

Flexion and extension views should not be obtained.

Chest

Clinical examination
- Inspect for bruising, lacerations, deformity, and movement.
- Inspect neck veins.
- Feel for tracheal deviation.
- Feel for tenderness, crepitus, and paradoxical movement.
- Percuss.
- Listen for breath sounds and added sounds.
- Listen for heart sounds.

Investigations (as indicated)
- ECG.
- Further chest radiographs.
- Special radiographs as indicated (e.g. tomogram, aortogram).
- CT scan.

Abdomen

Clinical examination
- Observe for movement.
- Inspect for bruising, lacerations, and swelling.
- Palpate for tenderness, rigidity, and masses.
- Auscultate for bowel sounds.

Rectal examination should only be performed if the result is going to alter management of the child. If necessary it should be done by the responsible surgeon so as to avoid unnecessary repetition of upsetting procedures. Vaginal examinations should not be performed on children.

Investigations (as indicated)
- Ultrasound.
- CT scan (double contrast).
- Diagnostic peritoneal lavage (rarely indicated).
- Intravenous urogram (pyelogram).

Pelvis

Clinical examination
- Inspect for bruising, lacerations, and deformity.
- Inspect the perineum.
- Inspect the external urethral meatus for blood.
- Press over the anterior iliac crests for elicited tenderness and abnormal mobility.

Investigations (as indicated)
- Bladder ultrasound.
- Retrograde urethrography.

Spine

Clinical examination

Proper spinal examination can only be carried out after the child has been log-rolled (see Chapter 24).

- Observe for swelling and bruising.
- Palpate for tenderness, bruising, swelling, and deformity.
- Assess motor and sensory function.

Investigations (as indicated)
- Radiographs.
- MRI scans.
- CT scans.

Extremities

Clinical examination
- Observe for bruising, swelling, and deformity.
- Palpate for tenderness. Crepitus and abnormal movement may be found (do not elicit deliberately as these are painful).
- Assess peripheral circulation – pulses and capillary return.
- Assess peripheral sensation – to touch and pin-prick.

Investigations (as indicated)
- Radiographs.
- Angiograms.

EMERGENCY TREATMENT

Emergency treatments are treatments that are necessary during the first hour or so of management. They are not as urgent as those that are performed to save life during the resuscitation phase, but are important nevertheless. Once the secondary survey has been completed an emergency treatment plan should be formed. This will include treatments for potentially life-threatening and limb-threatening injuries discovered during the secondary survey, and for more minor injuries discovered at the same time.

Emergency treatments are discussed in more detail in subsequent chapters.

CONTINUED MONITORING

Pulse, blood pressure, respiratory rate, oxygen saturation, pupil size and reactivity, and coma score should be measured and charted frequently (at least every 15 minutes). Urinary output must be recorded hourly. End-tidal CO_2 (in the ventilated child) provides useful additional information, and should be measured if possible.

Any deterioration should lead to immediate reassessment of the airway, breathing, and circulation, and appropriate resuscitative measures should be commenced.

DEFINITIVE CARE

Definitive care is the final part of the structured approach to trauma, and is often carried out by teams other than that which initially received the patient. Good notetaking and appropriate referral are essential if time is not to be lost. If definitive care is to be undertaken in a specialist centre then secondary transfer may be necessary at this stage.

Note-taking

The structured approach discussed in this chapter can provide a framework for the writing of notes. It is recommended that these should be set out as shown in Table 15.5.

Referral

Many teams may be involved in the definitive care of a seriously injured child. It is essential that referrals are made appropriately, clearly, and early. Guidance about which children to refer to which teams is given in subsequent chapters.

Transfer

Injured children may require transfer either within the hospital or to another centre. In either case thorough preparation of equipment, patient, and documentation is essential. Secondary transfer should not be undertaken until all life-threatening problems have been addressed, and the child is stable. Transport of children is discussed in more detail in Chapter 26.

15.5. Template for note-taking

```
Primary survey
    A
    B
    C
    D
    E

Resuscitation
    A
    B
    C

Secondary survey
    Head
    Face
    Neck
    Chest
    Abdomen
    Pelvis
    Spine
    Extremities
        Upper
        Lower
```

SUMMARY

The structured approach to initial assessment and management, discussed here, allows the professional to care for the seriously injured child in a logical, efficacious fashion.

Assessment of vital functions (airway, breathing, and circulation) is carried out first; resuscitation for any problems found is instituted immediately.

- Primary survey.
- Resuscitation.

A complete head-to-toe examination is then carried out, emergency treatment performed and finally referral to teams responsible for definitive care is made:

- Secondary survey.
- Emergency treatment.
- Definitive care.

CHAPTER

16

The child with chest injury

Following the establishment of a secure airway, the next most important consideration in the resuscitation of a child is the assessment of breathing. The child who has suffered multiple injuries may well have significant intrathoracic trauma that severely compromises respiration, and requires immediate treatment.

Substantial amounts of kinetic energy may be transferred through a child's chest wall with little or no external sign of injury. Furthermore, children have very elastic ribs which rarely fracture; thus a normal chest radiograph does not exclude major thoracic visceral disruption.

Thoracic injuries must be considered in all children who suffer major trauma. Some may be life threatening and require immediate resuscitative therapy during the primary survey and resuscitation, whereas others may be discovered during the secondary survey and be treated with appropriate emergency treatment at that stage. *The vast majority can be managed in the first hour by any competent doctor.* Practical procedures are described in detail in Chapter 24.

INJURIES POSING AN IMMEDIATE THREAT TO LIFE

Tension pneumothorax

This is a life-threatening emergency. Air accumulates under pressure in the pleural space; this, in turn, pushes the mediastinum across the chest and kinks the great vessels. This then compromises venous return to the heart and therefore cardiac output is reduced. The diagnosis is a clinical one. A radiograph that shows a tension pneumothorax should never have been taken.

Signs
- The child will be hypoxic and may be shocked.
- There will be decreased air entry and hyperresonance to percussion on the side of the pneumothorax.
- Distended neck veins may be apparent in thin children.
- Later the trachea will be deviated away from the side of the pneumothorax.

Resuscitation
- High-flow oxygen should be given through a reservoir mask.
- Immediate needle thoracocentesis should be performed to relieve the tension.
- A chest drain should be inserted urgently to prevent recurrence.

Air may be forced into the pneumothorax by positive pressure ventilation. Any patient with a pneumothorax will develop a tension pneumothorax if ventilated.

Massive haemothorax

Blood accumulates in the pleural space. This results from damage to the lung parenchyma with possible additional damage to pulmonary or chest wall blood vessels. The hemithorax can contain a substantial proportion of a child's blood volume.

Signs
- The child will be hypoxic and in shock.
- There will be decreased chest movement, decreased air entry, and decreased resonance to percussion on the side of the haemothorax.

Resuscitation
- High-flow oxygen should be given through a reservoir mask.
- Intravenous access should be established and volume replacement commenced.
- A relatively large chest drain should be inserted urgently.

Open pneumothorax

There is a penetrating wound in the chest wall with associated pneumothorax. The wound may be obvious, but it may be on the child's back, and will not be seen unless actively looked for.

Signs
- Air may be heard sucking and blowing through the wound.
- The other signs of pneumothorax will be present.

Resuscitation
- High-flow oxygen should be given through a reservoir mask.
- The wound should be occluded (on three sides only in order to allow air to escape during expiration).
- A chest drain should be inserted urgently.

Flail chest

The elasticity of the child's chest wall reduces the incidence of flail chest, on the one hand. On the other, the increased mobility means that children are badly affected by these injuries if they do occur, since the underlying lung injury tends to be worse. Anteroposterior or posteroanterior chest radiographs do not demonstrate rib fractures reliably and should not be relied upon in making the diagnosis.

Signs
- The child will be hypoxic.
- Abnormal chest movement associated with rib crepitus may be seen.
- Flail segments may not be seen on initial examination because reflex splinting of the segment occurs.

Resuscitation
- High-flow oxygen should be given through a reservoir mask.
- Tracheal intubation and ventilation should be considered.
- Adequate pain relief must be given; this is difficult to achieve in children because intercostal nerve blockade is dangerous in the uncooperative patient, and anaesthetic consultation may be required.

Cardiac tamponade

Cardiac tamponade can occur after both penetrating and blunt injury. The blood that accumulates in the fibrous pericardial sac reduces the volume available for cardiac filling during diastole. As more blood accumulates cardiac output is progressively reduced.

Signs
- The child will be in shock.
- There may be muffled heart sounds.
- There may be distended neck veins; this will not be apparent if significant hypovolaemia coexists.

Resuscitation
- High-flow oxygen should be given through a reservoir mask.
- Intravenous access should be established, and rapid volume replacement com-menced; this temporarily increases filling pressure.
- Emergency needle pericardiocentesis should be performed; removal of a small volume of fluid from within the pericardium can dramatically increase cardiac output.

SERIOUS INJURIES DISCOVERED LATER

Pulmonary contusion

Children have a high incidence of pulmonary contusion because of the mobility of the ribs. There may be no overlying fracture.This injury is usually the result of blunt trauma which ruptures pulmonary capillaries allowing blood to fill the alveoli, causing the child to become hypoxic.

Diagnosis is often by exclusion. "Consolidation" may be seen on chest radiograph, but this investigation may be normal. Treatment consists of the administration of high-flow oxygen, and artificial ventilation if necessary.

Tracheal and bronchial rupture

Frequently lethal, this presents as a pneumo- or haemopneumothorax, possibly with associated subcutaneous emphysema.

Resuscitation treatment is as described above. Continued significant air leaks after chest drain insertion strongly suggest this diagnosis. Definitive care requires referral to a cardiothoracic surgeon.

Disruption of great vessels

This is usually rapidly fatal. A child with this injury who survives to get to hospital has a tear in a vessel that has tamponaded itself.

The patient may be shocked and peripheral pulses may be poorly palpable. The diagnosis should be suspected if a widened mediastinum is seen on chest radiograph. A radiologist should be called to perform urgent angiography. Definitive treatment is by a cardiothoracic surgeon.

Ruptured diaphragm

This may occur following blunt abdominal trauma, and is more common on the left side. The child may be hypoxic due to pulmonary compression, and may have signs of hypovolaemia if intra-abdominal visceral injury has occurred. A chest radiograph often reveals abnormalities caused by the presence of abdominal contents. These may be non-specific, or can be diagnostic if bowel shadowing or an abnormal position for the nasogastric tube is present. A surgical referral should be made.

OTHER INJURIES

Simple pneumothorax

A self-limiting leak of air occurs. This causes partial lung collapse. Signs of hypoxia are rarely apparent. Clinically, decreased chest wall movement, diminished breath sounds, and hyperresonance may be found on the side of the pneumothorax. The diagnosis is usually made radiologically.

A chest drain should be inserted electively. If the patient is to be ventilated chest drain insertion *must* be undertaken urgently. In the ventilated patient a simple pneumothorax becomes a tension pneumothorax.

PRACTICAL PROCEDURES

Needle thoracocentesis, chest drain insertion, and pericardiocentesis are described in Chapter 24.

REFERRAL

Most immediately life-threatening chest injuries can be successfully managed by a competent doctor. However, cardiothoracic consultation may be required as a result of conditions uncovered by chest drainage and for serious injuries discovered during the secondary survey. The major reasons for referral are shown in the box.

Patients who require ventilation as part of the treatment of their chest injury (such as those with significant pulmonary contusion) will need transfer to a paediatric intensive care unit.

Indications for cardiothoracic surgical referral

Continuing massive air leak after chest drain insertion
Continuing haemorrhage after chest drain insertion
Cardiac tamponade
Disruption of the great vessels

SUMMARY

A clear airway must be established before attending to chest injuries

All patients should receive high-flow oxygen through a reservoir mask

Chest injuries are life threatening but most can be managed successfully by any doctor capable of performing the following techniques:

- Needle thoracocentesis
- Chest drain insertion
- Intubation and ventilation
- Fluid replacement
- Pericardiocentesis

Cardiothoracic surgical referral may be necessary once immediate management of life-threatening conditions has been carried out

17

The child with abdominal injury

Blunt trauma causes the majority of abdominal injuries in children. Most occur because of accidents on the roads, although a significant number happen during recreational activities. A high index of suspicion is necessary if some injuries are not to be missed.

The abdominal contents are very susceptible to injury in children for a number of reasons. The abdominal wall is thin and offers relatively little protection. The diaphragm is more horizontal than in adults, causing the liver and spleen to lie lower and more anteriorly. Furthermore the ribs, being very elastic, offer less protection to these organs. Finally, the bladder is intra-abdominal, rather than pelvic, and is therefore more exposed when full. Respiratory compromise can complicate abdominal injury because diaphragmatic irritation or splinting may occur – reducing the use of the diaphragm during breathing.

HISTORY

A precise history of the mechanism of injury may help in diagnosis. Rapid deceleration, such as experienced during road accidents, causes abdominal compression. The spleen and liver are at risk from such forces, and the duodenum may develop a large haematoma or may rupture at the duodenojejunal flexure. Direct blows, such as those caused by punching or impact with bicycle handlebars, injure underlying organs. Again the liver and spleen, being relatively exposed, are at risk. Finally, straddling injuries can cause perineal injury and may rupture the urethra.

ASSESSMENT OF THE INJURED ABDOMEN

Initial assessment and management must be directed to the care of the airway, breathing, and circulation as discussed in Chapter 15.

Examination

If shock is not amenable to fluid replacement during the primary survey and resuscitation, and no obvious site of haemorrhage exists, then intra-abdominal injury may be the cause of blood loss. The abdomen should be assessed urgently to establish whether early operative intervention is necessary. In other circumstances, the abdominal examination is carried out during the secondary survey.

The abdomen should be inspected for bruising, lacerations, and penetrating wounds. Major intra-abdominal injury can occur without obvious external signs, and visible bruising is therefore highly significant. Children with visible abdominal bruising, especially if associated with a lumbar spine fracture, have a high incidence of bowel perforation. A high index of suspicion and frequent repeated clinical assessment is appropriate in such cases. The external urethral meatus should be examined for blood.

Gentle palpation should be carried out. This will reveal areas of tenderness and rigidity. Care should be taken not to hurt the child because his or her continued cooperation is important during the repeated examinations that form an important part of management.

Rectal and vaginal examinations are mandatory in an adult with multiple injuries. In children every effort should be made to limit rectal examination to that performed by the surgeon who is going to operate on that child. Even then it should only be done if the result of the examination will alter the management. Vaginal examination should not be performed on children.

Aids to assessment

Both gastric and urinary bladder drainage may help the assessment by decompressing the abdomen.

Gastric drainage

Air swallowing during crying with consequent acute gastric dilatation is common in children. Early passage of a gastric tube of an appropriate size is essential. The tube should be aspirated regularly and left on free drainage at other times. A massively distended stomach can mimic intra-abdominal pathology needing laparotomy, and cause serious diaphragm splintage with consequent respiratory compromise.

Urinary catheterisation

Catheterisation of a child should only be performed if the child cannot pass urine spontaneously, or if continuous accurate output measurement is required. The route (urethral or suprapubic) will depend on factors related to signs of urethral, bladder, or intra-abdominal or pelvic injury (such as blood at the external meatus, or bruising in the scrotum or perineum). If a boy requires urethral catheterisation, urethral damage must be excluded first. The catheter should be silastic and as small as possible in order to reduce the risk of subsequent urethral stricture formation.

Investigations

Blood tests

Intravenous access will have already been secured during the primary survey and resuscitation, and at that time blood will have been drawn for baseline blood counts, urea and electrolytes, and cross-matching. An amylase estimation should be requested and can usually be performed on the sample sent for urea and electrolytes. Arterial blood gases should be sent if indicated. Repeated monitoring of blood parameters may be appropriate in some patients.

Radiographs
Views of the lateral cervical spine, chest, and pelvis will have been obtained during the course of the primary survey. Neither a normal chest radiograph

nor a normal pelvic radiograph excludes abdominal injury. A plain abdominal radiograph may be helpful to look for the position of the gastric tube, distribution of abdominal gas, presence of free gas, and soft tissue swellings including a full bladder. Renal injury may need investigation by intravenous urography. Blood at the external urethral meatus will require investigation using retrograde urethrography.

Computed tomography A double contrast CT scan of the abdomen (with intravenous and intragastric contrast) is the radiological investigation of choice in children. CT will alert the surgeon to solid organ rupture, free intraperitoneal contrast from a perforated viscus, the presence or absence of two functioning kidneys, and free intraperitoneal contrast from a ruptured bladder.

Ultrasound This may be readily available and give early information on free fluid and lacerations in the liver, spleen, or kidneys. A normal ultrasound early on does not exclude injury.

Diagnostic peritoneal lavage This should rarely be used in children, as the presence of intraperitoneal blood per se is not necessarily an indication for laparotomy. Once lavage fluid has been introduced, the peritoneum shows signs of irritation for up to 48 hours, and hence reduces the possibility of accurate repeated assessment. Peritoneal lavage should therefore only be carried out by the surgeon managing the case and will be needed only where facilities for imaging (CT and ultrasound) and for regular clinical reassessment are absent.

A lavage should be considered positive if the red cell count is over $100\,000/mm^3$, the white cell count over $500/mm^3$, or if enteric contents or bacteria are seen. Laboratory analysis gives the best sensitivity and specificity for this test. Bedside estimation is dangerously unreliable. This technique is described in Chapter 24.

DEFINITIVE CARE

Non-operative management

Until the early 1980s, both adult and paediatric patients with haemoperitoneum would undergo laparotomy. Damage to the spleen or liver would result in splenectomy or partial hepatectomy respectively. It has since been shown that the haemorrhage is often self-limiting, and many of these operations can therefore be avoided. As well as avoiding the morbidity associated with laparotomy, this approach also reduces the number of children at risk of overwhelming, potentially fatal sepsis following splenectomy.

For non-operative management to be undertaken the following are essential:

- Adequate observation and frequent monitoring.
- Precise fluid management.
- The immediate availability of a surgeon trained to operate on the paediatric abdomen (should this become necessary).

The need for clotting factors such as platelets, fresh frozen plasma, or cryoprecipitate must be monitored. Vigorous and early management of coagulopathy is indicated in order to improve clotting and hence achieve haemostasis.

Indications for operative intervention

Children whose circulation is not stable after replacement of 40 ml/kg of fluid are probably bleeding into the thoracic or abdominal cavities. In the absence of clear thoracic bleeding, urgent laparotomy may be necessary. All children with penetrating abdominal injuries and those with definite signs of bowel perforation will require urgent laparotomy.

A non-functioning kidney, as demonstrated on contrast studies, may have suffered renal pedicle injury. These require immediate exploration to ascertain whether the kidney can be saved. The warm ischaemia time for a kidney is only 45–60 minutes.

Indications for operative intervention following abdominal injury

Laparotomy
    Refractory shock
    Penetrating injuries
    Signs of bowel perforation
Renal exploration
    Non-functioning kidney

It is essential that the surgeon performing these procedures is competent to deal with paediatric trauma and can perform any reconstructive surgery that may be required.

SUMMARY

- The assessment and management of airway, breathing, and circulation must be carried out first. Abdominal assessment is only carried out at this stage if shock is refractory
- Abdominal assessment consists of careful observation and gentle, repeated palpation. Gastric and urinary drainage aid this assessment
- Abdominal CT scan is the investigation of choice. Diagnostic peritoneal lavage is rarely used in children
- Some children with visceral injury may be managed non-operatively if essential requirements are met. Others will need urgent operative intervention

CHAPTER
18

The child with trauma to the head

EPIDEMIOLOGY

Head injury is the most common single cause of trauma death in children aged 1–15 years. It accounts for 40% of deaths from injury.

The most common occurrence that causes death from head injury is a road traffic accident. Pedestrian children are the most vulnerable, followed by cyclists, and then passengers in vehicles. Falls are the second most common cause of fatal head injuries. In infancy the most common cause is child abuse.

PATHOPHYSIOLOGY

Brain damage may be from the primary or secondary effects of the injury.

Primary damage

- Cerebral lacerations.
- Cerebral contusions.
- Dural sac tears.
- Diffuse axonal injury.

Secondary damage

This may result from either the direct secondary effects of cerebral injury or from the cerebral consequences of associated injuries and stress:

- Ischaemia from poor cerebral perfusion secondary to raised intracranial pressure.
- Ischaemia secondary to hypotension and blood loss.
- Hypoxia from inadequate ventilation caused by loss of respiratory drive.
- Hypoxia from airway obstruction or thoracic injuries.
- Hypoglycaemia.
- Loss of metabolic homoeostasis.

- Hypothermia.
- Fever.
- Convulsions.

Raised intracranial pressure

Once sutures have closed at 12–18 months of age, the child's cranial cavity behaves like an adult's with a fixed volume. Cerebral oedema or haematomas increase the volume of the contents. Initial compensatory mechanisms include diminution of the total volume of cerebrospinal fluid and diminution in the pool of venous blood. When these mechanisms fail, volume increase leads to raised intracranial pressure. This causes an increased pressure gradient for the inflow of arterial blood and a fall in cerebral perfusion pressure.

Cerebral perfusion pressure = Mean arterial pressure –Mean intracranial pressure

Normal cerebral blood flow is 50 ml of blood per 100 g brain tissue per minute. A fall in cerebral perfusion pressure decreases cerebral blood flow. A flow of below 20 ml per 100 g of brain tissue per minute will produce ischaemia; this increases cerebral oedema and hence causes a further rise in intracranial pressure. A cerebral blood flow of below 10 ml/100 g/minute leads to electrical dysfunction of the neurones and loss of intracellular homoeostasis.

A generalised increase of intracranial pressure in the supratentorial compartment initially causes transtentorial (uncal), and later causes transforaminal (central) herniation (coning), and death. Unilateral increases in intracranial pressure secondary to haematoma formation cause ipsilateral uncal herniation. The third nerve is nipped against the free border of the tentorium, causing ipsilateral pupillary dilatation secondary to loss of parasympathetic constrictor tone to the ciliary muscles.

In childhood, the most common cause of raised intracranial pressure following head injury is cerebral oedema. Children are especially prone to this problem. They may, of course, also have expanding extradural, subdural, or intracerebral haematomas which will require surgical treatment.

Depending on the aetiology of the raised intracranial pressure, treatment is either aimed at preventing it rising further, or removing its cause (by surgical evacuation of haematomas).

There are special considerations in infants with head injuries. Their cranial volume can more easily increase because of unfused sutures. Therefore, large extradural or subdural bleeds may occur before neurological signs or symptoms develop. Such infants may show a significant fall in haemoglobin concentration. Additionally, the infant's vascular scalp may bleed profusely causing shock. In children over 1 year with shock associated with head injury, serious extracranial injury should be sought as the cause of the shock.

PATIENT TRIAGE

Head injuries vary from the trivial to the fatal. Triage is necessary in order to give more seriously injured patients a higher priority. Factors indicating a potentially serious injury are shown in the box.

Factors Indicating a potentially serious Injury

- History of substantial trauma such as involvement in a road traffic accident or a fall from a height
- A history of loss of consciousness
- Children who are not fully conscious and responsive
- Any child with obvious neurological signs/symptoms such as headache, convulsions, or limb weakness
- Evidence of penetrating injury

ASSESSMENT

Primary survey

The first priority is to assess and stabilise the airway, breathing, and circulation as discussed in Chapter 15. Head injury may be associated with cervical spine injury, and neck immobilisation must be achieved as previously described.

Pupil size and reactivity should be examined, and a rapid assessment of conscious level should be made. The latter consists of placing the child into one of four categories as shown.

A	**A**lert
V	Responds to **V**oice
P	Responds to **P**ain
U	**U**nresponsive

The history of the injury itself, and the child's course since the injury occurred, should be established from relevant personnel. Any other significant history can be obtained from parents or carers.

Secondary survey

The head should be carefully observed and palpated externally for bruises and lacerations to the scalp and for depressed skull fractures. Look for evidence of basal skull fracture such as blood or cerebrospinal fluid (CSF) from the nose or ear, haemotympanum, panda eyes, or Battle's sign (bruising behind the ear, over the mastoid).

The conscious level should be assessed using the relevant Children's Coma Scale if the child is less than 4 years old, and the Glasgow Coma Scale if the child is older than that. These scales are shown in Table 18.1. It should be noted that the Coma Scales reflect the degree of brain dysfunction *at the time of the examination*. Assessment should be repeated frequently.

The pupils should be examined for size and reactivity. A dilated non-reactive pupil indicates third nerve dysfunction; the cause is an ipsilateral haematoma until proven otherwise.

The fundi should be examined using an ophthalmoscope. Papilloedema may not be seen in acute raised intracranial pressure, but the presence of retinal haemorrhage may indicate abuse in a young infant with other unexplained injuries.

Motor function should be assessed. This includes examination of extraocular muscle function, facial and limb movements. Tone, movement, and reflexes should be assessed. Lateralising signs that indicate an intracranial bleed will be revealed in this way.

Investigations

Blood tests

Blood for haemoglobin, urea and electrolytes, and cross-match should have been taken during the primary survey and resuscitation. Arterial blood gases should be taken in head-injured patients, both to assess oxygenation and to measure $PaCO_2$.

Table 18.1. Glasgow Coma Scale and Children's Coma Scale

Glasgow Coma Scale (4–15 years)		Child's Glasgow Coma Scale (<4 years)	
Response	Score	Response	Score
Eye opening		*Eye opening*	
Spontaneously	4	Spontaneously	4
To verbal stimuli	3	To verbal stimuli	3
To pain	2	To pain	2
No response to pain	1	No response to pain	1
Best motor response		*Best motor response*	
Obeys verbal command	6	Spontaneous or obeys verbal command	6
Localises to pain	5	Localises to pain or withdraws to touch	5
Withdraws from pain	4	Withdraws from pain	4
Abnormal flexion to pain (decorticate)	3	Abnormal flexion to pain (decorticate)	3
Abnormal extension to pain (decerebrate)	2	Abnormal extension to pain (decerebrate)	2
No response to pain	1	No response to pain	1
Best verbal response		*Best verbal response*	
Orientated and converses	5	Alert, babbles, coos, words to usual ability	5
Disorientated and converses	4	Less than usual words spontaneous irritable cry	4
Inappropriate words	3	Cries only to pain	3
Incomprehensible sounds	2	Moans to pain	2
No response to pain	1	No response to pain	1

Radiology

A lateral view of the cervical spine, a chest radiograph, and a radiograph of the pelvis should have been taken during the primary survey.

Skull radiograph　　In severe head injury a skull radiograph may be superfluous as the information needed will be derived from the CT scan. The role of the skull radiograph in children's head injury is less clear than in adults. In adults the presence of a skull fracture increases the risk of developing a subdural haematoma in the conscious patient from 1:3000 to 1:40. However, in children the test is less specific. Indications for skull radiography are summarised in the box.

Indications for skull radiograph

- Loss of consciousness or amnesia at any time
- Neurological symptoms and signs
- CSF or blood from nose/ear
- Suspected penetrating injury or foreign body
- Scalp bruising or swelling
- Significant mechanism of injury
- Difficulty in assessing the patient
- Non-mobile infants (the likelihood of abuse is higher)
- Alcoholic intoxication

Computed tomography CT scanning and neurosurgical referral usually go hand in hand. The exception is the child with a head injury and a Glasgow Coma Score of 14 or less, who is about to undergo surgery for other serious injuries. A CT scan may be indicated in these cases, prior to surgery. Table 18.2 summarises the factors leading to the decision about whether or not to scan.

There is an increasing tendency to emulate US practice and perform a non-urgent CT scan on patients with a skull fracture but no signs/symptoms. A discussion of this area is outside the scope of this text. An area of concern especially in small children is the need, on occasion, to anaesthetise them for a CT scan if they are non-cooperative. This must only be done where skills and facilities are available for the anaesthetic care of young children.

Table 18.2. Guidelines for CT scanning of head-injured children

Coma	Fracture	Child's condition	CT scan
15	No	No signs	No
15	Yes	No signs	Consider
15	Yes	Signs/symptoms	Yes
13–14	No	No signs	Consider
13–14	Yes	No signs	Yes
<12	Yes/No	Signs/symptoms +/−	Yes

EMERGENCY TREATMENT

The initial aim of management of a child with a serious head injury is prevention of secondary brain damage. This is achieved by maintaining ventilation and circulation, and by avoiding raised intracranial pressure.

This can best be achieved by attention to the ABCs discussed earlier. The airway should be secured. Children with a Coma Score of 8 or less should be intubated and ventilated after rapid induction of anaesthesia. Capnogaphy must be used from the outset of intubation. Routine hyperventilation has not been shown to improve outcome and may adversely affect cerebral perfusion in areas of brain still responsive to changes in PCO_2. Normocapnia is now the aim. Hyperventilation is reserved for the patient with signs of significantly raised ICP such as transtentorial herniation. Shock should be treated vigorously to avoid hypoperfusion of the brain.

The withholding of analgesia may contribute to deterioration of the child's condition by leading to a rise in intracranial pressure, and may lead to misinterpretation of the conscious level. Following initial assessment, sufficient analgesia should be administered. Intravenous morphine, at an initial dose of 0·1–0·2 mg/kg, is ideal as the dose can be titrated against the child's response. Additionally the drug's effects can be rapidly reversed with naloxone if necessary. Local anaesthetic techniques such as femoral nerve block may also be used to good effect.

Management of specific problems

Deteriorating conscious level
If airway, breathing, and circulation are satisfactory, then a deteriorating conscious level is due to increased intracranial pressure; this may be due either to an intracranial haematoma or to cerebral oedema. Urgent neurosurgical referral and CT scan is indicated and the temporising manoeuvres shown in the box may be instituted.

187

> **Measures to increase cerebral perfusion temporarily**
>
> - Nurse in the 20° head-up position to help venous drainage
> - Ventilation to $Paco_2$ of 3·5–4·0 kPa (25–30 mmHg)
> - Infusion of intravenous mannitol 0·5–1 g/kg
> - Combat hypotension if present with colloid infusion

Signs of uncal or central herniation

These signs (discussed in Chapter 12) should lead to urgent institution of the measures in the box and neurosurgical referral.

Convulsions

A focal seizure should be regarded as a focal neurological sign. A general convulsion has less significance. Seizure activity raises intracranial pressure in both non-paralysed and paralysed patients. The diagnosis is difficult in the latter, but should be suspected if there is a sharp increase in heart rate and blood pressure, and dilatation of the pupils.

Seizures should be controlled if they have not stopped spontaneously within 5 minutes. The initial drugs of choice are diazepam or lorazepam (see Chapter 13). However, phenytoin should be used for prolonged or persistent convulsions as it has less sedative effect. The dose is 18 mg/kg intravenously over 20–30 minutes, with appropriate monitoring for rhythm irregularities and hypotension.

DEFINITIVE CARE

Neurosurgical referral

Indications for neurosurgical consultation are shown in the box.

> **Indications for referral to a neurosurgeon**
>
> - Deteriorating conscious level
> - Focal neurological signs
> - Evidence of depressed fracture
> - Evidence of penetrating injury
> - Evidence of basal skull fracture
> - Coma Score of less than 12

Secondary transfer

Transport of critically ill children is increasingly the responsibility of the receiving hospital. It is essential to secure the airway, ensure adequate ventilation, and maintain intravascular volume, temperature, and cerebral perfusion pressure if the child is to arrive in optimum condition. Quality of transfer is better than speed and as much time as necessary should be spent preparing the child (see checklist and Chapter 26).

Checklist for transfer

- Adequate sedation
- Full neuromuscular paralysis
- Intermittent positive pressure ventilation (IPPV) preferably by automatic paediatric ventilator
- Oximetry and capnography to monitor ventilation
- Adequate, secure vascular access
- Equipment box
- Heat conservation
- Full medical and nursing notes, charts, and radiographs
- Full parental information

SUMMARY

- Head injury causes primary brain damage. Secondary damage occurs because of the effects of hypoxia, and poor cerebral perfusion
- The first priority is assessment and management of the airway, breathing, and circulation
- A thorough examination including a mini-neurological examination should be carried out during the secondary survey; this involves assessment of external injury, conscious level, pupillary responses, fundi and motor functions
- Skull radiographs and CT brain scans should be performed if indicated
- The aim of management in the first hour is to prevent secondary damage; this is achieved by attention to airway, breathing, and circulation, and by prompt neurosurgical referral and transfer if indicated

19

The child with injuries to the extremities or the spine

EXTREMITY TRAUMA

INTRODUCTION

Skeletal injury accounts for 10–15% of all childhood injuries – of these 15% involve physeal disruptions. It is uncommon for extremity trauma to be life threatening in the multiply injured child. It is crucial to recognise and treat associated life-threatening injuries before assessing and managing the skeletal trauma. This chapter deals with problems from the perspective of multiple injury; the principles apply equally to individual injuries.

The differences between the mature and immature skeleton have a bearing on initial treatment and eventual outcome. Use of the principles usually applied to injuries of the mature skeleton will result in errors of both diagnosis and treatment. Children's bones are prone to a greater range of injury than those of adults. This is a reflection of the different mechanical properties of the immature skeleton, in particular the greater plasticity of bones and the presence of growth plates. These differences explain the occurrence of fractures unique to childhood. Greenstick and torus fractures occur because one or both cortices deform without fracturing. The growth plate is 2–5 times weaker than any other structure in the paediatric skeleton (including ligament and tendon), it is not surprising that it is commonly involved in fractures. The chance of fracture propagation is reduced and comminuted fractures are relatively rare. It should be remembered that children's bones can absorb more force than adults and this may result in an underestimation of the degree of trauma to associated soft tissues.

ASSESSMENT

Unless extremity injury is life threatening, evaluation is carried out during the secondary survey and treatment commenced during the definitive care phase. Single, closed, extremity injuries may produce enough blood loss to cause hypovolaemic shock, but this is not usually life threatening. Multiple fractures can, however, cause severe shock. Pelvic fractures are relatively uncommon in children – the energy that would have fractured a pelvis in an adult may have been transmitted to vessels within the pelvis of a child, leading to disruption and haemorrhage. Closed fractures of the femur may cause loss of approximately 20% of the intravascular volume into the thigh, and blood loss from open fractures can be even more significant. This blood loss begins at the time of the injury, and it can be difficult to estimate the degree of pre-hospital loss.

Primary survey

All multiply injured children should be approached in the structured way discussed in Chapter 15. Relevant history should be sought from relatives and pre-hospital staff. Extremity deformity and perfusion prior to arrival at hospital are especially important, and information concerning the method of injury is helpful.

Life-threatening injuries
These include the following:

- Crush injuries of the abdomen and pelvis.
- Traumatic amputation of an extremity.
- Massive open long-bone fractures.

They should be dealt with immediately and take precedence over any other extremity inury.

Crush injuries to the abdomen and pelvis　　Pelvic disruption can lead to life-threatening blood loss. The child will present with hypovolaemic shock; this may remain resistant to treatment until either the pelvic disruption is stabilised or the injured vessels are occluded.

Initial treatment during the primary survey and resuscitation phase consists of rapid fluid and blood infusions as discussed in Chapter 15. The diagnosis may be obvious if disruption is severe or if fractures are open. More often this cause of resistant hypovolaemia is discovered when the pelvic radiograph is taken.

Emergency orthopaedic opinion should be sought, and urgent external fixation of the pelvis should be considered. In some hospitals, radiographic identification and therapeutic embolisation of bleeding vessels may be attempted.

Traumatic amputation　　Traumatic amputation of an extremity may be partial or complete. Paradoxically, it is usually the former that presents the greatest initial threat to life. This is because completely transected vessels go into spasm whereas partially transected vessels do not. Blood loss can be large and the pre-hospital care of these injuries is critical; an exact history of this should be sought.

Once in hospital the airway should be cleared and breathing assessed as previously discussed. Two wide-bore cannulae should be inserted and rapid infusions should be commenced. Exsanguinating haemorrhage must be controlled. If local pressure and elevation are not sufficient, the application of a tourniquet should be considered. If this becomes necessary the tourniquet should be applied as distally as possible, and care should be taken to use a broad rather than a thin cuff. Orthopaedic pneumatic tourniquets are ideal but, if these are not available, a sphygmomanometer cuff inflated to above arterial pressure may be used. The time of application should be recorded, and emergency orthopaedic and plastic surgical opinions sought.

Reimplantation techniques are available in specialist centres. The success rate is improving, particularly in children. Urgent referral and transfer are necessary – the amputated part will only remain viable for 8 hours at room temperature, or for 18 hours if cooled. The amputated part should be cleaned, wrapped in a moist sterile towel, placed in a sterile, sealed plastic bag, and transported in an insulated box filled with crushed ice and water *in the same vehicle as the child*. Care should be taken to avoid direct contact between the ice and tissue.

If, after discussion with the specialist centre, it is decided that reimplantation is not appropriate, the amputated part should still be saved because it may be used for grafting of other injuries.

The child must be stabilised before transfer.

Massive, open, long-bone fractures   The blood loss from any long-bone fractures is significant; open fractures bleed more than closed ones because there is no tamponade effect from surrounding tissues. As a general rule an open fracture causes twice the blood loss of the corresponding closed fracture. Thus a single, open, femoral shaft fracture may result in 40% loss of circulating blood volume. This in itself is life threatening.

After airway and breathing have been assessed and treated, two relatively large-bore cannulae should be inserted and rapid infusion should be started. Exsanguinating haemorrhage should be controlled both by the application of pressure at the fracture site, and by correct splinting of the limb.

If haemorrhage cannot be controlled by these techniques, then emergency orthopaedic opinion should be sought. Angiography may be necessary to discover whether any major vessel rupture has occurred, and if such an injury is considered likely then a vascular surgical opinion should be obtained early.

Secondary survey

In a conscious child, inspection is usually the most productive part of the examination. Causing pain or eliciting crepitus in an injured extremity will only increase anxiety, ultimately making the child more difficult to manage.

The extremities should be inspected for discoloration, bruising, swelling, deformity, lacerations, and evidence of open fractures.

Next, *gentle* palpation should be undertaken to establish any areas of tenderness. Limb temperature and capillary refill should be assessed, and pulses sought – a Doppler flow probe should be used if necessary.

Finally, the active range of motion should be assessed if the child is cooperative. If there is an obvious fracture or dislocation, or the child refuses to move a limb actively, passive movement should be avoided.

Limb-threatening injury
The viability of a limb may be threatened by vascular injury, compartment syndrome, or by open fractures. These situations are discussed below.

Vascular injury   Assessment of the vascular status of the extremity is a vital step in evaluating an injury. Vascular damage may be caused by traction (resulting in intimal damage or complete disruption), or by penetrating injuries caused by either a missile or the end of a fractured bone. Brisk bleeding from an open wound or a rapidly expanding mass is indicative of active bleeding. Complete tears are less likely to bleed for a prolonged period due to contraction of the vessel. It should be remembered that nerves usually pass in close proximity to vessels and are likely to have been damaged along with the vessel.

193

The presence of a pulse, either clinically or on Doppler examination, does not rule out a vascular injury. *A diminished pulse should not be attributed to spasm.*

The signs of vascular injury are shown in the box.

> **Signs of vascular injury**
>
> * Abnormal pulses
> * Impaired capillary return
> * Decreased sensation
> * Rapidly expanding haematoma
> * Bruit

If these signs are present, urgent investigation and emergency treatment should be commenced. The fracture should be aligned and splints checked to ensure that they are not restrictive; if no improvement occurs a vascular surgeon should be consulted and angiography considered. Vascular damage may not always be immediately apparent so constant reassessment is therefore essential.

Compartment syndrome　If the interstitial pressure within a fascial compartment rises above capillary pressure, then local muscle ischaemia occurs. If this is unrecognised, it eventually results in Volkmann's ischaemic contracture.

Compartment syndrome usually develops over a period of hours and is most often associated with crush injuries. It may, however, occur following simple fractures. The classic signs are shown in the box.

> **Classic signs of compartment syndrome**
>
> * Pain, accentuated by passively stretching the involved muscles
> * Decreased sensation
> * Swelling
> * Weakness

Distal pulses only disappear when the intracompartmental pressure rises above arterial pressure; by this time irreversible changes have usually occurred in the muscle bed. Initial treatment consists of releasing constricting bandages and splints. If this is ineffective then urgent surgical fasciotomy should be performed.

Open fractures

Any wound within the vicinity of a fracture should be assumed to communicate with the fracture.

Open wounds are classified according to the degree of soft tissue damage, amount of contamination, and the presence or absence of associated neurovascular damage. Initial treatment includes removal of gross contamination, and covering of the wound with a sterile dressing. No attempt should be made to ligate bleeding points because associated nerves may be damaged as this is done. Bleeding should be controlled by direct pressure. Broad-spectrum antibiotics should be given, and tetanus immunisation status checked. Further management is surgical – debridement should be carried out within 8 hours.

Other injuries

Non-accidental injury

This must always be considered if the history is not consistent with the injury pattern. It is discussed in detail in Appendix C.

Fracture-dislocation

It is difficult to distinguish fractures and fracture-dislocations on clinical grounds. Radiology is often helpful, but in very young children, where ossification centres have not yet formed, an ultrasound examination or arthrogram may be necessary. In an older child (when some of the ossification centres are present), a comparative radiograph of the normal side may be helpful before more invasive investigations are considered. These investigations should be performed in the definitive care phase, unless there are vascular or neurological complications.

Dislocations

Dislocations, other than of the elbow and hip, are rare in children but, as for adults, may produce neurovascular injury that can result in permanent impairment. All dislocations should therefore be reduced as soon as possible.

Epiphyseal injuries

Fractures involving the epiphysis may be displaced or non-displaced. They should be managed by an orthopaedic surgeon.

EMERGENCY TREATMENT

Life-threatening problems identified during the primary survey in the multiply injured patient are managed first. Only then should attention be turned to the extremity injury. The specific management of complications such as vascular injury, compartment syndrome, traumatic amputation, and open wounds have been discussed earlier in this chapter.

Alignment

Severely angulated fractures should be aligned. Gentle traction should be applied to the limb to facilitate alingment, particularly when immobilising long-bone fractures. Splints should extend one joint above and below the fracture site. Perfusion of the extremity, including pulses, skin colour, temperature, and neurological status, must be assessed before and after the fracture is aligned. Radiographs, including arteriograms, should not be obtained until the extremity is splinted.

When aligning a fracture, analgesia is usually necessary. Entonox or intravenous opiates should be used. In femoral fractures, femoral nerve block is very effective – the technique is discussed in Chapter 24.

Immobilisation

Fractures (or suspected fractures) should be immobilised to control pain and prevent further injury. Splintage is a most effective way of controlling pain and subsequent doses of analgesia may be reduced. If pain increases after immobilisation, then an ischaemic injury and/or compartment syndrome must be excluded. Emergency splinting techniques for various injured extremities are described below.

Upper limb
Hand   Splinted in the position of function with the wrist slightly dorsiflexed and the fingers slightly flexed at all joints. This is best achieved by gently immobilising the hand over a large roll of gauze.

Forearm and wrist   Splinted flat on padded pillows or splints.

Elbow   Immobilised in a flexed position with a sling which may be strapped to the body.

Arm   Immobilised by a sling, which can be augmented with splints for unstable fractures. Circumferential bandages should be avoided as they may be the cause of constriction, particularly when swelling occurs.

Shoulder   Immobilised by a sling.

Lower limb
Femur   Femoral fractures should be treated in traction splints. Ipsilateral femoral and tibial fractures can be immobilised in the same splint. Excess traction may cause perineal injury and neurovascular problems, and should be avoided.

Tibia and ankle   Tibial and ankle fractures should be aligned and immobilised in padded box splints. Foot perfusion should be assessed before and after application of the splint.

SUMMARY

- Extremity trauma is rarely life threatening per se, unless exsanguinating haemorrhage ensues. Multiple fractures can cause significant blood loss
- The first priority is assessment of the airway, breathing, and circulation
- Full assessment of the extremities takes place during the secondary survey. Limb-threatening injuries should be identified at this stage and further investigation and management begun. Other injuries should be treated by splintage

SPINAL TRAUMA

Spinal injuries are rare in children which does not mean that they are unimportant. A high index of suspicion, correct management, and prompt referral are necessary in order to prevent exacerbation of underlying cord injury. Every severely injured child should be treated as though he or she has spinal injury until adequate examination and investigation exclude it.

INJURIES OF THE CERVICAL SPINE

Injuries to the cervical spine are rare in children. The upper three vertebrae are usually involved – injury is more common in the lower segments of an adult. The low incidence (0–2% of all children's fractures and dislocations) of bony injury is explained by the mobility of the cervical spine in children, which dissipates applied forces over a greater number of segments.

Radiographs

A lateral cervical spine radiograph will have been obtained during the primary survey. Injury must be presumed until excluded radiologically and clinically. Spinal injury may be present even with a normal radiograph. The development of the cervical vertebrae is complex. There are numerous physeal lines (which can be confused with fractures), and a range of normal sites for ossification centres. Pseudosubluxation of C2 on C3 and of C3 on C4 occurs in approximately 9% of children, particularly those aged 1–7 years. Interpretation of cervical radiographs can therefore be difficult even for the most experienced.

Indirect evidence of trauma can be detected by assessing retropharyngeal swelling. At the inferior part of the body of C3, the prevertebral distance should be one-third the width of the body of C2. This distance varies during breathing and is increased in a crying child. Cervical spine X-rays are discussed in more detail in Chapter 25.

Injury types

Atlantoaxial rotary subluxation is the most common injury to the cervical spine. The child presents with torticollis following trauma. Radiological demonstration of the injury is difficult, and computed tomography or magnetic resonance imaging may be necessary. Other injuries of C1 and C2 include odontoid epiphyseal separations and traumatic ligament disruption.

It should be noted that significant cervical cord injuries have been reported without any radiological evidence of trauma (see below).

Immediate treatment

Despite the rarity of fractures a severely injured child's spine should be securely immobilised until spinal injury has been excluded.

Cervical spine immobilisation techniques are described in Chapter 24.

INJURIES OF THE THORACIC AND LUMBAR SPINE

Injuries to the thoracic and lumbar spine are rare in children. They are most common in the multiply injured child. In the second decade, 44% of reported injuries result from sporting and other recreational activity. Some spinal injuries may result from non-accidental injury.

When an injury does occur, it is not uncommon to find multiple levels of involvement because the force is dissipated over many segments in the child's mobile spine. This increased mobility may also lead to neurological involvement without significant skeletal injury.

The most common mechanism of injury is hyperflexion and the most common radiographic finding is a wedge- or beak-shaped vertebra resulting from compression.

The most important clinical sign is a sensory level. Neurological assessment is difficult in children, and such a level may only become apparent after repeated examinations. Because of the difficulties of assessment, a child with multiple injuries should be assumed to have spinal injury, and should therefore be immobilised on a long spine board until investigations and examinations are complete. If injury is confirmed, further treatment is similar to that in adults. Unstable injuries may require open reduction and stabilisation with fusion.

If cord damage does occur, children can suffer the same complications as adults. In addition, late, progressive deformity to the spine may occur secondary to differential growth occurring around the injured segments.

SPINAL CORD INJURY WITHOUT RADIOLOGICAL ABNORMALITY

Spinal cord injury without radiological abnormality (SCIWORA) is said to have occurred when the spinal cord has been injured without an obvious accompanying injury to the vertebral column. It occurs almost exclusively in children (usually those younger than eight years). The cervical spine is affected more frequently than the thoracic spine. SCIWORA occurs in up to 55% of all paediatric complete cord injuries. Since the upper segments of the cervical spine have the greatest mobility, the upper cervical cord is most susceptible to this injury.

Children who are seriously injured should have immobilisation of the spine maintained until such time as a full neurological assessment can be carried out, since normal X-rays do not exclude a cord injury. If there is any doubt, MRI scans should be obtained.

SUMMARY

- Spinal injuries are rare in children
- Assessment can be difficult and significant cord damage can occur without fractures
- Spinal immobilisation must be appiied until such time as assessment is complete

CHAPTER

20

The burnt or scalded child

INTRODUCTION

Epidemiology

Each year some 50 000 burnt or scalded children attend emergency departments. Of these, 5000–6000 require hospital admission. In England and Wales in 1998, 20 children died from burns. Seventy per cent of those burnt are pre-school children, the most common age being between 1 and 2 years. Scalds occur mostly in the under-4s. Boys are more likely to suffer burns and serious scalds.

Most fatal burns occur in house fires and smoke inhalation is the usual cause of death. The number of deaths from burns has decreased because of a combination of factors. The move away from open fires, safer fireguards, smoke alarms and more stringent low flammability requirements for night clothes have all played a part. Non-fatal burns often involve clothing and are often associated with flammable liquids.

Scalds are usually caused by hot drinks, but bath water and cooking oil scalds are not uncommon. The improvement in survival following scalding (which followed improvements in treatment) has reached a plateau.

There is a strong link between burns to children and low socioeconomic status. Family stress, poor housing conditions, and over-crowding are implicated in this.

Pathophysiology

Two main factors determine the severity of burns and scalds – these are the temperature and the duration of contact. The time taken for cellular destruction to occur decreases exponentially with temperature. At 44°C, contact would have to be maintained for 6 hours, at 54°C for 30 seconds, and at 70°C epidermal injury happens within a second. This relationship underlies the different patterns of injury seen with different types of burn. Scalds generally involve water at below boiling point and contact for less than 4 seconds. Scalds that occur with liquids at a higher temperature (such as hot fat), or in children incapable of minimising the contact time (such as young infants and the handicapped), tend to result in more serious injuries. Flame burns can involve high temperatures and prolonged contact and consequently produce the most serious injuries of all.

It must be re-emphasised that the most common cause of death within the first hour

199

following burn injuries is smoke inhalation. Thus, as with other types of injury, attention to the airway and breathing is of prime importance.

PRIMARY SURVEY AND RESUSCITATION

When faced with a seriously burnt child it is easy to focus on the immediate problems of the burn, and forget the possibility of other injuries. The approach to the burnt child should be the structured one advocated in Chapter 15.

Airway and cervical spine

The airway may be compromised either because of inhalational injury, or because of severe burns to the face. The latter are usually obvious whereas the former may only be indicated more subtly. The indicators of inhalational injury are shown in the box.

Indications of inhalational injury

- History of exposure to smoke in a confined space
- Deposits around the mouth and nose
- Carbonaceous sputum

Since oedema occurs following thermal injury, the airway can deteriorate rapidly. Thus even suspicion of airway compromise, or the discovery of injuries that might be expected to cause problems with the airway at a later stage, should lead to immediate consideration of tracheal intubation. This procedure increases in difficulty as oedema progresses, and it is important to perform it as soon as possible. All but the most experienced should seek expert help urgently, unless apnoea requires immediate intervention.

If there is any suspicion of cervical spine injury, or if the history is unobtainable, appropriate precautions should be taken until such injury is excluded.

Breathing

Once the airway has been secured, the adequacy of breathing should be assessed. Signs that should arouse suspicion of inadequacy include: abnormal rate, abnormal chest movements, and cyanosis (a late sign). Circumferential burns to the chest may cause breathing difficulty by mechanically restricting chest movement.

All children who have suffered burns should be given high-flow oxygen. If there are signs of breathing problems then ventilation should be commenced.

Circulation

In the first few hours following injury signs of hypovolaemic shock are rarely attributable to burns. Therefore any such signs should raise the suspicion of bleeding from elsewhere, and the source should be actively sought. Intravenous access should be established with two cannulae during resuscitation and fluids started. If possible drips should be put up in unburnt areas, but eschar can be perforated if necessary. Remember that the intraosseous route can be used. Blood should be taken for haemoglobin, haematocrit, electrolytes and urea, and cross-matching at this stage.

Disability

Reduced conscious level following burns may be due to hypoxia (following smoke inhalation), head injury, or hypovolaemia. It is essential that a quick assessment is made during the primary survey as described in Chapter 15, because this provides a baseline for later observations.

Exposure

Exposure should be complete. Burnt children lose heat especially rapidly, and must be covered with blankets when not being examined.

SECONDARY SURVEY

As well as being burnt, children may suffer the effects of blast, may be injured by falling objects, and may fall while trying to escape from the fire. Thus other injuries are not uncommon and a thorough head-to-toe secondary survey should be carried out. This is described in Chapter 15. Any injuries discovered, including the burn, should be treated in order of priority.

Assessing the burn

The severity of a burn depends on its relative surface area and depth. Burns to particular areas may require special care.

Surface area
The surface area is usually estimated using burns charts. It is particularly important to use a paediatric chart when assessing burn size in children, because the relative surface areas of the head and limbs change with age. This variation is illustrated in Figure 20.1 and its accompanying table.

Another useful method of estimating relative surface area relies on the fact that the patient's palm and adducted fingers cover an area of approximately 1% of the body surface. This method can be used when charts are not immediately available, and is obviously already related to the child's size.

Note that the "rule of nines" cannot be applied to a child who is less than 14 years old.

Depth
Burns are classified as being superficial, partial thickness, or full thickness. The first causes injury only to the epidermis and clinically the skin appears red with no blister formation. Partial-thickness burns cause some damage to the dermis; blistering is usually seen and the skin is pink or mottled. Deeper (full-thickness) burns damage both the epidermis and dermis, and may cause injury to deeper structures as well. The skin looks white or charred, and is painless and leathery to touch.

Special areas
Burns to the face and mouth have already been dealt with above. Burns involving the hand can cause severe functional loss if scarring occurs. Perineal burns are prone to infection and present particularly difficult management problems.

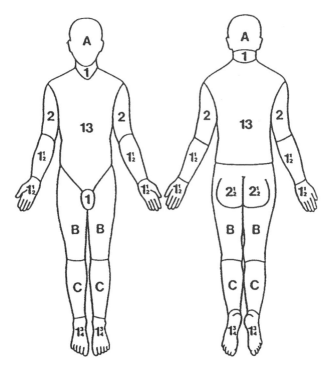

Figure 20.1. Body surface area (percent). (Reproduced courtesy of Smith & Nephew Pharmaceuticals Ltd)

Area indicated	Surface area at				
	0	1 year	5 years	10 years	15 years
A	9·5	8·5	6·5	5·5	4·5
B	2·75	3·25	4·0	4·5	4·5
C	2·5	2·5	2·75	3·0	3·25

EMERGENCY TREATMENT

Analgesia

Most burnt children will be in severe pain, and this should be dealt with urgently. Some older children may manage to use Entonox, but most will not. Any child with burns that are anything other than minor should be given intravenous morphine at a dose of 0·1 mg/kg as soon as possible. There is no place for administration of intramuscular analgesia in severe burns because absorption is unreliable.

Fluid therapy

Two cannulae should already have been sited during the primary survey and resuscitation and therapy for shock (20 ml/kg) commenced if indicated. Children with burns of 10% or more will require intravenous fluids as part of their burns care, in addition to their normal fluid requirement. The *additional* fluid (in ml) required per day to treat the burn can be estimated using the following formula:

$$\text{Percentage burn} \times \text{Weight (kg)} \times 4$$

and of this half should be given in the first 8 hours following the time of their burn. The fluid given is usually crystalloid. Remember that this is only an initial guide. Subsequent therapy will be guided by urine output, which should be kept at 1 ml/kg/h or more. Urethral catheterisation should therefore be performed as soon as is practicable.

Wound care

Infection is a significant cause of mortality and morbidity in burns victims, and wound care should start as early as possible to reduce this risk. Furthermore, appropriate wound care will reduce the pain associated with air passing over burnt areas.

Burns should be covered with sterile towels, and unnecessary re-examination should be avoided. Blisters should be left intact. Although cold compresses and irrigation with cold water may reduce pain, it should be remembered that burnt children lose heat rapidly. These treatments should only be used for 10 minutes or less, and only in patients with partial-thickness burns totalling less than 10%. Children should *never* be transferred with cold soaks in place.

DEFINITIVE CARE

Definitive care requires transfer to a paediatric burns facility. Criteria for transfer are shown in the box.

Criteria for transfer to a burns unit

- 10% partial- and/or full-thickness burns
- 5% full-thickness burns
- Burns to special areas

If in doubt discuss the child with the paediatric burns unit.

SUMMARY

- Initial assessment and management of the burnt child should be directed towards care of the airway, breathing, and circulation. Intubation and ventilation should be performed early if indicated
- Assessment of the area and depth of the burn should be undertaken during the secondary survey
- Fluid replacement should be used initially to treat shock. Additional fluids will be needed to treat the burn, and a guide to the amount required can be calculated. Urine output should be used as an indicator of the efficacy of treatment
- Specialist burns centres should be contacted, and transfer arranged if indicated

---

21

The child with an electrical injury or near drowning

ELECTRICAL INJURIES

INTRODUCTION

Epidemiology

Children account for 33% of all victims of electrical injuries; approximately 20% of reported electrical injuries are fatal. Over 90% result from accidents involving generated electricity.

Pathophysiology

The following factors determine the effects of an electric shock.

Current
Alternating current (AC) produces cardiac arrest at lower voltage than does direct current (DC). Whether electrocution is with AC or DC, the risk of cardiac arrest is greater with increasing size and duration of current passing through the heart; the current will be greater with low resistance and high voltage.

Lightning acts as a massive DC countershock which depolarises the myocardium and may lead to immediate asystole and death.

As current increases, the effects listed in the box may be seen.

Effect of increase in current

Above 10mA: tetanic contractions of muscles may make it impossible for the child to let go of the electrical source

50mA: tetanic contraction of the diaphragm and intercostal muscles leads to respiratory arrest which continues until the current is disconnected. If hypoxia is prolonged, secondary cardiac arrest will occur

Over 100mA: to several amps: primary cardiac arrest may be induced (defibrillators used in resuscitation deliver around 10 A)

50A to hundreds of amps: massive shocks cause prolonged respiratory and cardiac arrest, and more severe burns

---

Resistance

The resistance of tissues determines the path that the current follows. In general this is the path of least resistance from the entry point on the victim to the ground. Thus current preferentially flows down nerves and blood vessels, rather than through muscles, skin, tendon, fat, or bone. Electrocution of tissues with high resistance will generate most heat, and tissues tolerate this to varying degrees. Overall, nerves, blood vessels, skin, and muscle sustain most injury.

Water reduces skin resistance and thereby increases the current delivered to the body.

Voltage

High voltage ("tension") sources such as overhead electric power lines or lightning produce a higher current, and consequently cause more tissue damage than lower voltage sources.

MANAGEMENT

Before assessing or starting treatment it is essential that the child is disconnected from the electrical source.

Primary survey and resuscitation

The airway may be compromised by facial burns, and early management of such problems is essential (see Chapter 20). If the child is unconscious, the neck should be assumed to be broken and must be protected until injury is excluded. Other life-threatening injuries may occur due to secondary trauma and must be treated appropriately.

Secondary survey

Virtually any injury can occur. In particular, associated injuries can arise from being thrown from the source. Burns are common, and happen either because of the direct effects of the current (exit burns are often more severe than entry burns), or secondary to the ignition of clothing. The powerful tetanic contraction caused by the shock can cause fractures, dislocations, or muscle tearing.

LATE COMPLICATIONS

Cutaneous and deep tissue burns lead to fluid loss and oedema with dehydration. Myoglobinuria may arise if there is significant muscle breakdown. In such cases acute renal failure is a very real threat and a diuresis of *at least* 2 ml/kg/h must be maintained. Metabolic acidosis must be corrected with intravenous sodium bicarbonate because myoglobin is more soluble in alkaline urine.

REFERRAL

All children suffering from significant electrical burns should be discussed with the local Burns Unit; transfer to such specialist centres is usually indicated.

SUMMARY

- Cardiorespiratory arrest can occur
- Associated injuries may arise as a result of being thrown from the source
- Electrical burns may cause significant damage to deep structures. The extent of this damage may not be apparent on external examination
- All significant electrical burns should be discussed with burns centres

NEAR DROWNING

INTRODUCTION

Drowning is defined as death from asphyxia associated with submersion in a fluid. Near drowning is said to have occurred if there is any recovery (however transient) following a submersion incident.

Epidemiology

The incidence of survival from near drowning is unknown, but death from drownings and near-drowning is the third most common cause of accidental death in children in the UK (after road accidents and burns). In England and Wales 34 children died from drowning or near drowning in 1998. Children most commonly die in private swimming pools, garden ponds, and other inland waterways.

Pathophysiology

When a child is first submerged, apnoea occurs and the heart rate slows because of the diving reflex. As apnoea continues, hypoxia causes tachycardia, a rise in the blood pressure, and acidosis. Between 20 seconds and 2–5 minutes later a break point is reached, and breathing occurs. Fluid is inhaled and on touching the glottis causes immediate laryngeal spasm. Secondary apnoea eventually gives way to involuntary respiratory movements, and water, weeds, and debris enter the lungs. Bradycardia and arrhythmias follow, heralding cardiac arrest and death.

Children who survive because of interruption of this chain of events not only require therapy for near drowning, but also assessment and treatment of concomitant hypothermia, electrolyte imbalance, and injury (particularly spinal).

MANAGEMENT

Primary survey and resuscitation

The neck must be presumed to be injured, and the cervical spine should be immobilised until such injury is excluded. A history of diving is especially significant in this regard.

Following a significant near-drowning episode, the stomach is usually full of swallowed water. The risk of aspiration is therefore increased and tracheal intubation and gastric decompression must be performed early to protect the airway.

A deep body temperature reading (rectal or oesophageal) must be obtained as soon as possible. Hypothermia is common following near drowning, and adversely affects resuscitation attempts unless treated. Not only are arrhythmias more common but some, such as ventricular fibrillation, may be refractory at temperatures below 30°C. Resuscitation should not be discontinued until core temperature is at least 32°C or cannot be raised despite active measures.

Rewarming

External rewarming is usually sufficient if core temperature is above 32°C. Active core rewarming should be added in patients with a core temperature of less than 32°C, but beware "rewarming shock", which may result from hypovolaemia becoming apparent during peripheral vasodilatation. External and internal rewarming methods are shown in the box. Rhythm, pulse rate, and blood pressure monitoring should be undertaken. In severe hypothermia, admission to a high dependency area is necessary.

External rewarming

- Remove cold, wet clothing
- Supply warm blankets
- Infrared radiant lamp
- Heating blanket

Core rewarming

- Warm intravenous fluids to 39°C to prevent further heat loss
- Warm ventilator gases to 42°C to prevent further heat loss
- Gastric or bladder lavage with normal (physiological) saline at 42°C
- Peritoneal lavage with potassium-free dialysate at 42°C. Use 20 ml/kg cycled every 15 minutes
- Pleural or pericardial lavage
- Extracorporeal blood rewarming

Secondary survey

During the secondary survey, the child should be carefully examined from head to toe. Any injury may have occurred during the incident that preceded immersion; spinal injuries are particularly common.

Investigations

- Blood glucose.
- Arterial blood gases.
- Electrolytes.
- Baseline chest radiograph.
- Blood cultures.

Definitive care

Fever is common in the first few hours, but systemic infection should be suspected if a pyrexia develops after 24 hours. Once blood cultures have been taken, intravenous antibiotics can be started. The chosen agent should be effective against Gram-negative organisms. In children cefotaxime is used. Regular tracheal cultures, blood cultures, electrolytes, and white cell counts should be taken.

PROGNOSTIC INDICATORS

Immersion time

Most children who do not recover have been submerged for more than 3–8 minutes Details of the rescue are therefore vital.

Time to first gasp

If this occurs between 1 and 3 minutes after the start of basic cardiopulmonary support, the prognosis is good. If there has been no gasp after 40 minutes of full cardiopulmonary resuscitation, there is little or no chance of survival unless the child's respiration has been depressed (for example, by hypothermia or alcohol).

Rectal temperature

If this is less than 33°C on arrival, the chances of survival are increased because rapid cooling protects vital organs. Children cool quickly because of their large surface area/volume ratio.

Persisting coma

This indicates a bad prognosis.

Arterial blood pH

If this remains less than 7·0 despite treatment, the prognosis is poor.

Arterial blood $P\text{O}_2$

If this remains less than 8·0 kPa (60 mmHg), despite treatment, the prognosis is poor.

Type of water

Whether the water was salt or fresh has no bearing on the prognosis.

The decision to discontinue resuscitation attempts is particularly difficult in cases of drowning, and should be taken only after all the prognostic factors discussed above have been considered carefully.

OUTCOME

Seventy per cent of children survive near drowning when basic life support is provided at the waterside. Only 40% survive without early basic life support even if full advanced cardiopulmonary resuscitation is given in hospital.

Of those who do survive, having required full cardiopulmonary resuscitation in hospital, around 70% will make a complete recovery and 25% will have a mild neurological deficit. The remainder will be severely disabled or remain in a persisting vegetative state.

SUMMARY

- There is a high incidence of associated cervical spine injury especially during diving accidents
- Other associated injuries may arise during the incident leading to submersion
- Hypothermia should be actively sought and treated
- The decision to stop resuscitation should be taken after all prognostic indicators have been considered

CHAPTER

22

Practical procedures – airway and breathing

Procedures explained in this chapter

- Oropharyngeal airway insertion
    small child
    older child
- Nasopharyngeal airway insertion
- Orotracheal intubation
    infant/small child
    older child
- Surgical airway
    needle cricothyroidotomy
    surgical cricothyroidotomy
- Ventilation without intubation
    mouth-to-mask ventilation
    bag-and-mask ventilation

OROPHARYNGEAL AIRWAY INSERTION

If the gag reflex is present, it may be best to avoid the use of an oropharyngeal tube or other artificial airway, because it may cause choking, laryngospasm, or vomiting.

Small child

1. Select an appropriately sized Guedel airway (see Chapter 5).
2. Open the airway using the chin lift, taking care not to move the neck if trauma has occurred.
3. Use a tongue depressor or a laryngoscope blade to aid insertion of the airway "the right way up" (Figure 22.1).
4. Re-check airway patency.
5. If necessary, consider a different size from the original estimate.
6. Finally provide oxygen, consider ventilation by pocket mask or bag and mask.

Older child

1. Select an appropriately sized Guedel airway (see Chapter 5).
2. Open the airway using the chin lift, taking care not to move the neck if trauma has occurred.
3. Insert the airway concave upwards until the tip reaches the soft palate.
4. Rotate it through 180° (convex side upwards) and slide it back over the tongue.
5. Re-check airway patency.
6. If necessary, consider a different size from the original estimate.
7. Finally provide oxygen, consider ventilation by pocket mask or bag and mask.

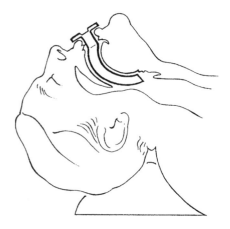

Figure 22.1. Oropharyngeal airway in situ

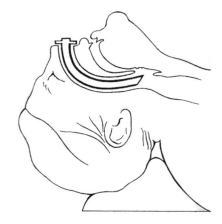

Figure 22.2. Nasopharyngeal airway in situ

NASOPHARYNGEAL AIRWAY INSERTION

Assess for any contraindications such as a base of skull fracture.

1. Select an appropriate size (length and diameter) (see Chapter 5).
2. Lubricate the airway with a water-soluble lubricant, and insert a large safety pin through the flange.
3. Insert the tip into the nostril and direct it posteriorly along the floor of the nose (rather than upwards).
4. Gently pass the airway past the turbinates with a slight rotating motion. As the tip advances into the pharynx, there should be a palpable "give".
5. Continue until the flange and safety pin rest on the nostril (Figure 22.2).
6. If there is difficulty inserting the airway, consider using the other nostril or a smaller size from the original estimate.
7. Re-check airway patency.
8. Finally provide oxygen, consider ventilation by pocket mask or bag and mask.

OROTRACHEAL INTUBATION

Infant or small child

1. Ensure that adequate ventilation and oxygenation by face mask are in progress.
2. Select an appropriate laryngoscope, and check the brightness of the light.

3. Select an appropriate tube size, but prepare a range of sizes, including the size above and below the best estimate (see Chapter 5).
4. Ensure manual immobilisation of the neck by an assistant if cervical spine injury is possible. Because of the relatively large occiput, it may be helpful to place a folded sheet or towel under the baby's back and neck to allow extension of the head. In the delivery suite, the design of the Resuscitaire allows the neonate's head to rest in the correct position (Figure 22.3).

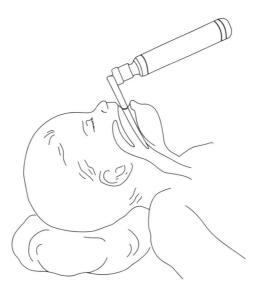

Figure 22.3. Orotracheal intubation – straight-blade laryngoscope technique

5. Hold the laryngoscope in the left hand, and insert it into the right-hand side of the mouth, displacing the tongue to the left. In the infant, it is sometimes useful to hold the laryngoscope with the left thumb, and index and middle fingers, leaving the little finger free to stretch down to press on the larynx to improve the view of the vocal cords (vocal folds). This is particularly useful if single handed.
6. In the "flat" baby being intubated by a relatively inexperienced doctor, it is often easiest to place the laryngoscope blade well beyond the epiglottis. The laryngoscope blade is placed down the right-hand side of the tongue into the proximal oesophagus. With a careful lifting movement, the tissues are gently tented up to "seek the midline". The blade is then slowly withdrawn until the vocal cords come into view. In some situations, it may be better to stay proximal to the epiglottis to minimise the risk of causing laryngospasm. This decision must be based on clinical judgement.
7. Insert the tracheal tube into the trachea, concentrating on how far the tip is being placed below the vocal cords. The tip should lie 2–4 cm below the vocal cords depending on age. Be aware that flexion or extension of the neck may cause migration downwards or upwards, respectively.
8. Check the placement of the tube by inspecting the chest for movement and auscultating the chest (including the axillae) and epigastrium.
9. If tracheal intubation is not achieved in 30 seconds, discontinue the attempt, ventilate and oxygenate by mask, and try again.
10. Once the tube is in place obtain a chest radiograph to confirm correct tube length.
11. Monitor expired CO_2 in the exhaled air by either colour change capnometry or end-tidal capnography.

Older child

1. Ensure that adequate ventilation and oxygenation by face mask are in progress.
2. Select an appropriate laryngoscope, and check the brightness of the light.
3. Select an appropriate tube size, but prepare a range of sizes, including the size above and below the best estimate (see Chapter 5).
4. Ensure manual immobilisation of the neck by an assistant if cervical spine injury is possible.
5. Hold the laryngoscope in the left hand, and insert it into the right-hand side of the mouth, displacing the tongue to the left.
6. Visualise the epiglottis, and place the tip of the laryngoscope in the vallecula.
7. Gently but firmly lift the handle towards the ceiling on the far side of the room being careful not to lever on the teeth (Figure 22.4).

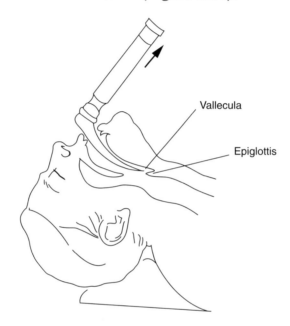

Figure 22.4. Orotracheal intubation – curved-blade laryngoscope technique

8. Insert the tracheal tube into the trachea, concentrating on how far the tip is being placed below the vocal cords (vocal folds). The tip should lie 2 cm below the vocal cords depending on age. If the tube has a "vocal cord level" marker, place this at the vocal cords. Be aware that flexion or extension of the neck may cause migration downwards or upwards, respectively.
9. In the adolescent, inflate the cuff to provide an adequate seal. In the pre-pubertal child do not use a cuffed tube.
10. Check the placement of the tube by inspecting the chest for movement and auscultating the chest (including the axillae) and epigastrium.
11. If tracheal intubation is not achieved in 30 seconds, discontinue the attempt, ventilate and oxygenate by mask, and try again.
12. Once the tube is in place obtain a chest radiograph to confirm correct placement.
13. Monitor expired carbon dioxide in the exhaled air by either colour change capnometry or end-tidal capnography.

Complications of tracheal intubation
These include:
- Oesophageal intubation (causing severe hypoxia if not immediately recognised).

- Endobronchial intubation, resulting in lung collapse and risk of pneumothorax.
- Severe hypoxia from a prolonged attempt to intubate.
- Airway injury from the laryngoscope, tube, or stylet (including direct trauma to the vocal cords), as well as chipping or loosening of the teeth.
- Neck strain by overextension, or exacerbation of a cervical spine injury with risk of neurological deterioration.

SURGICAL AIRWAY

Cricothyroidotomy is a "technique of failure". It is indicated if a patent airway cannot be achieved by other means. It must be performed promptly and decisively when necessary.

In children under the age of 12 years, needle cricothyroidotomy is preferred to surgical cricothyroidotomy. In the adolescent either technique can be used but the surgical technique allows better protection of the airway. The relevant anatomy is shown in Figure 22.5.

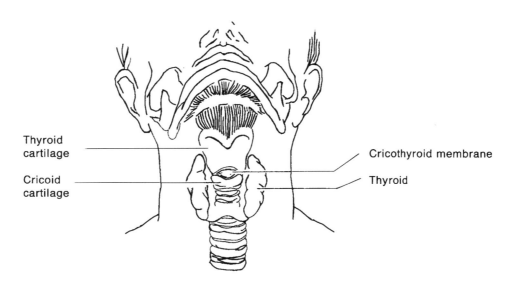

Figure 22.5. Surgical airway – relevant anatomy

In a very small baby, or if a foreign body is below the cricoid ring, direct tracheal puncture using the same technique can be used.

Needle cricothyroidotomy

This technique is simple in concept, but far from easy in practice. In an emergency situation the child may be struggling, and attempts to breathe or swallow may result in the larynx moving up and down:

1. Attach a cricothyroidotomy cannula-over-needle (or if not available, an intravenous cannula and needle) of appropriate size to a 5 ml syringe.
2. Place the patient in a supine position.
3. If there is no risk of cervical spine injury, extend the neck, perhaps with a sandbag under the shoulders.
4. Identify the cricothyroid membrane by palpation between the thyroid and cricoid cartilages.
5. Prepare the neck with antiseptic swabs.

217

6. Place your left hand on the neck to identify and stabilise the cricothyroid membrane, and to protect the lateral vascular structures from needle injury.
7. Insert the needle and cannula through the cricothyroid membrane at a 45° angle caudally, aspirating as the needle is advanced (Figure 22.6).

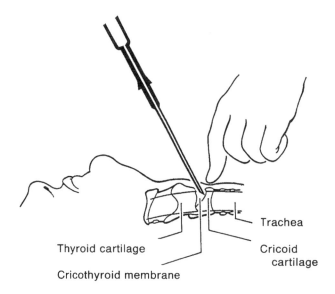

Figure 22.6. Needle cricothyroidotomy

8. When air is aspirated, advance the cannula over the needle, being careful not to damage the posterior tracheal wall. Withdraw the needle.
9. Re-check that air can be aspirated from the cannula.
10. Attach the hub of the cannula to an oxygen flowmeter via a Y-connector. Initially the oxygen flow rate (in litres) should be set at the child's age (in years).
11. Ventilate by occluding the open end of the Y-connector with a thumb for 1 second to direct gas into the lungs. If this does not cause the chest to rise the oxygen flow rate should be increased by increments of 1 litre, and the effect of 1 second's occlusion of the Y-connector reassessed.

Important notes

There are two common misconceptions about transtracheal insufflation. The first is that it is possible to ventilate a patient via a needle cricothyroidotomy using a self-inflating bag. The maximum pressure from a bag is approximately 4·41 kPa (45cm H_2O – the blow-off valve pressure) and this is insufficient to drive gas through a narrow cannula. In comparison, wall oxygen is provided at a pressure of 4 atmospheres (approximately 400kPa or 4000 cm H_2O). The second misconception is that expiration can occur through the cannula, or through a separate cannula inserted through the cricothyroid membrane. This is not possible. The intratracheal pressure during expiration is usually less than 2·9 kPa (30 cm H_2O – less than one-hundredth of the driving pressure in inspiration). Expiration must occur via the upper airway, even in situations of partial upper airway obstruction. Should upper airway obstruction be complete, it is necessary to reduce the gas flow to 1–2 l/min. This provides some oxygenation but little ventilation.

  Nevertheless, insufflation buys a few minutes in which to attempt a surgical airway.

12. Allow passive exhalation (via the upper airway) by taking the thumb off for 4 seconds.
13. Observe chest movement and auscultate breath sounds to confirm adequate ventilation.
14. Check the neck to exclude swelling from the injection of gas into the tissues rather than the trachea.
15. Secure the equipment to the patient's neck.
16. Having completed emergency airway management, arrange to proceed to a more definitive airway procedure, such as tracheotomy.

Surgical cricothyroidotomy

This should only be considered in the older child (12 years or over):

1. Place the patient in a supine position.
2. If there is no risk of neck injury, consider extending the neck to improve access. Otherwise, maintain a neutral alignment.
3. Identify the cricothyroid membrane.
4. Prepare the skin and, if the patient is conscious, infiltrate with local anaesthetic.
5. Place your left hand on the neck to stabilise the cricothyroid membrane, and to protect the lateral vascular structures from injury.
6. Make a small vertical incision in the skin, and press the lateral edges of the incision outwards, to minimise bleeding.
7. Make a transverse incision through the cricothyroid membrane, being careful not to damage the cricoid cartilage.
8. Insert a tracheal spreader, or use the handle of the scalpel by inserting it through the incision and twisting it through 90° to open the airway.
9. Insert an appropriately sized tracheal or tracheostomy tube. It is advisable to use a slightly smaller size than would have been used for an oral or nasal tube.
10. Ventilate the patient and check that this is effective.
11. Secure the tube to prevent dislodgement.

Complications of cricothyroidotomy
These include:

- Asphyxia.
- Aspiration of blood or secretions.
- Haemorrhage or haematoma.
- Creation of a false passage into the tissues.
- Surgical emphysema (subcutaneous or mediastinal).
- Pulmonary barotrauma.
- Subglottic oedema or stenosis.
- Oesophageal perforation.
- Cellulitis.

VENTILATION WITHOUT INTUBATION

Mouth-to-mask ventilation

1. Apply the mask to the face, using a jaw thrust grip, with the thumbs holding the mask. If using a shaped mask, it should be the right way up in children (Figure 22.7), or upside down in infants (Figure 22.8).

219

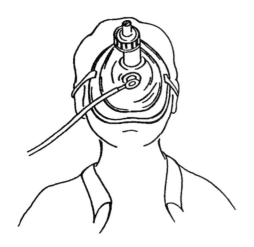

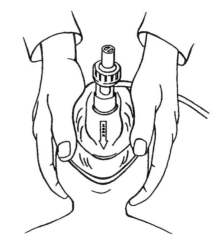

Figure 22.7. Mouth-to-mask ventilation in a child   **Figure 22.8.** Mouth-to-mask ventilation in an infant

2. Ensure an adequate seal.
3. Blow into the mouth port, observing the resulting chest movement.
4. Ventilate at 15–30 breaths/minute depending on the age of the child.
5. Attach oxygen to the face mask if possible.

Bag-and-mask ventilation

1. Apply the mask to the face, using a jaw thrust grip, with a thumb holding the mask (Figure 22.9).

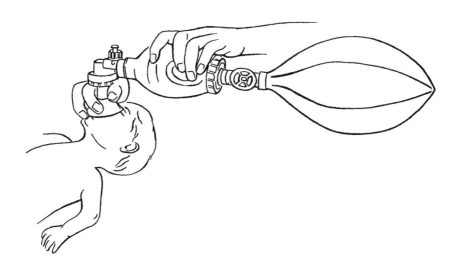

Figure 22.9. Bag-and-mask ventilation

2. Ensure an adequate seal.
3. Squeeze the bag observing the resulting chest movement.
4. Ventilate at 15–30 breaths/minute depending on the age of the child.

If a two-person technique is used, one rescuer maintains the mask seal with both hands, while the second person squeezes the self-inflating bag.

CHAPTER
23
Practical procedures – circulation

Procedures explained in this chapter

- Vascular access
    - peripheral venous access
        - upper and lower extremity veins
        - scalp veins
        - external jugular vein
        - venous cut-down
        - umbilical vein
    - central venous access
        - femoral vein
        - internal jugular vein
        - external jugular vein
        - subclavian vein
    - arterial puncture
    - intraosseous access
- Defibrillation

VASCULAR ACCESS

Access to the circulation is a crucial step in delivering advanced paediatric life support. Many access routes are possible; the one chosen will reflect both clinical need and the skills of the operator.

If fluids are to be given, infusion pumps or paediatric infusion sets must be used. This avoids inadvertent overtransfusion in small children.

Peripheral venous access

Upper and lower extremity veins
Veins on the dorsum of the hand, the elbow, the dorsum of the feet, and the saphenous

vein at the ankle can be used for cannulation. Standard percutaneous techniques should be employed if possible. Topical or injected local anaesthetic should be used whenever time allows.

Scalp veins

The frontal superficial, temporal posterior, auricular, supraorbital, and posterior facial veins can be used.

Equipment
- Skin cleansing swabs.
- Butterfly needle.
- Syringe and 0·9% saline.
- Short piece of tubing or bandage.

Procedure
1. Restrain the child.
2. Shave the appropriate area of the scalp.
3. Clean the skin.
4. Have an assistant distend the vein by holding a taut piece of tubing or bandaging perpendicular to it, proximal to the site of puncture.
5. Fill the syringe with 0·9% saline and flush the butterfly set.
6. Disconnect the syringe and leave the end of the tubing open.
7. Puncture the skin and enter the vein. Blood will flow back through the tubing.
8. Infuse a small quantity of fluid to see that the cannula is properly placed and then tape into position.

External jugular vein

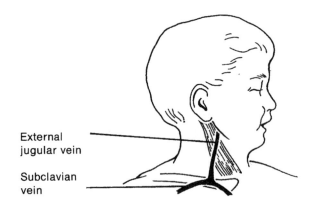

External
jugular vein

Subclavian
vein

Figure 23.1. The course of the external jugular vein

Equipment
- Skin cleansing swabs.
- Appropriate cannula.
- Tape.

Procedure
1. Place child in a 15–30° head-down position (or with padding under the shoulders so that the head hangs lower than the shoulders).
2. Turn the head away from the site of puncture. Restrain the child as necessary in this position.

3. Clean the skin over the appropriate side of the neck.
4. Identify the external jugular vein, which can be seen passing over the sternocleido-mastoid muscle at the junction of its middle and lower thirds (Figure 23.1).
5. Have an assistant place his or her finger at the lower end of the visible part of the vein just above the clavicle. This stabilises it and compresses it so that it remains distended.
6. Puncture the skin and enter the vein.
7. When free flow of blood is obtained, ensure no air bubbles are present in the tubing and then attach a giving set.
8. Tape the cannula securely in position.

Venous cut-down

If speed is essential, it may be more appropriate to use the intraosseous route for immediate access, and to cut down later for continued fluid and drug therapy.

Equipment
- Skin cleansing swabs.
- Lignocaine 1% for local anaesthetic with 2 ml syringe and 25-gauge needle.
- Scalpel.
- Curved haemostats.
- Suture and ligature material.
- Cannula.

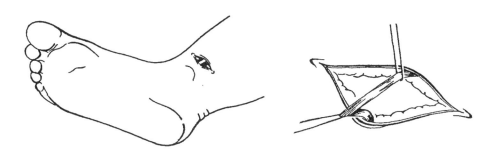

Figure 23.2.   Site of long saphenous cutdown and technique

Procedure
1. Immobilise the appropriate limb.
2. Clean the skin.
3. Identify the surface landmarks for the relevant vein. These are shown in Table 23.1.

Table 23.1.   Surface anatomy of the brachial and long saphenous veins

Child	Brachial	Saphenous (Figure 23.2)
Infant	One fingerbreadth lateral to the medial epicondyle of the humerus	Half a fingerbreadth superior and anterior to the medical malleolus
Small children	Two fingerbreadths lateral to the medial epicondyle of the humerus	One fingerbreadth superior and anterior to the medial malleolus
Older children	Three fingerbreadths lateral to the medial epicondyle of the humerus	Two fingerbreadths superior and anterior to the medial malleolus

223

4. If the child is responsive to pain, infiltrate the skin with 1% lignocaine.
5. Make an incision perpendicular to the course of the vein through the skin.
6. Using the curved haemostat tips, bluntly dissect the subcutaneous tissue.
7. Identify the vein and free 1–2 cm in length.
8. Pass a proximal and a distal ligature (Figure 23.2).
9. Tie off the distal end of the vein, keeping the ends of the tie long.
10. Make a small hole in the upper part of the exposed vein with a scalpel blade or fine-pointed scissors.
11. While holding the distal tie to stabilise the vein, insert the cannula.
12. Secure this in place with the upper ligature. Do not tie this too tightly and cause occlusion.
13. Attach a syringe filled with 0·9% saline to the cannula and ensure that fluid flows freely up the vein. If free-flow does not occur, then either the tip of the cannula is against a venous valve or the cannula may be wrongly placed in the adventitia surrounding the vein. Withdrawing the catheter will improve flow in the former case.
14. Once fluid flows freely, tie the proximal ligature around the catheter to help immobilise it.
15. Close the incision site with interrupted sutures.
16. Fix the catheter or cannula to the skin and cover with a sterile dressing.

Umbilical vein

Venous access via the umbilical vein is a rapid and simple technique. It is used during resuscitation at birth.

Equipment
• Skin cleansing swabs.
• Umbilical tape.
• Scalpel.
• Syringe and 0·9% saline.
• Catheter.

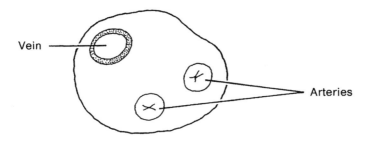

Figure 23.3. Umbilical cord cross-section

Procedure
1. Loosely tie the umbilical tape around the cord.
2. Cut the cord with a scalpel, leaving a 1 cm strip distal to the tape.
3. Identify the umbilical vein. Three vessels will be seen in the stump: two will be small and contracted (the arteries), and one will be dilated (the vein) (Figure 23.3).
4. Fill a French 5-gauge catheter with 0·9% saline.
5. Insert the catheter into the vein, and advance it approximately 5 cm.
6. Tighten the umbilical tape to secure the catheter. A purse-string suture may be used later to stitch the catheter in place.

Central venous access

Central access can be obtained through the femoral, internal jugular, external jugular, and (in older children) subclavian veins. The Seldinger technique is safe and effective. The femoral vein is often used as it is relatively easy to cannulate away from the chest during cardiopulmonary resuscitation. Central venous access via the neck veins is not without dangers, and may be difficult in emergency situations. The course of the central veins in the neck is shown in Figure 23.4.

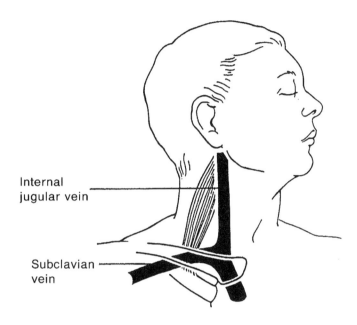

Internal jugular vein

Subclavian vein

Figure 23.4. The course of the central veins of the neck

Femoral vein

Equipment

- Skin cleansing swabs.
- Lignocaine 1% for local anaesthetic with 2 ml syringe and 23-gauge needle.
- Syringe and 0·9% saline.
- Seldinger cannulation set:
    syringe;
    needle;
    Seldinger guide wire;
    cannula.
- Suture material.
- Prepared paediatric infusion set.
- Tape.

Procedure

1. Place the child supine with the groin exposed and leg slightly abducted at the hip. Restrain the child's leg and body as necessary.
2. Clean the skin around the appropriate side.
3. Identify the puncture site. The femoral vein is found by palpating the femoral artery. The vein lies directly medial to the artery.

4. If the child is responsive to pain, infiltrate the area with 1% lignocaine.
5. Attach the needle to the syringe.
6. Keeping one finger on the artery to mark its position, introduce the needle at a 45° angle pointing towards the patient's head directly over the femoral vein. Keep the syringe in line with the child's leg. Advance the needle, pulling back on the plunger of the syringe all the time.
7. As soon as blood flows back into the syringe, take the syringe off the needle. Immediately occlude the end of the needle to prevent blood loss.
8. If the vein is not found withdraw the needle to the skin, locate the artery again, and advance as in (6) above.
9. Insert the Seldinger wire into the needle, and into the vein.
10. Withdraw the needle along the wire, ensuring that the wire is not dislodged from the vein.
11. Place the catheter over the wire and advance it through the skin, into the vein.
12. Suture the catheter in place.
13. Withdraw the wire, immediately occluding the end of the cannula to prevent blood loss.
14. Attach the infusion set.
15. Tape the infusion set tubing in place.

Internal jugular vein

Equipment
- Skin cleansing swabs.
- Lignocaine 1% for local anaesthetic with 2 ml syringe and 23-gauge needle.
- Syringe and 0·9% saline.
- Seldinger cannulation set: syringe; needle; Seldinger guide wire; cannula.
- Suture material.
- Prepared paediatric infusion set.
- Tape.

Procedure
1. Place the child in a 15–30° head-down position.
2. Turn the head away from the side that is to be cannulated and restrain the child as necessary.
3. Clean the skin around the appropriate side of the neck.
4. Identify the puncture site. This is found at the apex of the triangle formed by the two lower heads of the sternomastoid and the clavicle.
5. If the child is responsive to pain, infiltrate the area with 1% lignocaine.
6. Attach the needle to the syringe and puncture the skin at the appropriate place (see (4) above).
7. Direct the needle downwards at 30° to the skin; advance the needle towards the nipple, pulling back on the plunger of the syringe all the time.
8. As soon as the blood flows back into the syringe, take the syringe off the needle. Immediately occlude the end of the needle to prevent air embolism.
9. If the vein is not found withdraw the needle to the skin, and advance it again some 5–10° laterally.
10. Insert the Seldinger wire into the needle, and into the vein.
11. Withdraw the needle along the wire, ensuring that the wire is not dislodged from the vein.
12. Place the catheter over the wire and advance it through the skin, into the vein.
13. Suture the catheter in place.
14. Withdraw the wire, immediately occluding the end of the cannula to prevent air embolism.

15. Attach the infusion set.
16. Tape the infusion set tubing in place.
17. Obtain a chest radiograph in order to see the position of the catheter and to exclude pneumothorax.

External jugular vein

By using the Seldinger technique it is possible to obtain central venous access via the external jugular vein as described below. The anatomy is such that passage into the central veins can sometimes be more difficult compared to other approaches.

Equipment
• Skin cleansing swabs.
• Lignocaine 1% for local anaesthetic with 2 ml syringe and 25-gauge needle.
• Syringe and 0·9% saline.
• Seldinger cannulation set:
     syringe;
     needle;
     Seldinger guide wire (J wire);
     cannula.
• Suture material.
• Prepared paediatric infusion set.
• Tape.

Procedure
1. Place child in a 15–30° head-down position (or with padding under the shoulders so that the head hangs lower than the shoulders).
2. Turn the head away from the site of puncture. Restrain the child as necessary in this position.
3. Clean the skin over the appropriate side of the neck.
4. Identify the external jugular vein which can be seen passing over the sternocleidomastoid muscle at the junction of its middle and lower thirds.
5. Have an assistant place his or her finger at the lower end of the visible part of the vein just above the clavicle. This stabilises it and compresses it so that it remains distended.
6. Attach the needle to the syringe and puncture the vein.
7. As soon as free-flow of blood is obtained, take off the syringe and occlude the end of the needle.
8. Insert a J wire into the needle and into the vein.
9. Advance the J wire. There may be some resistance as the wire reaches the valve at the proximal end of the vein. Gently advance and withdraw the wire until it passes this obstacle.
10. Gently advance the wire.
11. Withdraw the needle along the wire, ensuring that the wire is not dislodged from the vein.
12. Place the catheter over the wire and advance it through the skin, into the vein.
13. Suture the catheter in place.
14. Withdraw the wire, immediately occluding the end of the cannula to prevent air embolism.
15. Attach the infusion set.
16. Tape the infusion set tubing in place.
17. Obtain a chest radiograph in order to see the position of the catheter and to exclude pneumothorax.

Subclavian vein

Equipment
- Skin cleansing swabs.
- Lignocaine 1% for local anaesthetic with 2 ml syringe and 23-gauge needle.
- Syringe and 0·9% saline.
- Seldinger cannulation set:
    syringe;
    needle;
    Seldinger guide wire;
    cannula.
- Suture material.
- Prepared paediatric infusion set.
- Tape.

Procedure
1. Place the child in a 15–30° head-down position.
2. Turn the head away from the site that is to be cannulated and restrain the child as necessary.
3. Clean the skin over the upper side of the chest to the clavicle.
4. Identify the puncture site. This is 1 cm below the mid-point of the clavicle.
5. If the child is responsive to pain, infiltrate the area with 1% lignocaine.
6. Attach the needle to the syringe and puncture the skin at the appropriate place (see (4) above).
7. Direct the needle under the clavicle, "stepping down" off the bone.
8. Once under the clavicle, direct the needle towards the suprasternal notch. Advance the needle, pulling back on the plunger of the syringe all the time, and staying as superficial as possible.
9. As soon as the blood flows back into the syringe, take the syringe off the needle. Immediately occlude the end of the needle to prevent air embolism.
10. If the vein is not found, slowly withdraw the needle, continuing to pull back on the plunger. If the vein has been crossed inadvertently, free-flow will often be established during this manoeuvre.
11. If the vein is still not found repeat (7) to (10) aiming at a point a little higher in the sternal notch.
12. Insert the Seldinger wire into the needle, and into the vein.
13. Withdraw the needle along the wire, ensuring that the wire is not dislodged from the vein.
14. Place the catheter over the wire and advance it through the skin, into the vein.
15. Suture the catheter in place.
16. Withdraw the wire, immediately occluding the end of the cannula to prevent air embolism.
17. Attach the infusion set.
18. Tape the infusion set tubing in place.
19. Obtain a chest radiograph in order to see the position of the catheter and to exclude pneumothorax.

Arterial puncture

Arterial cannulation is used to obtain blood samples for oxygen levels and acid–base balance. In children the radial and posterior tibial arteries are the preferred sites because collateral supply is good.

Radial artery puncture

Equipment
- Skin cleansing swabs.
- Heparinised syringe.
- Butterfly needle or needle.
- Gauze, pad, and tapes.

Procedure
1. Before using the radial artery check that an ulnar artery is present and patent. Occlude both arteries at the wrist then release the pressure on the ulnar artery; the circulation should return to the hand. (It will flush pink.) If this does not happen, do not proceed with a radial puncture on that side.
2. Keep the wrist hyperextended and restrained, and palpate the radial artery.
3. Clean the skin.
4. Insert the needle over the artery at 45° to the skin and advance it slowly. When the artery is punctured blood will be seen to pulsate into the syringe.
5. Collect the required amount of blood and withdraw the needle.
6. Compress the puncture site firmly for at least 5 minutes to prevent the formation of a haematoma.
7. Ensure that there are no air bubbles in the blood sample and either send it for analysis immediately or place it on ice if any delay is anticipated.

In very small babies a 23-gauge needle can be used to puncture the artery and blood collected (into a heparinised capillary tube) from the well of the needle.

Intraosseous transfusion

The technique of intraosseous transfusion is not new. It was used in the 1930s as a quick method of gaining vascular access (the only alternatives were to use a reusable, resharpened metal needle or to perform a venous cut-down). Because it is important to achieve vascular access quickly in many life-threatening situations, intraosseous infusion is again being recommended. Specially designed needles make this quick and easy. It is indicated if other attempts at venous access fail, or if they will take longer than 1·5 minutes to carry out. It is the recommended technique for circulatory access in cardiac arrest.

Equipment
- Alcohol swabs.
- An 18-gauge needle with trochar (at least 1·5 cm in length).
- A 5 ml syringe.
- A 20 ml syringe.
- Infusion fluid.

Procedure
1. Identify the infusion site. Fractured bones should be avoided, as should limbs with fractures proximal to possible sites. The landmarks for the upper tibial and lower femoral sites are shown below, and the former approach is illustrated in Figure 23.5.

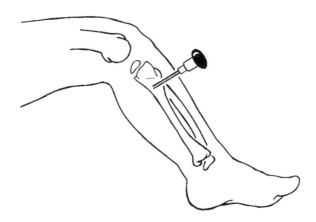

Figure 23.5. Tibial technique for intraosseous infusion

Surface anatomy for intraosseous infusions

Tibial	*Femoral*
Anterior surface, 2–3 cm below the tibial tuberosity	Anterolateral surface, 3 cm above the lateral condyle

2. Clean the skin over the chosen site.
3. Insert the needle at 90° to the skin.
4. Continue to advance the needle until a "give" is felt as the cortex is penetrated.
5. Attach the 5 ml syringe and aspirate or flush to confirm correct positioning.
6. Attach the filled 20 ml syringe and push in the infusion fluid in boluses.

DEFIBRILLATION

In order to achieve the optimum outcome defibrillation must be performed quickly and efficiently. This requires the following:

- Correct paddle position.
- Correct paddle placement.
- Good paddle contact.
- Correct energy selection.

Many defibrillators are available. Providers of advanced paediatric life support should make sure that they are familiar with those they may have to use.

Correct paddle selection

Most defibrillators are supplied with adult paddles attached (13 cm diameter, or equivalent area). Paddles of 4·5 cm diameter are suitable for use in infants, and ones of 8 cm diameter should be used for small children.

Correct paddle placement

The usual placement is anterolateral. One paddle is put over the apex in the midaxillary line, and the other is placed just to the right of the sternum, immediately below the clavicle (Figure 23.6).

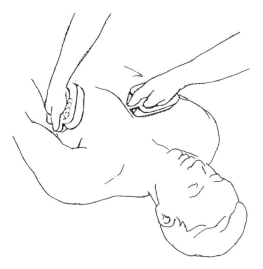

Figure 23.6. Standard anterolateral paddle placement

If the anteroposterior placement is used, one paddle is placed just to the left side of the lower part of the sternum, and the other just below the tip of the left scapula (Figure 23.7).

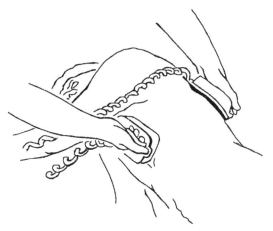

Figure 23.7. Anteroposterior paddle placement

Good paddle contact

Gel pads or electrode gel should always be used (if the latter, care should be taken not to join the two areas of application). Firm pressure should be applied to the paddles.

Correct energy selection

The recommended levels are shown in Chapters 6 and 11.

If the only device available is an AED, then energy levels are pre-set. This is suitable for a child over 8 years (25 kg) and may be used if no other options are available in younger children.

Safety

A defibrillator delivers enough current to cause cardiac arrest. The user must ensure that other rescuers are not in physical contact with the patient (or the trolley) at the moment the shock is delivered. The defibrillator should only be charged when the paddles are either in contact with the child or replaced properly in their storage positions.

Disconnect the oxygen supply to the patient.

Procedure

Basic life support should be interrupted for the shortest possible time (5–9 below)

1. Apply gel pads or electrode gel
2. Select the correct paddles
3. Select the energy required
4. Place the electrodes onto the pads of gel, and apply firm pressure
5. Press the charge button
6. Wait until the defibrillator is charged
7. Shout "Stand back!"
8. Check that.all other rescuers are clear
9. Deliver the shock

CHAPTER

24

Practical procedures – trauma

Procedures explained in this chapter

- Chest decompression
    needle thoracocentesis
    chest drain placement
- Pericardiocentesis
- Femoral nerve block
- Diagnostic peritoneal lavage
- Spinal care
    cervical spine immobilisation
    application of a cervical collar
    application of sandbags and tape
    log-rolling
- Helmet removal

NEEDLE THORACOCENTESIS

This procedure can be life saving and can be performed quickly with minimum equipment. It should be followed by chest drain placement.

Minimum equipment

- Alcohol swabs.
- Large over-the-needle intravenous cannula (16-gauge or larger).
- 20 ml syringe.

Procedure

1. Identify the second intercostal space in the mid-clavicular line on the side of the pneumothorax (the opposite side to the direction of tracheal deviation).

233

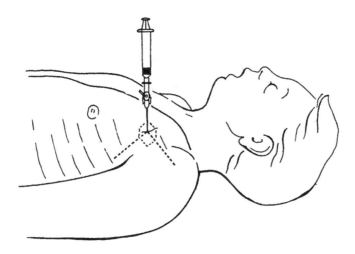

Figure 24.1. Needle thoracocentesis

2. Swab the chest wall with surgical preparation solution or an alcohol swab.
3. Attach the syringe to the cannula.
4. Insert the cannula vertically into the chest wall, just above the rib below, aspirating all the time (Figure 24.1).
5. If air is aspirated remove the needle, leaving the plastic cannula in place.
6. Tape the cannula in place and proceed to chest drain insertion as soon as possible.

If needle thoracocentesis is attempted, and the patient does not have a tension pneumothorax, the chance of causing a pneumothorax is 10–20%. Patients who have had this procedure must have a chest radiograph, and will require chest drainage if ventilated.

CHEST DRAIN PLACEMENT

Chest drain placement should be performed using the open technique described here. This minimises lung damage. In general, the largest size drain that will pass between the ribs should be used.

Minimum equipment

- Skin prep and surgical drapes.
- Scalpel.
- Large clamps × 2.
- Suture.
- (Local anaesthetic.)
- Scissors.
- Chest drain tube.

Procedure

1. Decide on the insertion site (usually the fifth intercostal space in the mid-axillary line) on the side with the pneumothorax (Figure 24.2).
2. Swab the chest wall with surgical prep or an alcohol swab.

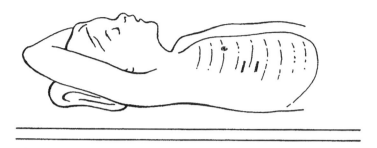

Figure 24.2. Chest drain insertion – landmarks

3. Use local anaesthetic if necessary.
4. Make a 2–3 cm skin incision along the line of the intercostal space, just above the rib below.
5. Bluntly dissect through the subcutaneous tissues just over the top of the rib below, and puncture the parietal pleura with the tip of the clamp.
6. Put a gloved finger into the incision and clear the path into the pleura (Figure 24.3). This will not be possible in small children.

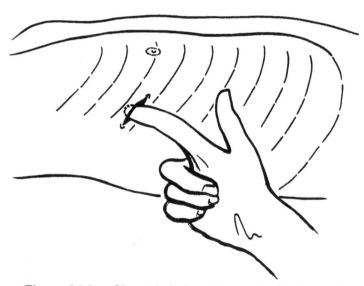

Figure 24.3. Chest drain insertion – clearing the path

7. Advance the chest drain tube into the pleural space during expiration.
8. Ensure the tube is in the pleural space by listening for air movement, and by looking for fogging of the tube during expiration.
9. Connect the chest drain tube to an underwater seal.
10. Suture the drain in place, and secure with tape.
11. Obtain a chest radiograph.

PERICARDIOCENTESIS

The removal of a small amount of fluid from the pericardial sac can be life saving. The procedure is not without risks and the ECG should be closely monitored throughout. An acute injury pattern (ST segment changes or a widened QRS) indicates ventricular damage by the needle.

Minimum equipment

- ECG monitor.
- (Local anaesthetic.)
- 20 ml syringe.
- Skin prep and surgical drapes.
- 6 inch over-the-needle cannula (16-gauge or 18-gauge).

Procedure

1. Swab the xiphoid and subxiphoid areas with surgical prep or an alcohol swab.
2. Use local anaesthetic if necessary.
3. Assess the patient for any significant mediastinal shift if possible.
4. Attach the syringe to the needle.
5. Puncture the skin 1–2 cm inferior to the left side of the xiphoid junction at a 45° angle (Figure 24.4).

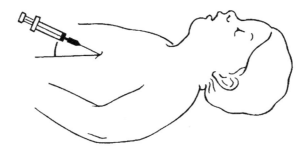

Figure 24.4. Needle pericardiocentesis — angle

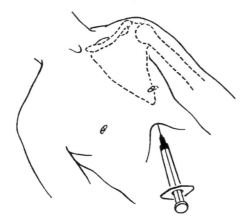

Figure 24.5. Needle pericardiocentesis — direction

6. Advance the needle towards the tip of the left scapula, aspirating all the time (Figure 24.5).
7. Watch the ECG monitor for signs of myocardial injury.
8. Once fluid is withdrawn, aspirate as much as possible (unless it is possible to withdraw limitless amounts of blood in which case a ventricle has probably been entered).
9. If the procedure is successful, remove the needle leaving the cannula in the pericardial sac. Secure in place and seal with a three-way tap. This allows later repeat aspirations should tamponade recur.

FEMORAL NERVE BLOCK

The femoral nerve supplies the femur with sensation and a block is useful in cases of femoral fracture. The technique may also be of benefit when analgesic agents would interfere with the management or assessment of other injuries. A long-acting local anaesthetic agent should be used so that radiographs and splinting can be undertaken with minimal distress to the child.

Equipment

- Antiseptic swabs to clean.
- Lignocaine 1%.
- A 2 ml syringe and 25-gauge needle.
- Syringe (5 or 10 ml) and 21-gauge needle.
- Bupivacaine 0·5% or Prilocaine 0·5%.

Table 24.1. Volume of bupivacaine (Marcain) needed

Bupivacaine volume (ml)	Age (years)
10	>12
5	5–12
1 per year	<5

Procedure

1. Move the fractured limb gently so that the femur lies in abduction and the ipsilateral groin is exposed.
2. Swab the groin clean with antiseptic solution.
3. Identify the femoral artery and keep one finger on it. The femoral nerve lies immediately lateral to the artery.
4. Using the 2 ml syringe filled with lignocaine and 25-gauge needle, infiltrate the skin just lateral to the artery. Aspirate the syringe frequently to ensure that the needle is not in a vessel.
5. Inject the bupivacaine around the nerve using the 21-gauge needle, taking care not to puncture the artery or vein.
6. Wait until anaesthesia occurs (bupivacaine may take up to 20 minutes to have its full effect).

DIAGNOSTIC PERITONEAL LAVAGE

The technique described here is designed to maximise the sensitivity and specificity of diagnostic peritoneal lavage. Special care should be taken when performing diagnostic peritoneal lavage in children, otherwise the unwary operator may be caught out by the relative thinness of the abdominal wall, the intra-abdominal position of the bladder, and the high incidence of acute gastric dilatation.

Equipment

- Antiseptic solution.
- Lignocaine 1% with epiephrine (adrenaline).
- Scalpel.
- Self-retaining retractors.
- Suture material.
- 500 ml sterile normal (physiological) saline (warmed).
- Sterile drapes.
- Syringe and needle.
- Artery forceps.
- Scissors.
- Peritoneal lavage catheter.
- Giving set.

Procedure

1. Ensure that the urinary bladder is catheterised and drained, and that a gastric tube has been passed to decompress the stomach.
2. Surgically prepare the abdomen with antiseptic solution and drapes.
3. Identify the site for incision – one-third of the way down from the umbilicus towards the pubis in the mid-line.
4. Anaesthetise the area to the peritoneum with 1% lignocaine and epinephrine.
5. Make a vertical incision through skin and subcutaneous tissue in the mid-line.
6. Incise the fascia.
7. Ensure haemostasis.
8. Apply two clips to the peritoneum and gently lift it away from underlying structures.
9. Using the scissors cut between the two clips – making a small hole in the peritoneum.
10. Insert the dialysis catheter through the hole, and gently advance it caudally into the pelvis.
11. Connect the dialysis catheter to a syringe and aspirate.
12. If blood is not aspirated, connect the catheter to the giving set and infuse 10 ml/kg of the warmed saline.
13. Remove any remaining saline from the bag.
14. If the patient is stable leave this fluid for 5–10 minutes, and then allow it to syphon out by placing the bag on the floor. This may take some time.
15. Send a sample of fluid to the laboratory for analysis.
16. Remove the lavage catheter and close the wound in layers.

CERVICAL SPINE IMMOBILISATION

All children with serious trauma must be treated as though they have a cervical spine injury. It is only when adequate investigations have been performed and a neuro-surgical or orthopaedic consultation obtained, if necessary, that the decision to remove cervical spine protection should be taken. In-line cervical stabilisation should be continued until a hard collar has been applied, and sandbags and tape or head blocks are in position as described below.

Two techniques are described. It is necessary to apply both to achieve adequate cervical spine control.

Once the collar is in place, the neck is largely obscured. Before placing the collar look for the following signs quickly and without moving the neck.

1. Distended veins.
2. Tracheal deviation.
3. Wounds.
4. Laryngeal crepitus.
5. Subcutaneous emphysema.

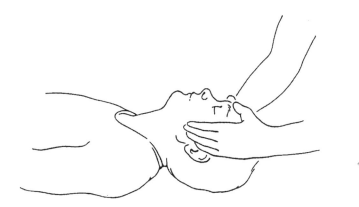

Figure 24.6. In-line cervical stabilisation

Application of a cervical collar

The key to successful, effective, collar application lies in selecting the correct size.

Minimum equipment
- Measuring device.
- Range of paediatric hard collars.

Method
1. Ensure in-line cervical stabilisation is maintained throughout by a second person.
2. Using the manufacturer's method, select a correctly sized collar.
3. Fully unfold and assemble the collar.
4. Taking care not to cause movement, pass the flat part of the collar behind the neck.
5. Fold the shaped part of the collar round and place it under the child's chin.
6. Fold the flat part of the collar with its integral joining device (usually Velcro tape) around until it meets the shaped part.
7. Reassess the correct fit of the collar.
8. If the fit is wrong, slip the flat part of the collar out from behind the neck, taking care not to cause movement. Select the correct size and recommence the procedure.
9. If the fit is correct secure the joining device.
10. Ensure that in-line cervical stabilisation is maintained until sandbags and tape or head blocks are in position.

Sandbags and tape

Equipment
- Two sandbags.
- Strong narrow tape.

Method
1. Ensure in-line cervical stabilisation is maintained by a second person throughout.
2. Place a sandbag either side of the head.
3. Apply tape across the forehead and securely attach it to the long spinal board.
4. Apply tape across the chin piece of the hard collar and securely attach it to the long spinal board.

> **Exceptions**
>
> Two groups of children cause particular difficulty. The first (and most common) is the frightened, uncooperative child; the second is the child who is hypoxic and combative. In both cases, overzealous immobilisation of the head and neck may paradoxically increase cervical spine movement. This is because these children will fight to escape from any restraint. In such cases a hard collar should be applied, and no attempt made to immobilise the head with sandbags and tape or head blocks.

LOG-ROLLING

In order to minimise the chances of exacerbating unrecognised spinal cord injury, non-essential movements of the spine must be avoided until adequate examination and investigations have excluded it. If manoeuvres that might cause spinal movement are essential (for example, during examination of the back in the course of the secondary survey) then log-rolling should be performed. The aim of log-rolling is to maintain the alignment of the spine during turning of the child. The basic requirements are an adequate number of carers and good control.

Method

1. Gather together enough staff to roll the child. In larger children four people will be required; three will be required in smaller children and infants.
2. Place the staff as shown in Table 24.2.
3. Ensure each member of staff knows what they are going to do as shown in Table 24.3.
4. Carry out essential manoeuvres as quickly as possible.

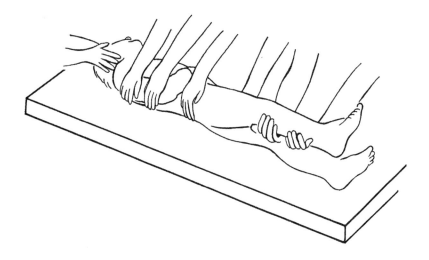

Figure 24.7.   Log-rolling a child (four-person technique)

Table 24.2. Position of staff in log-rolling

Staff member no.	Position of staff for	
	Smaller child and infant	Larger child
1	Head	Head
2	Chest	Chest
3	Legs and pelvis	Pelvis
4		Legs

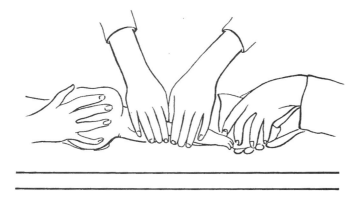

Figure 24.8. Log-rolling a small child or infant (three-person technique)

Table 24.3. Tasks of individual members of staff

Staff member – position	Task
Head	Hold either side of the head (as for in-line cervical stabilisation), and maintain the orientation of the head with the body in all planes during turning *Control the log-roll by telling other staff when to roll and when to lay the child back onto the trolley*
Chest	Reach over the child and carefully place both hands under the chest. When told to roll the child support the weight of the chest, and maintain stability. Watch the movement of the head at all times and roll the chest at the same rate
Pelvis and legs	*This only applies to smaller children and infants. If it is not possible to control the pelvis and legs at the same time get additional help immediately* Place one hand either side of the pelvis over the iliac crests. Cradle the child's legs between the forearms. When told to roll the child, grip the pelvis and legs and move them together. Watch the movement of the head and chest at all times, and roll the pelvis and legs at the same rate
Pelvis	Place one hand over the pelvis on the iliac crest and the other under the top of the far leg. When told to roll the child watch the movement of the head and chest at all times and roll the pelvis at the same rate
Legs	Support the weight of the far leg by placing both hands under it. When told to roll the child watch the movement of the chest and pelvis and roll the leg at the same rate

HELMET REMOVAL

Cycle or motorcycle helmets must be removed without causing cervical spine movements. This requires a minimum of two staff.

1. Obtain history of mechanism of injury.
2. Explain procedure to patient and parent(s).
3. Carry out brief neurological examination.
4. Demonstrate position of hands on each side of the helmet with thumbs on the mandible and fingers on the occipital ridge. Keep this position whilst an assistant removes the chin straps.
5. Direct the assistant to take control of the in-line stabilisation by holding the occipital ridge with one hand and placing the thumb and forefinger of the other hand along the mandible.
6. Gently remove the helmet spreading it laterally if necessary. Then resume in-line stabilisation with both thumbs on the mandible and fingers of both hands on the occipital ridge.
7. Ensure removal of any jewellery from the neck.
8. Place the patient in a cervical collar, sandbag and tape to the spinal board.*
9. Carry out a brief neurological exam again.

* A restless agitated child should not be sandbagged and taped or head-blocked because of the risk that their struggling may cause further cervical spine damage.

25

Interpreting trauma X-rays

INTRODUCTION

This chapter provides an overview of emergency imaging of the spine, chest and pelvis in children. It provides an introduction to interpretation for the doctor involved in managing paediatric trauma in the resuscitation room.

Radiological advice should be sought if there is any doubt that a film is normal. Discussing the film with an experienced emergency physician or trauma, orthopaedic or neurosurgeon may also help. An experienced emergency radiographer (technician) is a valuable asset to any department and, if they consider a film is abnormal, their comments should be carefully noted.

Radiography of a seriously injured child is technically challenging as access is often limited and films are often taken with a mobile machine. Equipment such as neck collars may obscure bony landmarks and the position in which the child is lying may cause difficulty in radiographic interpretation due to rotation.

The radiology department is not a place to leave a sick or unstable patient without adequate clinical supervision. Plain films are taken by a radiographer, who will not be able to supervise an ill patient. Complex investigations including ultrasound scanning, computed tomography (CT) or contrast studies take time, during which the child may deteriorate significantly without appropriate treatment.

Three standard trauma films are available to the emergency clinician:

1. Lateral cervical spine radiograph.
2. Chest radiograph.
3. Pelvic radiograph.

These three provide a basic screen for major injuries. They should only be taken after immediately life-threatening injuries have been identified and treated.

Viewing the film

Before reviewing any film, check the information shown over.

> - The name of the patient
> - The date and time that the film was taken
> - The orientation (side marker position).

View the film on a light box – not against the ceiling lights or a nearby window. Light boxes give uniform illumination and should be available in all resuscitation rooms.

The **ABCD** approach to radiographic interpretation is shown in the box below.

> **A**dequacy, **A**lignment and **A**pparatus
> **B**ones
> **C**artilage and soft tissues
> **D**isc spaces (in the spine), **D**iaphragm (in the chest)

CERVICAL SPINE

Cervical spine immobilisation should take place before any radiographs are performed. The standard film is a lateral radiograph, which may be supplemented by AP (lower cervical spine and odontoid peg views) when appropriate. If the child has an adequately fitted cervical collar for immobilisation, it is very difficult to get good quality AP views, including the odontoid peg. If sandbags rather than headblocks are used for immobilisation they may obscure bony landmarks.

Bony injury in itself is not the prime concern in spinal injury. The main risk is actual or potential injury to the cord. Any unstable fracture, if inadequately immobilised, may lead to progressive cord damage.

A lateral cervical spine film is often requested to "clear" the cervical spine, but a normal film may be falsely reassuring. The plain film only shows the position of the bones at the time the films was taken, and gives no idea of the magnitude of flexion and extension forces applied to the spine at the time of injury. The cord may be injured in a child without any apparent radiographic abnormality.

Unlike adult spines most paediatric cervical spine injuries occur either through the discs and ligaments, at the cranio-vertebral junction (C1, 2 and 3) or at C7/T1. The relatively large mass of the head, moving on a flexible neck with poorly supportive muscles, leads to injury in the higher cervical vertebrae.

Children develop three patterns of spinal injury:

1. Subluxation or dislocation without fracture
2. Fracture with or without subluxation or dislocation
3. SCIWORA

The last of these – SCIWORA (Spinal Cord Injury Without Radiographic Abnormality) is said to have occurred when radiographic films are totally normal in the presence of significant cord injury. If the film is normal in a conscious child with clinical symptoms (such as pain, loss of function or paraesthesia in a limb) then neck protection measures should be continued. In an unconscious child at high risk, a cord injury cannot be excluded until the patient is awake and has been assessed clinically, even in the presence of a normal cervical spine film. Adequate spinal precautions should be continued until the child is well enough to be assessed clinically, or magnetic resonance imaging has been carried out.

The most common site of a "missed" spinal injury is where a flexible part of the spine meets the fixed part. In the neck these are the cervico-cranial junction and the cervico-thoracic junction.

Adequacy

The whole spine should be viewed from the lower clivus down to the upper body of T1 vertebra. If the C7/T1 junction is not seen initially then gentle traction should be applied by pulling the arms down, holding them above the elbow joint. If the child is conscious they should be asked to relax their shoulders as traction is applied. If the child is on a spinal board then this must be stabilised by an assistant.

Alignment

See Figure 25.1.

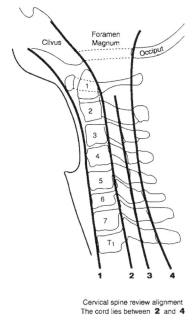

Cervical spine review alignment
The cord lies between **2** and **4**

Figure 25.1. Lateral cervical spine showing anatomy and four review lines

The four lines shown in Figure 25.1 are reviewed. These are:

1. Anterior vertebral line.
2. Posterior vertebral line (anterior wall of the spinal canal).
3. Facet line.
4. Spino-laminar line (posterior wall of the spinal canal).

The continuity of these lines should be maintained, no matter what the degree of flexion or extension seen on the neck film. There should be no 'steps' or angulation.

The spinal cord lies in the canal between the posterior vertebral (2) and the spino-laminar (4) line. The former should line up with the clivus and the latter with the back of the foramen magnum.

Bones

The outline of each vertebra should be reviewed in turn. Fracture lines going through the cortex, vertebral bodies, laminae, or spinous processes should be sought.

The spaces between the facet joints and the gaps between adjacent spinous processes should be similar (Figure 25.2).

The joint between the odontoid peg and the anterior arch of the atlas should be less than 3 mm in a child. This is illustrated in Figure 25.3.

The gap between the posterior arch of C1 and the spinous process of C2 may be slightly larger than the gaps at the other levels in flexion. The base of the odontoid peg may not be completely fused onto the body of the axis (C2) in a small child, but the orientation of the odontoid peg should always be perpendicular to the body of C2.

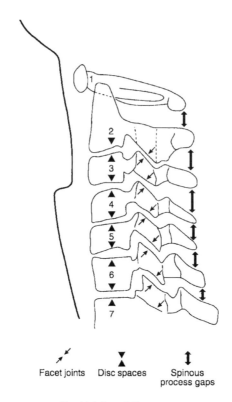

Figure 25.2. Lateral cervical spine showing disc spaces, facet joints and spinous process spaces

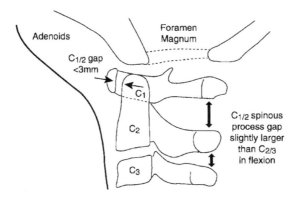

Figure 25.3. C1/2 anatomy in the older child

In adolescence ring apophyses are seen related to the vertebral bodies as shown in Figure 25.4. These are sometimes a site for fracture separation from the vertebral body. The appearances of the apophyses at each level should be compared with the vertebra above and below.

Cartilage and soft tissues

Abnormal widening of the prevertebral soft tissues may indicate a haematoma due to cervical spine injury. There may however be a significant spinal injury with normal soft tissues – thus the absence of soft tissue swelling does not exclude major bony or ligamentous injury. When a child is intubated, it is difficult to assess prevertebral soft tissue swelling. Small children have large adenoids which are seen as well demarcated soft tissue swelling at the base of the clivus. This is shown in Figure 25.5.

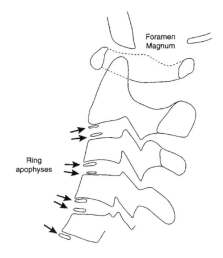

They are parallel to the vertebral end plates
and with equal spacing from the vertebrae.

Figure 25.4. Ring apophyses in the adolescent spine

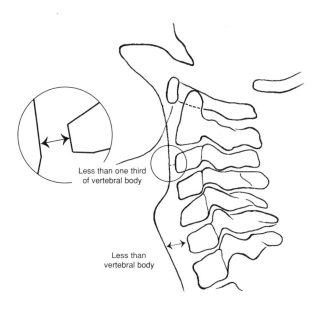

Figure 25.5. Lateral cervical spine – soft tissues

Acceptable soft tissue thicknesses are:

• Above the larynx – less than one third of the vertebral body width and
• Below the larynx – not more than one vertebral body width.

Below the level of the larynx the prevertebral soft tissues become progressively *narrower* towards the cervico-thoracic junction. If the prevertebral soft tissues are wider at C7 than at the C5 level then this suggests trauma at the C7/T1 level.

Any soft tissue swelling outside these limits should be regarded as abnormal and neck protection measures maintained until a further clinical and radiological opinion can be obtained. In small children the soft tissues may appear abnormally wide if the film is taken with the infant lying in flexion – if in doubt maintain the neck protection and ask for advice.

Discs

The height of the vertebral disc should be compared from C2/3 to C7/T1. The discs should all be of similar height as shown earlier in Figure 25.2.

Flexion and extension cervical spine films should never be performed in the acute trauma situation. Further imaging is obtained when the patient is stable, including CT to assess the bones or magnetic resonance imaging (MRI) for the spinal cord.

AP films of the cervical spine may be taken. The films should be reviewed using the same system as was used for the lateral cervical spine film:

Figure 25.6 shows five lines of alignment to assess. The spinal cord lies between lines 2 and 4.

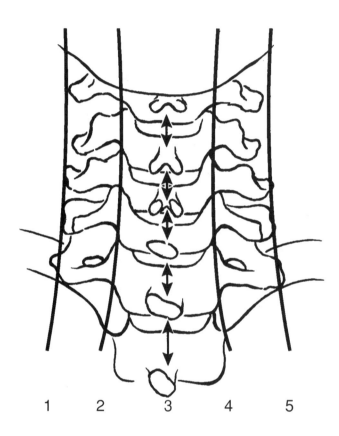

Figure 25.6. AP cervical spine showing anatomy and five review lines, discs and spinous processes

Chest radiograph

Adequacy and alignment

Adequacy can be assessed by considering both penetration and the depth of inspiration.

The film should be sufficiently penetrated to just visualise the disc spaces of the lower thoracic vertebrae through the heart shadow. At least five anterior rib ends should be seen above the diaphragm on the right side. An expiratory film may mimic consolidation.

Alignment – Can be assessed by ensuring that the medial ends of both clavicles are equally spaced about the spinous processes of the upper thoracic vertebrae as shown in

248

Figure 25.7. Abnormal rotation may create apparent mediastinal shift. The trachea should be equally spaced between the clavicles.

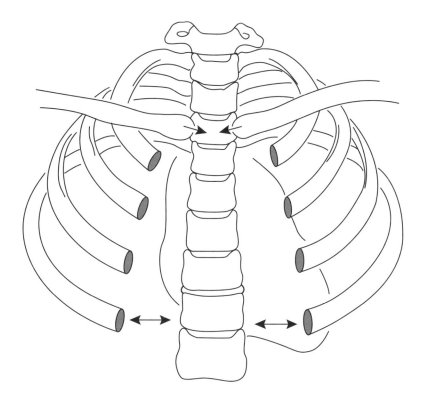

Figure 25.7. Assessing rotation – straight chest film

Apparatus

Check the position of any apparatus including:

- Tracheal tube
- Central venous lines
- Chest drains

Misplacement of the tracheal tube (ETT) should be evident clinically, but may be seen on a chest film if you look for it. Do this first when reviewing any CXR on an intubated patient. Malposition of an ETT can result in reduced ventilation and hypoxia.

The ideal position for an ETT is below the clavicles and at least 1cm above the carina. To find the carina, identify the slope of the right and left main bronchi – the carina is where the two lines meet in the midline.

Bones

The posterior, lateral and anterior aspects of each rib must be examined in detail. This can be done by tracing out the upper and lower borders of the ribs from the posterior costochondral joint to where they join the anterior costal cartilage at the mid-clavicular line. The internal trabecula patten can then be assessed.

The ribs in children are soft and pliable and only break when subjected to considerable force. Even greater force is required to fracture the first rib or to break multiple ribs. Consequently, presence of these fractures should stimulate you to look for other sites of injury both inside and outside the chest.

Finish assessing the bones by inspecting the visible vertebrae, the clavicles, scapulae and proximal humeri.

Thoracic spine injuries may be overlooked on a chest radiograph. Abnormal flattening of the vertebral bodies, widening of the disc spaces, or gaps between the spinous processes or pedicles may be seen. On the AP views increased vertical or horizontal distances between the pedicles or spinous processes on the AP views indicates an unstable fracture as shown in Figure 25.8

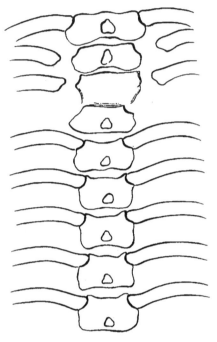

Figure 25.8. Vertical fracture of the thoracic spine

If there are rib fractures in the first three ribs, these may be associated with major spinal trauma and great vessel injury.

Cartilage and soft tissues

Lungs

In a well-centred film, the lungs should appear equally black on both sides.

Compare the left and right lungs in the upper third, middle third and lower third of the chest.

Check that the lungs go all the way out to the rib cage – i.e. there is no pleural effusion or pneumothorax. A black lung on one side may be due to a pneumothorax or air trapping. A white lung on one side may be due to collapse, pulmonary haemorrhage, contusion or an effusion (including haemothorax).

On the supine film, blood or fluid lies posteriorly giving a generalised greyness to the lung, rather than the typical meniscus sign seen on the erect film. At the apex of each lung, an effusion displacing the lung down (apical cap) may indicate spinal injury or major vessel damage.

A suspected tension pneumothorax should be treated clinically in the emergency situation, without confirmatory X-ray. On a supine film air in a simple pneumothorax rises anteriorly and may only be evident by an abnormal blackness or "sharpness" of the diaphragm or cardiac border. The standard appearances of a pneumothorax where there is a sharp lung edge and the vessels fail to extend to the rib cage and the lung edges, may not occur in the supine film.

The heart

The cardiac outline should lie one third to the right of midline and two thirds to the left of midline. If the film is not rotated, then mediastinal shift is either due to the heart being pushed from one side or pulled from the other. For example mediastinal shift to the left may be due either to a pneumothorax, air trapping or effusion on the right side, or to collapse of the left lung.

All trauma radiographs are taken in the supine position, often using portable X-ray machines. The tube is near to the patient and the heart is anterior with the film posterior. The heart in this situation appears abnormally magnified (widened) and the cardio-thoracic ratio is difficult to assess on supine AP films.

The mediastinal cardiac outline should be clear on both sides. Any loss of definition suggests consolidation (de-aeration) of adjacent lungs. A "globular" shape to the heart may suggest a pericardial effusion. Tamponade is managed clinically not radiologically. A cardiac echo is useful in equivocal cases.

The upper mediastinum

In the teenager the mediastinum should appear as narrow as in an adult. In children under the age of 18 months, the normal thymus may simulate superior mediastinal widening (above the level of the carina). A normal thymus may touch the right chest wall, left chest wall, left diaphragm or right diaphragm making it very difficult to exclude mediastinal pathology. Fortunately, mediastinal widening due to aortic dissection or spinal trauma is very rare in small children.

In cases of doubt, where there is a normal clinical examination, an opinion from a radiologist should be sought. In the older child involved in trauma, mediastinal widening may mean aortic dissection or major vessel, or spinal injury. Ultrasound, CT or angiography may be required to resolve this, when the child is stable.

Diaphragms

The cardiophrenic angles and costophrenic angles should be clear on both sides. The diaphragms should be clearly defined on both sides and the left diaphragm should be clearly visible behind the heart. Loss of definition of the left diaphragm behind the heart suggests left lower lobe collapse, an abnormal hump suggests diaphragmatic rupture and an elevated diaphragm suggests effusion, lung collapse or nerve palsy.

At the end of the systematic ABCD review of the X-ray check again in the key areas shown in box below.

- Behind the heart (left lower lobe consolidation or collapse)
- Apices for effusions, pneumothorax, rib fractures and collapse/consolidation
- Costophrenic and cardiophrenic angles – fluid or pneumothorax
- Horizontal fissure – fluid or elevation (upper lobe collapse)
- Trachea for foreign body (and ETT)

Pelvis

A single, anteroposterior pelvic view is usually taken. As with other films this can be reviewed using the ABC approach.

Adequacy and alignment

Rotation of the pelvic film causes great difficulty in interpretation. In a non-rotated pelvic film the tip of the sacrum and spine will be aligned with the symphysis pubis.

The whole of the pelvis from the top of the iliac crests to the ischial tuberosities should be included, as should both hips with the femoral necks shown to the level of the trochanters.

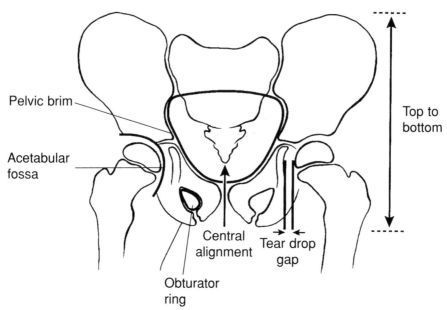

Figure 25.9. Normal straight pelvis in a young child

Bones

The pelvis is made up from the sacrum, innominate bones (iliac wings), ischium and pubic bones. These come together to form an Y-shaped cartilage in the floor of the acetabulum. In young children the joint between the ischium and the pubis (ischiopubic synchondrosis) is commonly seen and may simulate a fracture.

The pelvis is reviewed as a series of rings including the pelvic brim, the two obturator rings and both acetabular fossae. These should be smooth and symmetrical in a well centred film. They are illustrated in Figure 25.9. The femoral necks must be checked for fracture and symmetry of the "tear drop" gap.

Cartilage and soft tissues

Minor degrees of rotation, hip flexion or hip rotation will distort the fat plane and make assessment of soft tissue displacement difficult. Abnormal widening of the obturator fat pad may indicate a pelvic side wall haematoma.

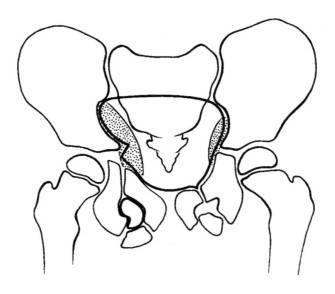

Figure 25.10. Multiple pelvic fractures

The paediatric pelvis is held together by cartilage. Separation through the cartilage of the sacroiliac joint, the symphysis pubis or the "Y" cartilage of the acetabular floor may occur without apparent bony injury. Comparison of both hips and sacroiliac joints on a well-centred film may show this. On a well-centred film the distance between the femoral head and floor of the acetabular "tear drop" should be symmetrical – it is abnormal in effusion or dislocation.

If further assessment is needed a CT scan is performed when the patient is stabilised. Angiography may be needed for vessel injury, or cystourethrography to assess associated urethral or bladder damage.

26

Transport of children

INTRODUCTION

Sick or injured children may initially be taken to a unit which can offer adequate resuscitation or stabilisation but is unable to offer further acute or long-term medical management. Such children must be transported to another hospital or department. Critically ill children transferred by untrained personnel have been shown to suffer largely preventable transfer-related morbidity. In the United Kingdom a standard of practice for the transport of critically ill children has been set by the Paediatric Intensive Care Society. This may involve specialised paediatric transfer teams which are usually based at a paediatric intensive care unit. These teams can be contacted in the event of requests for transfer of a child to a paediatric intensive care facility or specialised facility such as a neurosurgical or burns unit. Often a patient needs to be transported from the Emergency department to another department within the same hospital. Not surprisingly, such transfers are also associated with a high incidence of serious transport-related adverse events.

The basic principles of good transport should be applied to all sick children moved within or between hospitals, whether or not a specialised team is involved.

It is essential to evaluate, resuscitate and stabilise a child's condition before moving him or her. Whatever the injury or illness the airway must be secured and ventilation must be adequate. Intravenous access must be established and fluids and/or life-saving drugs given. Proper evaluation requires a thorough examination to show whether any orthopaedic, surgical or medical procedures should be carried out prior to transportation. Baseline haematological and biochemical samples should be taken when the intravenous lines are placed and essential imaging should be carried out at this time.

The staff at the receiving hospital or department must be contacted prior to arranging transport. They must be clearly told what has happened, the state of the child, the treatment received and what transport facilities and staff are needed. Both teams can then decide if the child is stable enough for transport and whether the referring or receiving hospital will provide the staff to supervise transfer.

Joint management by the referring hospital and transport team should commence immediately since successful initial resuscitation and stabilisation is crucial to ultimate outcome. It must be stressed that this initial role is, and must remain, the responsibility of the referring unit and should be provided at a senior level in conjunction with advice given by the receiving hospital staff.

Equipment

Dedicated transport equipment for monitoring and therapy should be available in the Emergency department. Familiarity with such equipment is a prerequisite for all emergency staff who are involved in the transport of a critically ill child. A list of essential equipment is shown in the box.

Paediatric resuscitation equipment

Airway
1. Oropharyngeal airway sizes 000, 00, 0, 1, 2, 3
2. Tracheal tubes sizes 2·5–7·5 mm uncuffed (in 0·5-mm steps) and 7·5 cuffed
3. Laryngoscopes:
   - straight paediatric blades
   - adult curved blade
4. Magill forceps
5. Yankauer sucker
6. Soft suction catheters
7. Needle cricothyroidotomy set

   Breathing
1. Oxygen masks with reservoir
2. Self-inflating bags (with reservoir)
   - 240 ml infant size
   - 500 ml child size
   - 1600 ml adult size
3. Face masks
   - infant – circular 01, 1, 2
   - child – anatomical 2, 3
   - adult – anatomical 4, 5
4. Catheter mount and connectcors
5. Ayre's T-piece

Circulation
1. ECG monitor – defibrillator (with paediatric paddles)
2. Non-invasive blood pressure monitor (with infant- and child-sized cuffs)
3. Pulse oximeter (with infant- and child-sized probes)
4. Intravenous access requirements
   - Intravenous cannulae (as available) 18–25 g

- Intraosseous infusion needles 16–18 g
- Graduated burette
- Intraveous giving sets
- Syringes 1–50 ml
5. Intravenous drip monitoring device
6. Cut-down set

Fluids
- 0·9% saline
- Hartmann's solution or Ringer's lactate
- 4% dextrose and 0·18% saline
- 5% dextrose
- Colloid
- 4·5% albumin

Drugs
- Epinephrine (adrenaline) 1:10 000
- Epinephrine (adrenaline) 1:1000
- Atropine 0·6 or 1 mg/ml
- Sodium bicarbonate 8·4%
- Dopamine 40 mg/ml
- Dobutamine
- Lignocaine 1%
- Amiodarone
- Dextrose 5% and 10%
- Calcium chloride 10%
- Frusemide 20 mg/ml
- Mannitol 10% or 20%
- Antibiotics – penicillin, gentamicin, ampicillin, ceftazidime, cefotaxime

Miscellaneous
- Stick test for glucose
- Chest drain set

The ability to monitor and record the vital functions shown in the box is essential during transport.

- ECG and heart rate
- Oxygen saturation
- Non-invasive blood pressure
- Temperature (core and peripheral)
- Invasive pressure
- End-tidal CO_2
- Respiratory rate

All the equipment must be kept in a constant state of readiness and be checked at frequent intervals. Batteries must be capable of supporting full function for a period of at least twice the maximum anticipated length of the transfer.

THE TRANSFER

Airway and breathing

Whatever the injury or illness the airway must be secured and ventilation must be adequate. Tracheally intubated patients should be ventilated mechanically rather than manually. Portable mechanical ventilators which function solely on pipe/cylinder oxygen pressure allow the setting, delivery, and measurement of peak inspiratory pressures, positive end-expiratory pressure, minute ventilation, fractional inspired oxygen concentration and respiratory rate. Only some of the new models of portable ventilators offer a low pressure/disconnect alarm and therefore the capnogram on the end-tidal CO_2 monitor provides a useful alarm as well as a monitor of ventilation. With the use of portable suction machines, adequate tracheal toilet can be carried out and a condenser humidifier will reduce the chance of tube blockage.

The use of appropriate sedative agents and muscle relaxants is necessary for the comfort and safety of all intubated children during transfer. These agents reduce the chance of accidental extubation. However, the tracheal tube must be of the appropriate length and size and be well secured. Secure fixation of nasal tubes is much easier and is the preferred technique providing there are no contraindications (such as coagulopathy or suspected base of skull fracture).

A fully pressurised, size E oxygen cylinder contains approximately 600 l of gas and is the most practical portable means of carrying oxygen.

Calculate the amount of oxygen required for the journey using the following formula:

$$(PSI \times 0.3)/\text{flow l/min} = \text{minutes of oxygen available}$$

e.g. A size E cylinder reads 2000 PSI and oxygen flow is set at 4 l/min $(2000 \times 0.3)/4 = 150$ minutes of oxygen available.
Always allow at least twice as much oxygen as the estimated journey time requires.

Circulation

Battery powered syringe pumps capable of holding syringes up to 50 ml and performing accurately at all infusion rates are indispensable for transfer. Two secure intravenous access points are the minimum number required. Children with established

257

or potential haemodynamic instability will require central venous access. Large bore (5 or 7 Foley) multi-lumen central venous catheters facilitate measurement of central venous pressure, rapid administration of colloid and the administration of vasoactive agents or irritant solutions (bicarbonate, potassium, calcium) into the central circulation.

Central venous cannulation should only be atttempted by skilled personnel. The subclavian route should be avoided in the presence of coagulopathy. Insertion of neck lines should be avoided in patients with raised intracranial pressure, or potential spinal injury.

The aim of the treatment of shock is to optimise the perfusion of critical vascular beds and to prevent and correct metabolic abnormalities arising from cellular hypoperfusion. To this end, besides attention to ABC, other important therapeutic measures – such as inotropic support, the correction of metabolic derangements (hypoglycaemia, acidosis, severe electrolyte derangements) – may be required.

All critically ill children who are ventilated and are haemodynamically unstable should have blood pressure monitored invasively.

Disability

The transfer of the comatosed child requires consideration, especially in the context of head injuries. Coma is the sign of significant "brain failure" and requires emergency treatment to prevent secondary central nervous system damage. Full assessment and initial management of ABC and seizures along APLS guidelines take precedence over the need to get the patient to the CT or MRI scanner.

Exposure

Children become cold very quickly, particularly if seriously ill. Adequate steps must be taken to ensure that hypothermia does not occur. Blankets or duvets should cover all exposed parts and all infused fluids should be warmed.

Documentation

All procedures should be documented.

The child's notes, radiographs, charts and any cross-matched blood should be taken to the receiving unit. Results of investigations that become available after the child has left should be communicated to the receiving unit immediately.

Parents

Parents must be kept fully informed of the situation. If clear explanations are given as to why and where a child is being taken it lessens their anxiety and increases their cooperation.

SUMMARY

Meticulous attention to initial assessment and resuscitation together with appropriate emergency treatment will reduce the chance of transport-related morbidity and mortality. Critically ill and injured children can be transferred by a specialised paediatric transport team with minimal related complications. A check list is shown in the box.

Checklist prior to transporting a child

1. Is the airway protected and ventilation satisfactory? (substantiated by blood gases, pH and pulse oximetry if possible).
2. Is the neck properly immobilised?
3. Is there sufficient oxygen available for the journey?
4. Is vascular access secure and will the pumps in use during transport work by battery?
5. Have adequate fluids been given prior to transport?
6. Are fractured limbs appropriately splinted and immobilised?
7. Are appropriate monitors in use?
8. Will the child/baby be sufficiently warm during the journey?
9. Is documentation available? Include:
   child's name
   age
   date of birth
   weight
   radiographs taken
   clinical notes
   observation charts
   neurological observation chart
   the time and route of all drugs given
   fluid charts
   ventilator records
   results of investigations
10. Has the case been discussed with the receiving team directly?
11. Have plans been discussed with the parents?

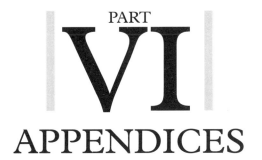

PART

VI

APPENDICES

APPENDIX

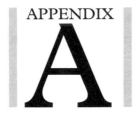

Acid–base balance

ACIDOSIS

Acidosis is a common problem in sick children. Under normal circumstances the blood pH is tightly controlled between 7·35 and 7·45. Although this sounds like very little variation, it has to be remembered that there is a logarithmic relationship between pH and hydrogen ion concentration ($[H^+]$). Thus a pH rise from 7·35 to 7·45 represents a fall in $[H^+]$ from 45 to 35 nmol/l. By the time the pH has fallen to 7·1 the $[H^+]$ has doubled to 80 nmol/l. Many buffers exist to protect against the pH changes that occur as H^+ production increases in sepsis, injury, poor perfusion, and catabolism, or if there is failure to excrete normal acids produced.

It is easy to get confused by the complexities of the inter-relationships between buffering systems (red blood cells, plasma proteins and bicarbonate) but the practical management of a patient with acidosis can be simplified by the application of straightforward rules.

Acidosis is the result of a pathological change and correction will occur if the original pathology is dealt with. Practical intervention to maintain the circulation and treat shock will improve acidosis. With normal renal function and bicarbonate production most acidoses will correct themselves, providing the underlying cause of the acidosis is being treated. Thus intervention is only required if the pH has fallen so low that it has an effect on the ability of the cells to function normally. This level is arbitrary, but is taken as a pH below 7·15.

The acid/alkali balance equation

In the blood, bicarbonate reacts with hydrogen ions to produce CO_2 and water:

$$H^+ + HCO_3 = H_2O + CO_2$$

These four substances are in balance. Thus increased removal of CO_2, by hyperventilation for example, will shift the equation to the right and remove hydrogen ions. This will improve acidosis in the short term but will use up bicarbonate. Retention of CO_2 will lead to a worsening of acidosis by preventing incorporation of produced hydrogen ions into water, at least until bicarbonate production is increased to provide extra buffer.

Acidosis with a low or normal CO_2 is thus *metabolic* in origin and is due to increased production of or failure to excrete hydrogen ions.

Acidosis with a high CO_2 is *respiratory*. Often a mixed picture occurs.

Figure A.1 shows the relationship between pH and bicarbonate concentration at different levels of CO_2. It can be seen that at a given bicarbonate concentration the pH falls as the CO_2 rises. Also, it can be seen that at lower pH levels small falls in bicarbonate concentration produce dramatic reductions in pH. Similarly at low pHs small amounts of bicarbonate cause large shifts in pH. The nearer the pH gets to normal the larger the amount of bicarbonate needed to produce any change.

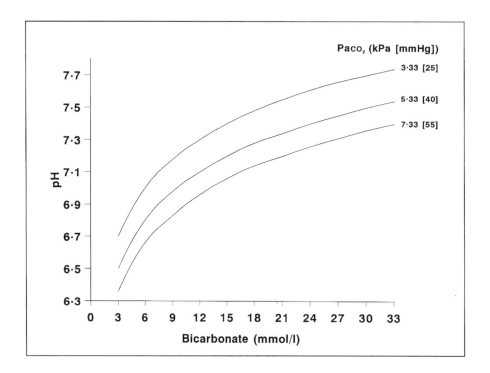

Figure A.1.   The relationship between pH, bicarbonate, and carbon dioxide

In a clinical situation complex calculations of the amount of bicarbonate needed are unnecessary. Since correction is only going to be attempted at a pH of below 7·15, then a single dose of 2·5 mmol/kg (2·5 ml/kg of 8·4% $NaHCO_3$) should be given. This is based on the knowledge that bicarbonate will quickly be distributed about the extracellular and intracellular fluids – about 600 ml/kg. Thus a dose of 2·5 mmol/kg will raise the serum bicarbonate by just over 4 mmol/l. Re-examination of Figure A.1 shows that this rise in serum bicarbonate will usually take the pH to greater than 7·15. If the pH is rechecked after this dose has been given and significant correction has not occurred then it is because of the presence of a high acid load or high acid production rates. The dose should be repeated. When correcting an acidosis the serum calcium and potassium should be monitored carefully. Correction of acidosis reduces the ionised calcium and may produce symptomatic hypocalcaemia. Although the serum potassium is often high in the face of acidosis, correction will cause it to fall because of intracellular movement and supplementation may be required. Continued use of sodium bicarbonate will lead to hypernatraemia.

ALKALOSIS

Alkalosis is a much rarer problem. The two major causes are hyperventilation and vomiting.

Hyperventilation can be a manifestation of an acute anxiety problem. The CO_2 can fall quite markedly, causing a significant rise in pH which is often enough to produce hypocalcaemic tetany. Use of a rebreathing bag is an excellent initial treatment. Although psychological causes are the most common, aspirin poisoning may cause hyperventilation and salicylate levels should be measured if this is suspected.

Severe vomiting causes alkalosis in two ways. First there is direct loss of acid from the stomach. Secondly, severe hypovolaemia may be induced by vomiting. This causes hyperaldosteronism in an attempt to promote salt and water retention which, in turn, leads to increased renal potassium and hydrogen ion loss, with bicarbonate retention. This exacerbates the alkalosis. Volume expansion with normal saline promotes correction. Congenital hypertrophic pyloric stenosis is a good example of this pathophysiological process in action.

ANALYSIS OF AN ARTERIAL BLOOD GAS (ABG)

The proper interpretation of an ABG sample requires clinical history, examination, knowledge of treatments given, and other laboratory investigations. In emergencies, when much of the data is lacking, interpret the findings with caution.

What is the pH? (normal 7·36–7·44)

Is there an acidosis or alkalosis? If the pH is near normal it may be due to respiratory or metabolic compensation. This compensation is never complete, so if the pH is near normal it will still always tell you if the child has a compensated acidosis (pH slightly lower than normal) or a compensated alkalosis (pH slightly higher than normal).

What is the $Pa\text{CO}_2$? (normal 4·7–6·0 kPa, 35–45 mmHg)

This is a good indicator of ventilatory adequacy because it is inversely proportional to alveolar minute volume (Respiratory rate × alveolar tidal volume). When the pH is known it can be used to determine if there are primary or compensatory ventilatory changes.

A higher than normal $Pa\text{CO}_2$ indicates under-ventilation.

A lower than normal $Pa\text{CO}_2$ indicates over-ventilation.

What is the base excess? (normal ± 2)

A positive base excess indicates a metabolic alkalosis. A negative base excess indicates a metabolic acidosis. A negative base excess is only treated if it is more negative than −6 and the pH is low.

Bicarbonate and base excess are *calculated* by blood gas analysers using the Henderson Hasselbach equation. These results must always be interpreted cautiously in clinical situations

What is the $Pa\text{O}_2$? (normal 10·6 kPa, >80 mmHg in air)

The partial presssure of oxygen in arterial blood sample must be interpreted in the light of the inspired oxygen concentration and the pressure of its delivery.

There is a fall of about 7·5 kPa between the $P\text{O}_2$ at the mouth and in the alveoli. For example, inspiring 30% O_2 from an oxygen mask would give an alveolar concentration 20–25·5 kPa.

An easy method for blood gas interpretation

Step 1

Assess the pH. Is it raised >7·44 (alkalosis) or lowered <7·36 (acidosis)? This is the overall status of the patient, regardless of compensatory mechanisms.

Step 2

	Acidosis	Alkalosis
Respiratory	CO_2 ↑	CO_2 ↓
Metabolic	Base excess ↓ or Bicarbonate ↓	Base excess ↑ or Bicarbonate ↑

Look at the CO_2 on the chart above.

- If the CO_2 provides a cause for the abnormal pH, i.e. low pH and high CO_2 (acidosis) and high pH with low CO_2 (alkalosis), then the overall picture is a *respiratory* acidosis or alkalosis.
- If the CO_2 does not provide a cause for the pH, it is *compensating* for a *metabolic* abnormality.

Step 3

Confirm your findings by looking at the base excess of bicarbonate.

- If the base excess provide a cause for the abnormal pH, i.e. low pH with negative base excess (acidosis) and high pH with positive base excess (alkalosis), the overall picture is a *metabolic* acidosis or alkalosis.
- If the base excess does not provide a cause for the pH, it is compensating for a *respiratory* abnormality.

Example

In a patient with shock, showing sighing respirations:

pH	7·24
P_{CO_2}	31
HCO_3	14
BE	−8

- The pH is low, showing acidosis.
- The P_{CO_2} does not provide a cause for the abnormal pH (a low CO_2 indicates a respiratory alkalosis, not an acidosis) therefore it is compensating for a metabolic acidosis.
- The base excess accounts for the abnormal pH (a negative base excess indicates a metabolic acidosis).
- Therefore, the patient is acidotic. He or she has a metabolic acidosis which is being partially compensated by a respiratory alkalosis.

Precautions when taking an arterial blood sample

The taking of arterial blood samples is described in Chapter 23. Certain errors must be avoided:

- Ensure an adequate sample and avoid bubbles. The dead space in the syringe will allow CO_2 and O_2 to diffuse in or out of the sample. Seal the syringe with a plastic cap for the same reasons.
- Avoid excess heparin. Fill the dead space of a 2 ml syringe and attached needle with 1/1000 heparin. A pre-heparinised syringe is preferable.
- Minimise metabolism in the sample. Delay in analysis allows O_2 consumption and CO_2 generation to continue in the syringe sample. If delay of more than a few minutes is anticipated store the sample on ice.

B

Fluid and electrolyte management

INTRODUCTION

Fluid and electrolyte management is an essential part of both the immediate and the ongoing care of all sick children. In this Appendix we will look at the following:

- Normal requirements.
- Dehydration.
- Diabetic ketoacidosis.
- Hypervolaemia (fluid overload).
- Specific electrolyte problems.

NORMAL REQUIREMENTS

Volume

Blood volume is about 100 ml/kg at birth, falling to about 80 ml/kg at one year. Total body water varies from just under 800 ml/kg in the neonate to about 600 ml/kg at one year, after this it varies little. Of this about two-thirds (400 ml/kg) is intracellular fluid, the rest being extracellular fluid. Thus initial expansion of vascular volume in a state of shock can be achieved with relatively small volumes of fluid: 20 ml/kg will usually suffice. However, this volume is only a fraction of that required to correct dehydration if the fluid has been lost from all body compartments; 20 ml/kg is 2% of body weight. Clinically, dehydration which is distributed across the fluid compartments rather than being restricted to the vascular compartment is not detectable until it is greater than 5% (50 ml/kg).

Much is spoken about normal fluid requirements, although in truth there is no such thing. We are all aware as adults that if we drink little we do not get dehydrated and if we drink excessively we merely diurese. Healthy children's kidneys are just as capable of maintaining fluid balance. Fluids in neonates are often prescribed upon the basis of 150 ml/kg/day but this is not related to fluid needs but is merely the volume of standard formula milk required to give an adequate protein and calorie intake. What is required clinically is a simple means of prescribing fluid such that patients are maintained well hydrated and passing reasonable quantities of urine. It should be possible to modify this formula to take account of the need for rehydration of dry patients, and prevention of overhydration in patients in whom renal function is impaired or in whom there is a reason to keep the patient underhydrated (for example, meningitis, cerebral oedema). Fluid requirement can be divided into four types:

1. For replacement of *insensible losses* through sweat, respiration, gastrointestinal loss etc.
2. For replacement of *essential urine output*, the minimal urine output to allow excretion of urea etc.
3. Extra fluid to maintain a modest state of diuresis.
4. Fluid to replace *abnormal losses* such as blood loss, severe diarrhoea, diabetic polyuria losses etc.

A formula for calculating normal fluid requirement is given in Table B.1 below. It is useful because it is simple, can be applied to all age ranges and is easily subdivided. The formula gives total fluid requirements, that is, types 1 + 2 + 3 above.

Table B.1. Normal fluid requirements

Body weight	Fluid requirement per day	Fluid requirement per hour
First 10 kg	100 ml/kg	4 ml/kg
Second 10 kg	50 ml/kg	2 ml/kg
Subsequent kg	20 ml/kg	1 ml/kg

For example: a 6 kg infant would require 600 ml per day
a 14 kg child would require 1000 + 200 = 1200 ml per day
a 25 kg child would require 1000 + 500 + 100 = 1600 ml per day

Electrolytes

To speak of normal electrolyte requirements is as artificial as speaking of normal fluid requirements. There are obligatory losses of electrolytes in stools, urine, and sweat, and these require replacement. Any excess is simply excreted in the urine. Table B.2 gives electrolyte "requirements" if there are not excessive losses from any compartment. These "requirements" represent quantities that if given maintain homeostasis without recourse to the various hormonal and renal tubular mechanisms for maintaining the extracellular fluid composition.

Table B.2. Normal water, electrolyte, energy

Body weight	Water (ml/kg/day)	Sodium (mmol/kg/day)	Potassium (mmol/kg/day)	Energy (kcal/day)	Protein (g/day)
First 10 kg	100	2–4	1·5–2·5	110	3·00
Second 10 kg	50	1–2	0·5–1·5	75	1·5
Subsequent kg	20	0·5–1	0·2–0·7	30	0·75

Intravenous fluids are available in a variety of electrolyte compositions. In particular, there are a number of different strengths of dextrose and saline (often as a mixture in the same bag) – the concentration of sodium being expressed in mmol/l on the side of the infusion bag, as well as a percentage. Always check the sodium concentration in mmol/l is actually what you require and take great care to specify the concentration of both the dextrose and the saline (if a dextrose/saline solution is being used) when writing the prescription to avoid ambiguity. Tables B.3 and B.4 show the composition of commonly available fluids.

Table B.3. Commonly available crystalloid fluids

Fluid	Na$^+$ (mmol/l)	K$^+$ (mmol/l)	Cl$^-$ (mmol/l)	Energy (kcal/l)	Other
Isotonic crystalloid fluids					
Saline 0·9%	150	0	150	0	0
Saline 0·45%, dextrose 2·5%	75	0	75	100	0
Saline 0·18%, dextrose 4%	30	0	30	160	0
Dextrose 5%	0	0	0	200	0
Saline 0·18%, dextrose 4%, 10 mmol KCl/500 ml					
Hartmann's solution	131	5	111	0	Lactate
Hypertonic crystalloid solutions					
Saline 0·45%, dextrose 5%	75	0	75	200	0
Dextrose 10%	0	0	0	400	0
Saline 0·18%, dextrose 10%	30	0	30	400	0
Dextrose 20%	0	0	0	800	0

Table B.4. Commonly available colloid fluids

Colloid solutions	Na$^+$ (mmol/l)	K$^+$ (mmol/l)	Ca^{2+} (mmol/l)	Duration of actions (hours)	Comments
Albumin 4·5%	150	1	0	6	Protein buffers H$^+$
Gelofusine	154	<1	<1	3	Gelatine
Haemaccel	145	5	12·5	3	Gelatine
Pentastarch	154	0	0	7	Hydroxyethyl starch

DEHYDRATION

Dehydration is the result of abnormal fluid losses from the body which are greater than the amount for which the kidneys can compensate. The natural mechanisms for compensation have the primary aim of maintaining circulating volume and blood pressure at all cost. Thus the majority of patients with dehydration maintain their central circulation satisfactorily. Loss of central circulatory homeostasis constitutes hypovolaemic shock and is dealt with in Chapter 10.

The major causes of dehydration in children are gastrointestinal disorders and diabetic ketoacidosis. Some renal disorders (polyuric tubulopathy with urinary tract infection, polyuric chronic renal failure and diabetes insipidus) might also present in this way. Depending on the source of fluid losses and the quantities of electrolytes lost dehydration can be divided into three types:

1. Isotonic dehydration – sodium and water lost in proportion to each other.
2. Hyponatraemic dehydration – proportionately more sodium lost than water.
3. Hypernatraemic dehydration proportionately more water lost than sodium.

In all three types there is usually a total body deficit of salt and water. Between the three types the relative amounts of salt and water loss vary. Table B.5 shows the symptoms and signs of dehydration and gives a guide towards the assessment of the degree of dehydration. On the whole, the more severe the dehydration the more likely that hypovolaemia will be a problem; most patients with more than 10% dehydration are hypovolaemic at presentation. However, speed of fluid loss is important. Slow, prolonged losses can give rise to massive dehydration without hypovolaemia, similarly acute, severe loss can present as hypovolaemia without apparent significant dehydration. The latter is not infrequently the case in acute gastroenteritis in infants where acute fluid loss into the bowel causes hypovolaemia and the patient can present even before any diarrhoea has occurred.

Table B.5. Symptoms and signs of dehydration

Sign/symptoms	Mild <5%	Moderate 5–10%	Severe >10%	Notes/caveats
Decreased urine output	+	+	+	Beware watery diarrhoea making nappies appear "wet"
Dry mouth	+/−	+	+	Mouth breathers are always dry
Decreased skin turgor	−	+/−	+	Beware the thin, use several sites
Tachypnoea	−	+/−	+	Metabolic acidosis and pyrexia worsen this
Tachycardia	−	+/−	+	Hypovolaemia, pyrexia and irritability cause this

Management of dehydration

Mild dehydration (<5%) can usually be managed with oral rehydration if vomiting is not a major problem. Oral rehydration fluids are better absorbed if they contain a small amount of sodium and glucose in addition to water. Commercial preparations contain, for example, 35–50 mmol of sodium per litre when made up as instructed.

Moderate and severe dehydration will require more accurate replacement of fluid loss and although oral rehydration may often be possible, intravenous therapy may be needed.

For fluid balance purposes, as the body is mostly water, a weight loss of 1 kg equals a fluid loss of 1 litre, as one millilitre of water weighs one gramme. Thus fluid loss or gain can be measured easily by weighing the patient. The child's fluid deficit can be worked out from the child's weight and/or a clinical assessment of the percentage dehydration if the initial weight is not available. For example, a 10 kg child is 7·5% dehydrated. How much fluid will the child need for rehydration and what sodium concentration will be required?

The child will need maintenance + replacement of deficit. Calculate them separately and add them up.

Step 1
What is the fluid deficit?
$$7 \cdot 5\% \text{ of } 10\,\text{kg} = 0 \cdot 75 \text{ kg} = 750\,\text{g}$$
$$750\,\text{g is the weight of } 750\,\text{ml fluid}$$

A convenient formula to remember is:

Percentage dehydration × Weight in kg × 10 = Fluid deficit (ml)

Thus the fluid deficit is 750 ml. The fluid deficit is essentially made up from (roughly) 0·9% saline (which has 150 mmol/l) since it is mainly extracellular fluid that has been lost which has a sodium concentration of approximately 140 mmol/l.

Step 2

The child also needs maintenance fluids. These can be worked out in the normal way. A 10 kg child will need 10 × 100 ml/day for normal maintenance (Table B.1) = 1000 ml. The sodium required for maintenance (Table B.2) will be approximately 3 mmol/kg × 10 kg = 30 mmol/day.

In total, then, the child needs 1000 ml maintenance plus 750 ml replacement of losses, totalling 1750 ml, for adequate rehydration.

If we were following the sums exactly we should put up two drips – one of 750 ml with sodium of 140 mmol/l and another of 1000 ml with 30 mmol of sodium. As fluid balance is not often an exact science (ongoing losses, clinical estimations etc.), it is usually more convenient to pick one intravenous fluid with a sodium concentration somewhere between the two and give the total volume using this. The fluid which fits this specification best in this case is 0·45% saline, which has 75 mmol/l. This can be changed to fluid containing more or less sodium depending on subsequent serum sodium results. To make it isotonic 0·45% saline is usually made up with 2–5% dextrose. Beware of using IV fluids with no dextrose in small children as they may become hypoglycaemic. Careful reassessment and re-estimation of weight and electrolytes is essential for further fluid adjustment.

In patients with a low or normal sodium, lost fluid can be replaced over 24 hours. In hypernatraemic patients, it must be replaced over at least 48 hours and sometimes longer depending on the severity – the higher the sodium the slower the rehydration must be. If the sodium and water are corrected too rapidly in the extracellular space, water will pour into cells, and if this happens in the brain, cerebral oedema and even death may occur. Aim to bring down the serum Na in a hypernatraemic patient by no more than 5 mmol per day, for example, in an infant who presents with a Na of 170 mmol/l, the Na should be no less than 165 mmol/l by the next day. In these patients, the electrolytes should be checked 4-hourly, at least initially.

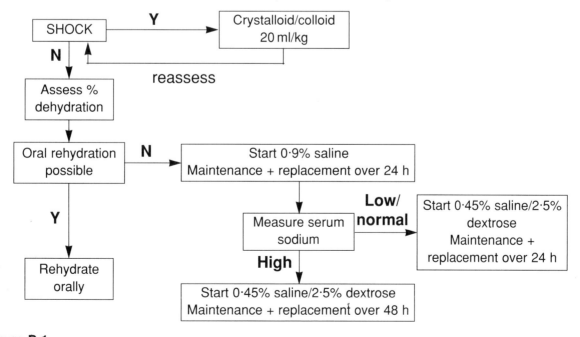

Figure B.1.

The very sick child

In the very sick child it may be uncertain whether normal homeostatic mechanisms will work. The patient may be progressing into renal failure and be oliguric or inappropriately polyuric. In such cases the best management is to:

- Catheterise the patient.
- Calculate and replace deficit, over 24 hours, with normal saline.
- Calculate insensible losses and replace with 0·18% saline, 4% dextrose.
- Measure urine output and replace ml for ml on an hourly basis with 0·18% or 0·45% saline with dextrose according to the plasma electrolytes.

This technique is applicable to all patients with all conditions in all states of hydration. Moreover, subsequent measurement of urinary electrolytes can allow exact tailoring of IV fluids to maintain normal serum electrolytes.

DIABETIC KETOACIDOSIS (DKA)

DKA is a special case in which a relative or absolute lack of insulin leads to an inability to metabolise glucose. This leads to hyperglycaemia and an osmotic diuresis.

Once urine output exceeds the ability of the patient to drink, dehydration sets in. In addition, without insulin, fat is used as a source of energy leading to the production of large quantities of ketones and metabolic acidosis. There is initial compensation for the acidosis by hyperventilation and a respiratory alkalosis but, as the condition progresses, the combination of acidosis, hyperosmolality, and dehydration leads to coma. DKA is often the first presentation of diabetes; it can also be a problem in known diabetics who have decompensated through illness, infection or non-adherence to their treatment regimes.

History

The history is usually of weight loss, abdominal pain, vomiting, polyuria, and polydipsia, though symptoms may be much less specific in under-5-year-olds who also have an increased tendency to ketoacidosis.

Examination

Children are usually severely dehydrated with deep and rapid (Kussmaul) respiration. They have the smell of ketones on their breath. Salicylate poisoning and uraemia are differential diagnoses to be excluded. Infection often precipitates decompensation in both new and known diabetics, and must be sought.

Management

Assess
- **A**irway.
- **B**reathing.
- **C**irculation.

Give 100% oxygen and place on a cardiac monitor. Hypokalaemia can cause dysrhythmias.

Site IV infusion and begin fluid replacement. If shock is present, treat as discussed in Chapter 10, although patients with DKA are likely to require only one fluid bolus. Beware of giving too much fluid as this may precipitate cerebral oedema.

Take blood for:

- Bicarbonate/blood gases.
- Urea and electrolytes, creatinine, calcium, albumin.
- Glucose.
- Culture.
- Haemoglobin and differential white cell count.

Take urine for:

- Culture.
- Sugar.
- Ketones.

Fluids

Children with DKA will have lost a great deal of sodium, whatever their initial measured plasma sodium. Normal saline is the correct initial fluid. The principles of fluid management outlined above work as well for DKA as for any other cause of dehydration. However, because of the hyperglycaemia it is often best not to give dextrose initially. Thus, having calculated deficit, maintenance, and 24-hour requirement, this can initially be given all as normal saline, switching to 0·45% saline or 0·18% saline with dextrose once the blood sugar has fallen. With the osmotic diuresis, which will persist until the blood sugar falls, calculated fluid requirements will be an underestimate and ongoing fluid replacement should be recalculated 4 hourly to take into account excess fluid losses. Potassium should be added to the fluids (20–40 mmol/l initially) once a urine output has been confirmed. There is a loss of potassium in DKA and, additionally, the use of insulin will drive potassium into cells, further lowering the plasma potassium.

Insulin

Insulin should be given by continuous infusion. The initial dose is 0·1 units/kg/hour. Once the blood sugar falls to less than 10 mmol/l, glucose must be added to the IV. Do not stop using insulin. This is the child's prime requirement. Administer the insulin by separate line. Add 25 units of soluble insulin to 50 ml saline. This solution is 0·5 unit/ml: 0·1 units/kg/hour is equal to $0·05 \times$ weight in kg, as ml/hour. Thus a 20-kg child would have 2 ml/hour, a 35 kg child 3·5 ml/hour. This often needs decreasing when blood sugar starts to fall. In a very young diabetic (under 5 years), start with the smaller dose.

Acidosis

The acidosis of DKA is initially compensated for by hyperventilation. Once the blood pH falls below 7·1, CNS depression can occur and this can prevent compensation. Acidosis will nearly always resolve with correction of fluid balance and cessation of ketosis following insulin therapy. Bicarbonate should be avoided unless the blood pH is less than 7·0, or less than 7·1 and not improving after the first few hours of fluid and insulin therapy. Many formulas exist relating the base excess to the child's weight and the bicarbonate requirement. However, because of the logarithmic relationship between $[H^+]$ and pH a dose of 2·5 ml/kg of 8·4% $NaHCO_3$ will correct the pH to 7·2 or 7·3 in all cases. This should be administered slowly over 2 hours by infusion. Recheck the pH after the first hour and stop the infusion if the pH is above 7·15 as the rest will correct naturally.

Other treatments

A nasogastric tube is essential as acute gastric dilatation is a complication. Depending on the level of consciousness, bladder catheterisation may be required. Antibiotics may be indicated.

Monitoring progress

Use a flow sheet to record vital signs, neurological status, input and output of fluids, blood results and insulin infusion rates. Record urine ketones and glucose. Initially, whilst IV insulin is in use, check blood sugar, biochemistry and acid–base status 2-hourly.

Regular, frequent (i.e. initially half-hourly) assessment of conscious level by the Glasgow Coma Score is required to recognise early cerebral oedema. This complication of diabetic ketoacidosis is uncommon but may be devastating. It is not confined to children with severe illness. Early recognition of reduced conscious level should lead to measures to reduce raised intracranial pressure, and transfer to intensive care for intracranial pressure monitoring.

Complications

Major complications of diabetic ketoacidosis	
Cerebral oedema	Prevent by slow normalisation of sugar and hydration over 36–48 hours; monitor GCS; treat with mannitol and hyperventilation. Inform neurosurgeons. ?CT scan. ?Monitor ICP
Cardiac dysrhythmias	Usually secondary to electrolyte disturbances, particularly potassium
Acute renal failure	Uncommon because of high osmotic urine flow

All of these complications require intensive monitoring on an intensive care unit.

HYPERVOLAEMIA

Hypervolaemia in children is uncommon and is usually due to either cardiac or renal failure. Occasionally water intoxication due to deliberate ingestion of water or excessive administration of desmopressin (DDAVP) may be the cause.

Signs of hypervolaemia include raised venous pressure, a triple rhythm on auscultation of the heart, and pulmonary crackles. Hypertension may be present, particularly in fluid overload of renal origin. Treatment of hypervolaemia is initially with diuretics. These may be ineffective, particularly in renal failure, in which case urgent dialysis may be needed. Oxygen may be required and in severe cases positive pressure ventilation may be needed to maintain adequate oxygenation because of pulmonary oedema.

ß-blockers are contraindicated in hypervolaemia, because of the risk of cardiac failure.

Water intoxication will usually present as convulsions from cerebral oedema and hyponatraemia. Treatment is along the usual lines for patients with convulsions and coma (Chapters 12 and 13). Severe fluid restriction will be necessary, and if hyponatraemia is severe (<120 mmol/l), fluids ought to be given as 0·9% saline. Diuretics, particularly mannitol, which causes a free water diuresis and reduces cerebral oedema, are sometimes of value.

Mild oedema may occur in any of these conditions. Severe oedema does not, and when present, is usually a manifestation of a low serum albumin, most commonly nephrotic syndrome. This is important as patients with nephrotic syndrome are intravascularly fluid depleted and diuretics are contraindicated.

SPECIFIC ELECTROLYTE PROBLEMS

Sodium is the major extracellular cation. Its movement is inextricably linked to that of water. Disorders of sodium balance are, therefore, those of over- and under-hydration, and are dealt with in the section on fluid balance.

Potassium

Unlike sodium, potassium is mainly an intracellular ion and the small quantities measurable in the serum and extracellular fluid represent only a fraction of the total body potassium. However, the exact value of the serum potassium is important as cardiac arrhythmias can occur at values outside of the normal range. The intracellular potassium acts as a large buffer to maintain the serum value within its normal narrow range. Thus hypokalaemia is usually only manifest after significant total body depletion has occurred. Similarly, hyperkalaemia represents significant total body overload, beyond the ability of the kidney to compensate. The exception to both these statements is the situation in which the cell wall pumping mechanism is breached. A breakdown of the causes of hyper- and hypokalaemia is given in Table B.6.

Table B.6. Causes of hypo- and hyperkalaemia

Hypokalaemia	Hyperkalaemia
Diarrhoea	Renal failure
Alkalosis	Acidosis
Volume depletion	Adrenal insufficiency
Primary hyperaldosteronism	Cell lysis
Diuretic abuse	Excessive potassium intake

Hypokalaemia

Hypokalaemia is rarely a great emergency. It is usually the result of excessive potassium losses from acute diarrhoeal illnesses. As total body depletion will have occurred, large amounts are required to return the serum potassium to normal. The fastest way of giving this is with oral supplementation. In cases where this is unlikely to be tolerated, IV supplements are required. However, strong potassium solutions are highly irritant and can precipitate arrhythmias, thus the concentration of potassium in IV solutions ought not to exceed 80 mmol/l when given centrally except on intensive care units. Fortunately this is not usually a problem as renal conservation of potassium aids restoration of normal serum levels.

Patients who are alkalotic, hyperglycaemic (but not diabetic), or are receiving insulin from exogenous sources will have high intracellular potassium stores. Thus hypokalaemia in these cases is the result of a redistribution of potassium rather than potassium deficiency and treatment of the underlying causes is indicated.

Hyperaldosteronism is a cause of hypokalaemic alkalosis. Patients with this condition will have salt and water retention and will be hypertensive on presentation. Secondary hyperaldosteronism is the body's natural response to hypovolaemia and salt deficiency and is thus a common cause of hypokalaemic alkalosis. As there is primary salt and water deficiency the patient is not usually hypertensive. The most common causes are diarrhoeal illness and salt-losing conditions such as cystic fibrosis. External loss of fluid from intestinal ostomies or drains are other causes. Although potassium replacement is required in this condition the main thrust of therapy has to be with salt and water replacement to re-expand the circulation and cut down on aldosterone production.

Hyperkalaemia

Hyperkalaemia is a dangerous condition. Although the normal range extends up to 5·5 mmol/l it is rare to get arrhythmias below 7·5 mmol/l. The most common cause of hyperkalaemia is renal failure – either acute or chronic. Hyperkalaemia can also result from potassium overload, loss of potassium from cells due to acidosis or cell lysis, hypoaldosteronism and hypoadrenalism.

The immediate treatment of hyperkalaemia is shown schematically in Figure B.2. If there is no immediate threat to the patient's life because of an arrhythmia then a logical sequence of investigation and treatment can be followed. Beta-2 stimulants, such as salbutamol, are the immediate treatment of choice. They act by stimulating the cell wall pumping mechanism and promoting cellular potassium uptake. They are best administered by nebuliser. The dose to be given is shown in Table B.8. The serum potassium will fall by about 1 mmol/l with these dosages.

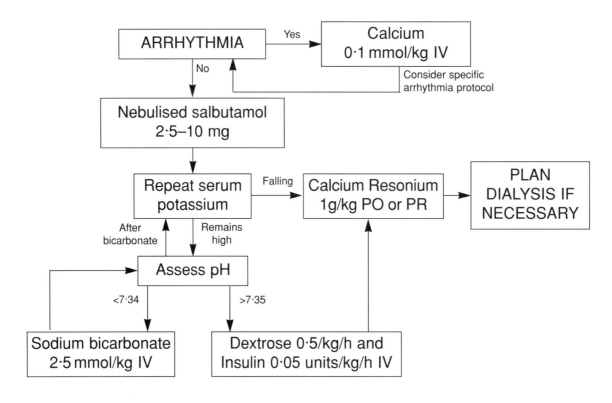

Figure B.2. Algorithm for the management of hyperkalaemia

Table B.8. Salbutamol dose by age

Age (years)	Salbutamol dose (mg)
≤2·5	2·5
2·5–7·5	5
>7·5	10

Sodium bicarbonate is also effective at rapidly promoting intracellular potassium uptake. The effect is much greater in the acidotic patient (in whom the hyperkalaemia is likely to be secondary to movement of potassium out of the cells). The dosage is the same as that used for treating acidosis and 2–5ml/kg of 8–4% $NaHCO_3$ is usually effective. It is mandatory to also check the serum calcium, since particularly in patients with profound sepsis or renal failure, hyperkalaemia can be accompanied by marked hypocalcaemia. The use of bicarbonate in these situations can provoke a crisis by lowering the ionised calcium fraction, precipitating tetany, convulsions or hypotension and arrhythmias.

Insulin and dextrose are the classic treatment for hyperkalaemia. They are not, however, without risks. It is very easy to precipitate hypoglycaemia if monitoring is not adequate. Large volumes of fluid are often used as a medium for the dextrose and, particularly in the patient with renal failure, hypervolaemia and dilutional hyponatraemia can then be a problem. Many patients are quite capable of significantly increasing endogenous insulin production in response to a glucose load and this endogenous insulin is just as capable of promoting intracellular potassium uptake. It thus makes sense to start treatment with just an intravenous glucose load and then to add insulin as the blood sugar rises. The initial dosage of glucose ought to be 0·5/kg/hour, i.e. 2·5 ml/kg/hour of 20% dextrose. Once the blood sugar is above 10 mmol/l, insulin can be added if the potassium is not falling. The dosage of insulin is initially half that used in diabetic ketoacidosis, i.e. 0·05 units/kg/hour. This can then be titrated according to the blood sugar.

The above treatments are the fastest means of securing a fall in the serum potassium but all work through a redistribution of the potassium into cells. Thus the problem is merely delayed rather than treated in the patient with potassium overload. The only ways of removing potassium from the body are with dialysis or ion exchange resins such as calcium resonium. If it is anticipated that the problem of hyperkalaemia is going to persist then the use of these treatments ought not to be delayed. Dialysis can only be started when the patient is in an appropriate environment. Ion exchange resins can be used at the outset. The dosage of calcium resonium is 1 g/kg as an initial dose either orally or rectally, followed by 1 g/kg/day in divided doses.

In an emergency situation where there is an arrhythmia (heart block or ventricular arrhythmia) the treatment of choice is intravenous calcium. This will stabilise the myocardium but will have no effect on the serum potassium. Thus the treatments discussed above will still be necessary. The dosage is 0·5 ml/kg of 10% Ca gluconate (i.e. 0·1 mmol/kg Ca). This dose can be repeated twice. With a very high potassium, more than one treatment can be used simultaneously.

Calcium

Some mention of disorders of calcium metabolism is relevant as both hyper- and hypocalcaemia can produce profound clinical pictures.

Hypocalcaemia

Hypocalcaemia can be a part of any severe illness, particularly septicaemia. Other specific conditions that may give rise to hypocalcaemia are severe rickets, hypoparathyroidism, pancreatitis, or rhabdomyolysis, and citrate infusion (in massive blood transfusions). Acute and chronic renal failure can also present with severe hypocalcaemia. In all cases hypocalcaemia can produce weakness, tetany, convulsions, hypotension, and arrhythmias. Treatment is that of the underlying condition. In the emergency situation, however, intravenous calcium can be administered. As most of the above conditions are associated with a total body depletion of calcium and as the total body pool is so large, acute doses will often only have a transient effect on the serum calcium. Continuous infusions will also often be required, and must be given through a central venous line as calcium is so irritant in peripheral veins. In renal failure, high serum phosphate levels may prevent the serum calcium from rising. The use of oral phosphate binders or dialysis may be necessary in these circumstances.

Hypercalcaemia

Hypercalcaemia usually presents as long-standing anorexia, malaise, weight loss, failure to thrive and vomiting. Causes include hyperparathyroidism, hypervitaminosis D or A, idiopathic hypercalcaemia of infancy, malignancy, thiazide diuretic abuse and skeletal disorders. Initial treatment is with volume expansion with normal saline. Following this, investigation and specific treatment are indicated.

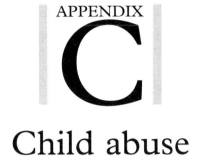

APPENDIX
C
Child abuse

INTRODUCTION

All those working with children have an impulse to deny that human beings will harm their young. Health care workers will come into contact with:

1. Children who have been abused by adults or by other children.
2. Children who have abused other children.
3. Adults who were abused as children.

In any group of staff some may have been abused themselves. If these survivors have had support following the abuse, they will be able to recognise and help abused children. If they have residual problems arising out of their own abuse, they may become disturbed and need help themselves if approached by children or adults whose experiences reflect their own.

Historical

The standard of care of children has varied over the centuries. Up to the nineteenth century, children were used in industry in a manner that today we would classify as abuse. In Victorian times beating children as a means of discipline was accepted by most social groups. Today, corporal punishment is forbidden in schools but the laws of the UK allow parents to administer physical punishment to children within limits.

A good working definition is that a child is considered to be abused if he or she is treated by an adult or by another child in a way that is unacceptable in a given culture at a given time.

The extremes of physical abuse were described in 1962 by Kempe, an American paediatrician, as the battered baby syndrome – multiple bruises, intracranial haemorrhages, fractures, and internal injuries in children under the age of 1 year.

Since 1962 we have gradually recognised many more forms of abuse. Present classifications are as follows.

Classification of child abuse

Neglect

Neglect means the persistent or severe neglect of a child, or the failure to protect a child from exposure to any kind of danger, including cold or starvation, or extreme failure to carry out important aspects of care, resulting in the significant impairment of the child's health or development, including non-organic failure to thrive. There are at least 20 areas of care in which children may be neglected.

Physical injury

This is actual or probable physical injury to a child, or failure to prevent physical injury (or suffering) to a child, including deliberate poisoning, suffocation, and Munchhausen's syndrome by proxy.

Sexual abuse

This is the involvement of dependent, developmentally immature children, and adolescents in sexual activities which they do not truly comprehend, to which they are unable to give informed consent or which violate the social taboos of family roles. There are many types of sexual abuse:

- Touching, fondling, or licking of genitals or breasts.
- Masturbation of child by adult or adult by child; or of an adult in the presence of the child.
- Body contact with the adult genitals including rubbing or simulated intercourse by the adult against or between thighs, buttocks, or elsewhere.
- Heterosexual or homosexual intercourse with actual or attempted vaginal, anal, or oral penetration.
- Exhibitionism (the display of genitals).
- Involvement in pornography, including photography and erotic talk.
- Involvement in prostitution, male or female.
- Other varieties of sexual exploitation.

Most of these abusive acts will leave no physical signs on the victim.

Emotional abuse

This is described actual or probable severe adverse effect on the emotional and behavioural development of a child caused by persistent or severe emotional ill treatment or rejection. All abuse involves some emotional ill treatment. This category should be used where it is the main or sole form of abuse.

Grave concern

This is described in children whose situations do not currently fit the above categories, but where social and medical assessments indicate that they are at significant risk of abuse. These could include situations where another child in the household has been harmed or the household contains a known abuser.

Organised abuse

This characteristically involves multiple perpetrators, involves multiple victims, and is a form of organised crime. There are three sub-sections. The first is paedophile and/or pornographic rings. The second is cult-based ritualistic abuse in which the abuse has spiritual or social objectives. The third is pseudoritualistic abuse in which the degradation of children is the end rather than the means.

Presentations of physical abuse

- Head injuries - fractures, intracranial injury.
- Fractures of long bones
    - single fracture with multiple bruises;
    - multiple fractures in different stages of healing, possibly with no bruises or soft tissue injury;
    - metaphyseal or epiphyseal injuries, often multiple.
- Fractured ribs. Spinal injuries.
- Internal damage.
- Burns and scalds – "glove and stocking" appearance.
- Cold injury – hypothermia, frostbite.
- Poisoning – drugs or household substances. Suffocation.
- Cuts and bruises - imprints of hands, sticks, whips, belts, bites, etc. may be present.

Presentations of sexual abuse

- Disclosure by child.
- Suspicion by third party because of behaviour of child, especially changes in behaviour. These include: insecurity; fear of men; sleep disorders; mood changes, tantrums, aggression at home; anxiety, despair, withdrawal, secretiveness; poor peer relationships; lying, stealing, arson; school failure; eating disorders: anorexia, compulsive overeating; running away, truancy; suicide attempts, self-poisoning, self-mutilation, abuse of drugs, solvents, alcohol; unexplained acquisition of money; sexualised behaviour: drawings with a sexual content; knowledge of adult sexual behaviour shown in speech, play, or drawing; apparently sexual approaches; promiscuity.
- Symptoms such as sore bottom, vaginal discharge, bleeding per rectum, inflamed penis which caregiver believes is due to sexual abuse.
- Symptoms as above and/or signs, e.g. unexplained perineal tear and/or bruising, torn hymen, perineal warts, but doctor is the first person to suspect abuse.
- Sexually transmitted disease.
- Faecal soiling or relapse of enuresis.
- Child (usually adolescent girl) presents frequently with a variety of problems including: recurrent abdominal pain, overdose of drugs, reluctance to go home.
- Pregnancy but girl refuses to name the putative father or even indicate the category, e.g. boyfriend, casual acquaintance.

ASSESSMENT

The child who has disclosed abuse, or who is the subject of suspected abuse, will be overwhelmed by the number of professional people who are involved in the assessment of the situation. If the disclosure or suspicion arises in a nursery or school, then teachers and health visitors/school nurses will make preliminary enquiries and referrals. In all intra-familial abuse, social workers will speak to the child and the family. They will be responsible for the safety of the child, for ongoing care of the family, and for any subsequent civil proceedings. All child abuse is criminal activity so police officers will interview the alleged victim, the alleged offender, and any other witnesses to the incidents. In most areas of the UK good liaison exists between social workers and police officers so joint interviews are done to minimise the number of times the child will have to relate the details of the incident(s). Whenever possible, these interviews are recorded on video-tape to be used as evidence. Under the Criminal Justice Act 1991, video-tapes can be used as evidence in chief for children under the age of 14 years, provided that the child is available for cross-examination.

Medical assessment will be carried out by a paediatrician with forensic training or jointly by a police surgeon and a paediatrician. If the child has severe psychological disturbance or psychiatric symptoms, then a psychologist and/or psychiatrist will also see the child and the family. The basic medical assessment should follow the pattern used for all other diagnostic problems.

Details of medical assessment

History

Full details of the history of the incident(s) should be obtained from the child and the caregivers. If social workers and police officers have previously talked to the child, then taking this history from them may be appropriate, especially for alleged sexual offences. Frequent repetition of the details can be very disturbing to the child.

Systemic enquiry is then done for the cardiovascular system, respiratory system, gastrointestinal tract (remember to ask about soiling), urogenital system (remember to ask about wetting), central nervous system, musculoskeletal system, skin, and behaviour.

Personal history must start with pregnancy, birth, the neonatal period, and subsequent developmental milestones. Then details of immunisations, drug history, and allergies are obtained. Information on the child's performance at nursery or school should include social factors.

Enquiries are made about previous illnesses and injuries with dates of attendance at hospital or at the surgery of the family doctor. Whenever possible, past records should be obtained and relevant information should be extracted.

The traditional family history should include details of the natural parents, all cohabitees and any other people who regularly care for the child, e.g. relatives, childminders. Parental illness should be discussed, particularly psychiatric illness. Then the names, ages, and medical histories of all siblings and half-siblings are obtained. Any miscarriages, stillbirths, or deaths of siblings are discussed sensitively. Familial illnesses which are particularly important are inherited skin or blood disorders.

Examination

The general examination starts while the history is being taken. During that time the doctor observes the affect of the child, the relationships between child/mother/father/others present and any behavioural problems. If the child is reluctant to be examined, then playing with toys or the doctor's stethoscope often breaks the ice. No child should be examined against his or her will as this constitutes an assault. Sometimes a child who refuses to be examined one day will come back quite cheerfully another day. Examination under anaesthesia is rarely required.

Each child is examined from head to toe rather than in systems. Height and weight are checked, as is head circumference in babies. Careful notes are made of all normal and abnormal findings, including any marks on clothing, e.g. tears, blood stains. All marks, contusions, abrasions, and lacerations must be measured. Drawings must be made. If an abnormality is found that has not been discussed previously in the history, then further questions are asked – most undisclosed events are recent minor childhood accidents or previous ones that have left scars. When the upper part of the body has been examined, the child is asked to put the clothes back on to that area before taking the clothes off the abdomen and legs. Finally, the genitalia and anal region are examined. This method minimises the embarrassment of the sensitive child.

Investigations

During the examination, specimens needed for forensic investigation will be taken by a police surgeon or a paediatrician with forensic experience. These are relevant when there has been contact within 7 days of the examination. Swabs for microbiological investigation will be taken if there is a vaginal discharge or if threadworms may be present. Investigations for sexually transmitted diseases are done 2 weeks after the last alleged offence if oral, vaginal, or anal intercourse has taken place.

If bruises are found, then organic disease may be present with or without abuse, so haematological investigations are needed. Venous blood is taken for full blood count, bleeding, and clotting studies.

Radiograph interpretation

Occasionally old rib fractures may be seen on a chest X-ray. Posterior rib fractures in adjacent ribs are very suggestive of non-accidental injury due to abnormal squeezing or compression of the chest. Recent rib fractures, unless displaced, may be difficult to detect radiographically and may only be seen in the healing phase. Small children's ribs are relatively pliable compared to adults and will tend to bend rather than fracture with compressive forces. It is exceptionally unusual to fracture a child's ribs during cardio-pulmonary resuscitation in a child with a normal skeleton. The presence of a rib fracture, recent or healed, is a significant finding. Metaphyseal fractures seen in the shoulders on a CXR, are significant.

Skull fractures may occur in small infants who fall from a significant height onto a hard floor, but are rarely seen when a child rolls off a sofa onto a carpeted floor. Femoral and humeral fractures occur infrequently in domestic accidents in infants. The history always needs to be correlated with the clinical and radiographical findings.

In suspected non-accidental injury the child should be protected from further assault and further assessment made. In physical abuse of children under the age of 2 years this involves a full skeletal survey. A skeletal survey can only be performed after adequate explanation to the child's carers and does not normally need to be performed in the emergency situation. The components of a skeletal survey are shown in the box.

- Front and lateral skull films
- Lateral whole spine
- CXR
- AP views of all the long bones
- AP views of lumbar spine, pelvis and hips
- Supplemented with lateral views of the metaphyses where there is any suspected abnormality or clinical symptoms
- Neurocranial imaging (e.g. CT and/or MRI) as appropriate to the child's symptoms

Diagnosis

Classic pointers to the diagnosis of inflicted injury are:

- There is delay in seeking medical help or medical help is not sought at all.
- The story of the "accident" is vague, is lacking in detail, and may vary with each telling and from person to person. Innocent accidents tend to have vivid accounts that ring true.
- The account of the accident is not compatible with the injury observed.
- The parents' affect is abnormal. Normal parents are full of anxiety for the child who has been injured. Abusing parents tend to be more preoccupied with their own problems – for example, how they can return home as soon as possible.
- The parents' behaviour gives cause for concern. They may become hostile, rebut accusations that have not been made, or leave before the consultant arrives.
- The child's appearance and his interaction with his parents are abnormal. He may look sad, withdrawn, or frightened. There may be visible evidence of a failure to

thrive. Full-blown frozen watchfulness is a late stage and results from repetitive physical and emotional abuse over a period of time.

- The child may disclose abuse. Always make a point of talking to the child in a safe place in private if the child is old enough to be separated from the parents. Interviewing the child as an outpatient may fail to let the child open up as he is expecting to be returned home in the near future. He may disclose more in the safety of a foster home.

At the end of the medical assessment the diagnosis may be clear. More often the doctor has a differential diagnosis which includes abuse. Discussion then takes place between the social workers, health care workers, and police officers who have information about the family to balance the probabilities of abuse having occurred. In familial abuse a child protection conference will be held as soon as possible. In the meantime it may be necessary to arrange for the child to be taken to a place of safety (see "Emergency Protection Orders").

MANAGEMENT

All child protection work is based on cooperation between families, social workers, police officers, health care workers, and educationalists. This multi-agency approach is to ensure that all aspects of the care of the family are considered when decisions are being made. Certain decisions in management must be made by one profession, e.g. only a doctor can decide on the treatment required for fracture, only a police officer can decide the charge that is appropriate for the alleged offence. However, whenever possible, unilateral decisions are avoided in the best interests of the child and the family.

Some doctors are reluctant to share information with other professionals because of the ethical consideration of confidentiality. However, the Annual Standards Committee of the Council of the General Medical Council in November 1987 expressed the view that, if a doctor has reason for believing that a child is being physically or sexually abused, not only is it permissible for the doctor to disclose information to a third party but it is a duty of the doctor to do so. This is still the stance of the General Medical Council.

When the diagnosis is one of child abuse then the decisions to be made on management are the following:

- Does the child need admission for treatment of the injuries?
- Will the child be safe if returned home?
- If the child needs protection from an abuser who is in his or her own home, how can this be done?
- What support/protection is needed for the rest of the family?

If the alleged abuser is not in the same household as the child and the caregivers can protect the child, then he or she can return home. If the alleged abuser is in the same household as the child but is in custody, then the child will still be safe at home with another caregiver. When a person is charged and is allowed bail, one condition must be that he or she lives away from the household of the child. If this is not done then alternative care will be needed for the child.

Whenever there is a disclosure or suspicion of abuse, then the whole family needs support. Siblings may have been at risk of injury and so will need to be assessed. Spouses may be ambiguous in their loyalties to the child and to the alleged abuser. The child will need much support to withstand the stress of the investigation, especially if there are subsequent legal proceedings.

The details of management of these many facets are decided in the child protection conference. In this all the professional people meet with the family to collate information and to produce a plan of care.

286

MEDICOLEGAL ASPECTS

Health care professionals must be familiar with the medicolegal aspects of their work. The most important are the following:

- Emergency Protection Orders, Child Assessment Orders, Residence Orders, Police Protection Orders.
- Consent to examination.
- Writing of statements and reports for criminal and civil proceedings.
- Presentation of evidence.

Emergency Protection Order (EPO)

The Emergency Protection Order (Children Act 1989, sections 44 and 45) replaced the Place of Safety Order. It may be made for a maximum of 8 days with a possible further extension of up to 7 days. An application for discharge of that order may be made. The court may only make the order if it is satisfied that there is reasonable cause to believe that the child is likely to suffer significant harm if either he is not removed to another place or if his removal from a safe place (such as a hospital) is not prevented. Another clause is that, in the case of an application made by a Social Services Department or the NSPCC, the applicant "has reasonable cause to suspect that a child is suffering or is likely to suffer significant harm" and enquiries which are being made with respect to the child "are frustrated by access to the child being unreasonably refused" and the applicant believes that access is required as a matter of urgency.

Child Assessment Order (CAO)

This Order (Children Act 1989, section 43) addresses those situations where there is good cause to suspect that a child is suffering or is likely to suffer significant harm but is not at immediate risk, and the applicant believes that an assessment (medical, psychiatric, or other) is required. If the parents are unwilling to cooperate, the Social Services Department or the NSPCC can apply for a Child Assessment Order. The Order has a maximum duration of 7 days from the date on which it comes into effect. The court will direct the type and nature of the assessment that is to be carried out, and whether the child should be kept away from home for the purposes of the assessment. A child of reasonable understanding may refuse to have this assessment. Lawyers suggest that a child of reasonable understanding is a normal child of 10 years of age or more.

Residence Order

A Residence Order states with whom the child is to live. It has the effect of ending any care order and gives parental responsibility to the person with the order.

Police Protection Order

A constable has powers (Children Act 1989, section 46) to take a child "into Police protection" for up to 72 hours. This power can be used to prevent the removal of a child from hospital.

Consent to examination

Consent for all examinations that are for evidential purposes must be obtained from a person with parental responsibility. In the Children Act 1989 (section 3), parental responsibility is defined as "all the rights, duties, powers, responsibilities and authority which by law a parent has in relation to the child and his property". Those with parental responsibility are specified in the Children Act 1989 (section 2). This can be summarised as in the box.

Parental responsibility
- Parents married at time of birth both have parental responsibility which continues after separation or divorce
- An unmarried mother has parental responsibility
- An unmarried father can apply to obtain parental responsibility; he can be appointed a guardian or if he can prove paternity then he can have the same legal position as if married
- Person in whose favour a Residence Order has been made – this is for the duration of the Order
- Appointed Guardian
- Local Authority while a Care Order is in force
- Person who applied for an Emergency Protection Order

When more than one person has parental responsibility, each of them can act alone and without the other in meeting that responsibility. Parents do not lose parental responsibility if a Care Order or an Emergency Protection Order is in force. Parents lose parental responsibility with an Adoption Order. Parental responsibility can be delegated to a person acting on their behalf, e.g. while they are on holiday.

To cover emergency situations, those caring for a child who do not have parental responsibility may do what is reasonable in all the circumstances for the purpose of safeguarding or promoting the child's welfare.

Consent from the child or young person is needed if that person is of sufficient understanding to make an informed decision. Lawyers suggest that in a normal child this would be at age 10 years. The Gillick ruling (1986) allows an individual under the age of 16 years to submit to examination and treatment without the parents being informed, provided that is the wish of the child or young person.

Court reports

When preparing a written report on a child for the court all health care professionals should keep in mind that the written report may be used in subsequent court appearances. Therefore, the report should be confined to the facts. Whenever possible, objective and measurable evidence of the child's health and development should be presented. Where subjective views must be given they should reflect balanced professional judgement. If the report is comprehensive and comprehensible, then the health care professional may not be called to give verbal evidence in person. Always keep a copy of the report and a photocopy of the original notes if they have to be filed in a general filing system. All court personnel will ask for the original notes to be produced, but if these have gone missing then a photocopy may be acceptable. For the health care professional this is essential for good evidence.

Statements

The purpose of a statement is to provide the court with an informative and relevant account of the medical assessment of the child. The statement will give details of the persons involved, the observations, and the findings. Information given by another person should not be included unless this has been requested. In many areas, the Crown Prosecution Service wish statements to record all information although hearsay may be excluded before presentation to the court.

A statement is a professional document. It should be well written in good basic English. Technical terms should be avoided or, if quoted, should be followed immediately by appropriate lay terms. Most statements will be for the prosecution and a printed statement form will be provided. The standard sequence of writing a statement is as shown in the box.

Sequence for writing a statement

1. Full name with surname in capitals
2. Qualifications
3. Occupation
4. Name of person requesting the assessment
5. Date, time, and place of the assessment
6. Name of person who was examined
7. Name of persons present
8. Details of the relevant history – if general history taken produced nothing significant then make a general comment including the sight of the detailed notes
9. Details of examination – if joint examination then specify who did each part
10. Investigations
11. Opinion on findings
12. The time at which examination ended

Each page must be signed at the bottom and the final page must be signed on the line below the completion of the writing. Any alterations must be initialled.

Always keep a copy of the statement.

Presentation of evidence

Dress in a professional manner. Arrive early in court. Take along all notes relevant to the case. Revise these on the day before the court proceedings. With permission from the magistrate or judge, you may refer to contemporaneous notes. However, revision helps to put the whole picture of the incident into the forefront of your mind so that you can find the appropriate notes more quickly.

When giving evidence stay calm even if the barrister becomes abusive. Do not be persuaded to answer questions which are outside your knowledge or experience.

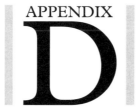

APPENDIX

D

Childhood accidents and their prevention

INTRODUCTION

Child accident and, injury prevention is important because of the following:

- On average, one to two children die in accidents every day.
- Accidents are the most common cause of death among children aged 1 to 14 years.
- Accidents cause a third of deaths of children aged between 10 and 14 years.
- Accidents result in about 10 000 children being permanently disabled annually.
- Accidents cause one child in five to attend an accident and emergency department every year.
- Accidents lead to one-fifth of all hospital paediatric admissions.

To put it another way, accidental injury to children leads to about 500 deaths, 120 000 hospital admissions and about 2 million Accident and Emergency department attendances in England and Wales every year.

This is the bad news about children's accidents. The good news is that they may often be prevented. This is because accidents are predictable. They are closely linked to the child, his or her circumstances, and development. There are measures available that can prevent accidents completely or diminish their impact measures that are applicable to a variety of fields.

RISK FACTORS

Who is most at risk? There are definite predisposing factors which enable high-risk groups to be identified.

Sex

Boys are more frequently injured than girls. The difference emerges at age 1–2 years. How much of this difference is innate and how much cultural is a subject for speculation. Girls may mature more rapidly in terms of perception and coordination.

291

Age

Children's accidents are intimately related to development. Take falls as an example. A newborn baby can only fall if dropped, or if a parent falls holding the baby. An older baby can wriggle and roll off a changing table or a bed. A crawling baby can climb upstairs and fall back. A small child can climb and fall out of a window. An older child can climb a tree, or fall in a playground. Knowledge of development helps in anticipation of dangers. Exposure to different circumstances also varies with age. Children under 5 years experience accidents at home. School-age children experience accidents at school, sport, and play, and are especially at risk of accidental deaths as pedestrians and cyclists.

Social class

As with so many other health problems, accidents are linked to inequalities in environments. Children in social class V, derived from head of household's occupation, are twice as likely to die from an accident as children in social class I and, for some accident types, such as burns, the chances are six times higher.

This does not mean that working-class parents care less about their children than middle-class parents, or that they do not know about accident risks. It may mean that there are many other pressures – overcrowding, lack of money, poor housing – and there is less power – owning one's own home, being able to afford safety equipment – to make changes for safety.

The provision of safe places for children to play is more difficult for lower income families.

Psychological factors

Accidents are more common in families where there is stress from mental illness, marital discord, moving home, and a variety of similar factors.

Ethnic origin

On the whole, social class is more important than ethnic origin in determining accident risk.

ACCIDENT PREVENTION

How can injuries be prevented? There are a number of basic principles.

Accidents can be prevented completely. This is termed "primary prevention". An example is a fireguard preventing access to an open fire. The harm caused by an accident can be minimised. This is "secondary prevention". For example, a seat belt can reduce injury even if a car crash occurs. Finally, rapid attention to an injury can reduce mortality and morbidity. This is "tertiary prevention". Examples are cold water on burns and scalds, or pressing on a laceration.

There are three main approaches to accident prevention. These are the following.

Education

Increasing knowledge about a problem and the solutions, to change attitudes and eventually behaviour. This does not just mean the family's behaviour but the behaviour of the whole community. For example: driving at or below the speed limit and avoiding "short cuts" through residential areas.

Engineering

Safe design of products and the environment, including the architecture of the home. Installation and upkeep of proven safety devices like smoke alarms. The use of cycle helmets.

Enforcement

The role of legislation, regulations, and standards in accident prevention.

Countermeasures can be active, i.e. a conscious decision to use them has to be taken every time. This could be putting pans on the back hobs of the cooker. They can be passive, i.e. built in to the product. For example, junior formulations of paracetamol are sold in small bottles that do not contain a lethal dose

How can individuals participate in reducing children's injuries? There are a variety of things they can do.

Be informed
This can be at a personal level. Organisations such as the Child Accident Prevention Trust, the Royal Society for the Prevention of Accidents can provide information.

Set a good example
Wear your seat belt. Drive carefully past schools. Consider your own home and family with safety in mind.

Take opportunities
Can you offer safety advice to a family after an accident has happened? Do you know possible preventive strategies for that accident type?

Can you photograph that injured child in that setting, and use it to support a family in improving their household, or a neighbourhood in a media campaign?

Collaborate with others
Be prepared to participate in working groups and campaigns. You have special expertise and influence to offer.

Children's accidents and injuries are the major public health problem to children in Britain today. Every one should learn more about them and have something to offer in reducing their toll.

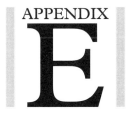

Dealing with death

As already stressed the outcome for attempted resuscitation for cardiorespiratory arrest in childhood is poor. This is particularly so in out of hospital arrest and in the case of "cot death" where the infant is usually not discovered until resuscitation is impossible.

Unless there has been a clear written and agreed "do not resuscitate" (DNR) order, resuscitation should be undertaken. Parental presence during the procedure is becoming increasingly common, this should be a decision for both parents and staff. If parents are present during resuscitation then a member of staff must be available exclusively for their support.

Breaking the news

Telling the parents that their child is dead is a difficult task, usually undertaken by senior staff. Once the patient has been certified dead do not keep the parents waiting in false hope. A direct and sympathetic approach is best. On entering the room sit down with the parents, having ensured that you know the child's name. The news should be broken sympathetically but without euphemisms to the parents. If it is appropriate and you feel comfortable doing it you can show sympathy by holding the parent's hand or putting an arm around them. Usually the parents will turn away towards each other for a while but may wish to ask questions about the cause of death and what they should do now. If you are asked about the cause of death answer as simply and honestly as you can, making it clear that some answers are not yet available.

A check list is then invaluable for ensuring that procedures or information are not forgotten. In the event of cot death or suspicious death there are usually local procedures concerning immediate postmortem sampling. Ensure that these are followed.

Sympathetic and sensitive support of the family by emergency department or paediatric staff can do much to help the process of adjustment to the bereavement. Encourage the family to spend time with their dead child, touching and holding. Facilitate their return to see their child on subsequent days. Accept their obvious distress as natural and support them in this. Each institution will have its own bereavement support programme: ensure that you are familiar with local resources and that the family are contacted for support and medical advice following any postmortem examination.

At the end of a shift spent coping with the sudden death of a child staff will be under great stress. They should be supported in this work by being taught about it beforehand and by staff counselling sessions afterwards.

The child

- Full and thorough examination
- Core temperature
- Wrap child in clean warm clothes for parents to see and hold

The parents

- Explain that the child (use name) has died
- Gently get as full a history as possible
- Ask if they would like a priest/religious leader present
- Ask if they want any close relative to be contacted
- Encourage the parents to see and hold the child
- Let them know if a postmortem examination needs to be carried out and ensure that they understand all that they wish to know about the procedure and have given their written consent where appropriate
- Let them know that police are always informed of sudden unexpected deaths and will need to ask a few simple questions of the carers
- Ask what address the family will be going to on leaving hospital
- Arrange transport from hospital to home and if alone make sure they are accompanied on the journey and not left alone at home
- Be gentle, unhurried, calm and careful
- Do not guess at the diagnosis

Obtain details of

- Child's and parents' names
- Child's date of birth
- Address at which death occured
- Time of arrival in department
- Time last seen alive
- Usual address if different from above

Inform

- GP – advise of child's death and give address to which parents will be going from hospital
- Health visitor
- Social worker
- Any relative as requsted by the family
- Coroner – who will need to know the full name and address and DOB of child, time of arrival, place of death, brief recent history, any suspicious circumstances

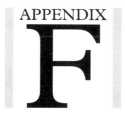

APPENDIX F

Management of pain in children

In general, children, especially very young ones, are under-treated for pain. They receive fewer, smaller doses of opiate drugs and instead are prescribed less powerful analgesics than adults. The reasons for this include:

- Fear of the harmful side effects.
- Failure to accept that children, especially infants, feel pain like adults.
- Fear of inducing addiction.
- The child's fear of receiving intramuscular injections.

Inadequate analgesia can be detrimental in the critically ill child. Bronchoconstriction and increases in pulmonary vascular resistance caused by pain can lead to hypoxia.

RECOGNITION AND ASSESSMENT OF PAIN

There are four main ways in which we recognise that a child is in pain:

- A description from the child or parent.
- Behavioural changes such as crying, guarding of the injured part, facial grimacing.
- Physiological changes such as pallor, tachycardia and tachypnoea, which are observed by the clinician.
- An expectation of pain because of the pathophysiology involved, e.g. fracture, burn or other significant trauma.

The purpose of pain assessment is to establish, as far as possible, the degree of pain experienced by the child so as to select the right level of pain relief. Additionally, re-assessment using the same pain tool will indicate whether the pain management has been successful or whether further analgesia is required. The ideal pain assessment tool would be simple and quick to use, have been validated and would give reliable reproducible results which took account of both patient and observer data. To date, no pain tool fulfils all these criteria. The following are two pain scales for older and for younger children and a combination of these is shown in Figure F.1.

1. *The pain ladder.* Suitable for children of 8 years and older.
2. *Faces scale.* These are for children from 4 to 8 years.

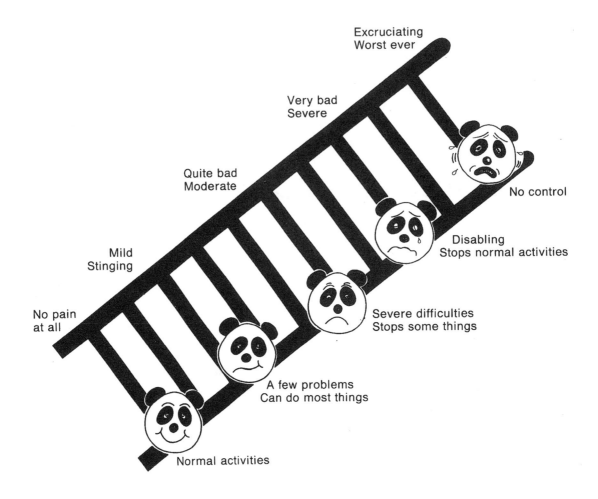

Figure F.1.   Continued pain scale

PAIN MANAGEMENT

Environment

The Emergency department and the treatment room on the paediatric ward are frightening places for children. Negative aspects of the environment should be removed or minimised. This includes an overly "clinical" appearance and evidence of invasive instruments. An attractive, decorated environment with toys, mobiles and pictures should be substituted.

Preparation

Except in a life-threatening emergency or when dealing with an unconscious child, an explanation of the procedure to be undertaken and the pain relief planned should be given to the child and his parents. If time permits, they should contribute to the pain management plan by relating previous pain experiences and successful relief measures.

Physical treatments: supportive and distractive techniques

The presence of parents during an invasive procedure on their child is important. In one study almost all children between the ages of 9 and 12 reported that "the thing that helped most" was to have a parent present during a painful procedure. As well as being present, parents need some guidance on how to help their child during the procedure. Studies suggest that talking to and touching the child during the procedure is both soothing and anxiety-relieving. Other distractive strategies include:

- Looking at pop-up books.
- Listening through headphones to stories or music.
- Blowing bubbles.
- Video or interactive computer game.
- Moving images projected on a nearby wall, e.g. fish swimming, birds flying.
- Presence of transitional objects (comforters), e.g. favourite blanket, soft toy.

Pharmacological treatment

Local anaesthetics: topical
Emla (Eutectic mixture of local anaesthetics) This is a mixture of lignocaine 2·5% and prilocaine 2·5% which is applied under an occlusive dressing over the site planned for venesection or cannulation.

- Takes 45–60 minutes to be effective.
- Irritates the skin if left on for more than 2 hours.
- Can be toxic if swallowed.
- Can only be used on intact skin.
- Can induce vasoconstriction lasting approximately 15 minutes after the cream is removed.
- The analgesia produced lasts for about an hour.
- Can cause sensitisation on repeated exposure.

Ametop gel This contains amethocaine base 4%.

- Used under an occlusive dressing.
- Analgesia achieved after 30–45 minutes.
- Anaesthesia remains for 4–6 hours after removal of gel.
- Slight erythema, itching, and oedema may occur at site but capillary vessels may be dilated making venesection easier.
- Not to be applied on broken skin, mucous membranes, eyes or ears.
- Can cause sensitisation on repeated exposure.

Local anaesthetics: infiltrated
Lignocaine 1% lignocaine is used for rapid and intense sensory nerve block.

- The onset of action is significant within 2 minutes and is effective for up to 2 hours.
- Often used with epinephrine (adrenaline) to prolong the duration of sensory blockade and limit toxicity by reducing absorption – epinephrine concentration 5 μg/ml. Epinephrine containing local anaesthetic should not be used in areas served by an end artery such as a digit.
- Maximum dose given locally 3 mg/kg.

Bupivacaine This local anaesthetic is used at a concentration of 0·5% when longer-lasting local anaesthesia is required.

- The onset of anaesthesia is up to 15 minutes but its effects last up to 8 hours.
- Maximum dosage is 2 mg/kg.

Prilocaine   This local anaesthetic is associated with lower toxicity than bupivacaine. Its concentration is 0·5%.

Local anaesthetics are manufactured to a pH of 5 (to improve shelf life) and can be painful for this reason. A buffered solution and the use of smaller needles will lessen the pain associated with infiltration, but local epinephrine cannot then be used as it is inactivated by the bicarbonate buffer.

The suggested upper limits given are for local anaesthetics without the addition of epinephrine. Direct intra-arterial or intravenous injection of even a fraction of these doses may result in systemic toxicity or death.

Overdose or inadvertent circulatory injection of local anaesthetics results in cardiac arrhythmias and convulsions. Resuscitative facilities and skills must therefore be available where these drugs are injected.

Non-opiate analgesics

These drugs are analgesic, anti-pyretic, and anti-inflammatory to varying degrees.

Paracetamol   Paracetamol is probably the most widely used analgesic in paediatric practice. It is thought to work through inhibiting cyclo-oxygenase in the central nervous system, but not in other tissues so that it produces analgesia with no anti-inflammatory effect. It does not cause respiratory depression. It has a bad taste which has to be disguised. It is very dangerous in overdose but very safe in the recommended dose.

Non-steroidal anti-inflammatory drugs (NSAID)   These are anti-inflammatory and anti-pyretic drugs with moderate analgesic properties. They are less well tolerated than paracetamol, causing gastric irritation, platelet disorders and bronchospasm. They should therefore be avoided in children with a history of gastric ulceration, platelet abnormalities, and significant asthma. Their advantage is that they are especially useful for post-traumatic pain because of the additional anti-inflammatory effect. Ibuprofen is given by mouth and if rectal administration is necessary then diclofenac can be used.

Opiate analgesics

Morphine   Morphine is the standard for analgesia against which all other opiates are measured. When small doses are administered, analgesia occurs without loss of consciousness. It produces peripheral vasodilatation and venous pooling, but in single doses has minimal haemodynamic effect in a supine patient with normal circulating volume. In hypovolaemic patients it will contribute to hypotension but this is not a contraindication to its use and merely an indication for cardiovascular monitoring and action as appropriate. Opiates produce a dose-dependent depression of ventilation primarily by reducing the sensitivity of brain stem respiratory centres to hypercarbia and hypoxia. This means that the patient who has received a dose of an opiate requires observation and/or monitoring and should not be discharged home until the effects of the opiate are clearly significantly reduced. The nausea and vomiting produced in adults by morphine seems to be less common in children.

Parenteral morphine should always be given intravenously. The therapeutic effects and side effects are much more easily controlled with the IV or intraosseous route than with intramuscular injection.

Codeine   Oral codeine is almost always prescribed in combination with paracetamol for the treatment of moderate pain. It is a less potent opiate than morphine but similarly has less effects on the central nervous system. Codeine must not be given intravenously as it can cause profound hypotension.

Opiate antagonists

Naloxone Naloxone is a potent opiate antagonist. It antagonises the sedative, respiratory depressive, and analgesic effects of opiates. It is rapidly metabolised and is best given parenterally because of its rapid first pass extraction through the liver following oral administration. Following IV administration naloxone reverses the effects of opiates virtually immediately. Its duration of action, however, is much shorter than the opiate agonist. Therefore, repeated doses or an infusion may be required if continued opiate antagonism is wanted.

Entonox Nitrous oxide is a colourless, odourless gas that provides analgesia in sub-anaesthetic concentrations. It is supplied as a 50% mixture with oxygen to prevent hypoxia. Most devices act on a demand principle, i.e. the gas is only delivered when the patient inhales and applies a negative pressure. The patient has to be awake and cooperative to be able to inhale the gas; this is an obvious safeguard with the technique.

Because nitrous oxide is inhaled and has a low solubility in blood, its onset of effect is very rapid. It takes 2–3 minutes to achieve its peak effect. For the same reason, the drug wears off over several minutes enabling patients to recover considerably quicker than if they received narcotics or sedatives. Laryngeal protective reflexes do not always remain intact.

Nitrous oxide is therefore most suitable for procedures where short-lived intense analgesia is required, e.g. dressing changes, suturing, needle procedures such as venous cannulation, lumbar punctures and for pain relief during splinting or transport.

Entonox can be used by children as young as 5 years of age if they are well supported. The black rubber masks that are used are unacceptable to some children but a mouthpiece can overcome some of these problems.

Toxicity in the emergency situation is not a problem, but prolonged exposure to high concentrations can cause bone marrow depression and neuronal degeneration.

Entonox must not be used in children with possible intracranial or intrathoracic air since replacement of the air by Entonox may increase pressure.

Sedative drugs

In addition to analgesics, psychotropic drugs may also be useful when undertaking lengthy or repeated procedures. Sedatives relieve anxiety and not pain. They may reduce the child's ability to communicate discomfort and therefore should not be given in isolation. The problems associated with the use of sedatives are those of side effects (usually hyperexcitability) and the time required for the child to be awake enough to be allowed home if admission is not necessary.

Midazolam This is an amnesic and sedative drug. It can be given orally or intranasally. It has an onset time of action of 15 minutes and recovery occurs after about an hour. In some cases there is respiratory depression necessitating monitoring of respiratory rate and depth and pulse oximetry. A few children become hyperexcitable with this drug. Its action can be reversed by flumazenil intravenously.

SPECIFIC CLINICAL SITUATIONS

Severe pain

Children in severe pain (e.g. major trauma, femoral fracture, significant burns, displaced or comminuted fractures etc.) should receive IV morphine at an initial dose of 0·1–0·2 mg/kg infused over 2–3 minutes. A further dose can be given after 5–10 minutes if sufficient analgesia is not achieved. The patient should be monitored using pulse oximetry and electrocardiography.

301

Analgesic	Pain severity	Single dose	Duration of effect	Common side effects	Comments
Morphine IV	Moderate to severe	Over 1 yr: 0·1–0·2 mg/kg 3 months to 1yr: 0·05–0·1 mg/kg 0–3 mth: 0·025 mg/kg	4 hr	Respiratory depression Hypotension	Monitor respiration and pulse oximetry ECG
Morphine oral	Moderate	Over 1yr: 0·2–0·4 mg/kg Under 1 yr: 0·1–0·2 mg/kg	4 hr		Observe respiration
Codeine	Mild to moderate	Oral 1–1·5 mg/kg	4–6 hr		Avoid in patients <1yr Do not give IV
Paracetamol	Mild	Over 3 months: 15 mg/kg orally or rectally	4–6 hr		Avoid in liver impairment
Ibuprofen	Mild to moderate	5 mg/kg	4–6 hr	Avoid in asthmatics	Not recommended for patients <10 kg
Diclofenac	Moderate	1 mg/kg orally or rectally	8 hr	Avoid in asthmatics	Not for patients under the age of 1yr
Midazolam	Not analgesic	0·5 mg/kg orally		Respiratory depression Hyperexcitability	Monitor Sao_2

Head injuries

There is often concern about giving morphine to a patient who has had a head injury and who could therefore potentially lose consciousness secondary to the head injury. If the patient is conscious and in pain then the presence of a potential deteriorating head injury is not a contraindication to giving morphine. First, an analgesic dose is not necessarily a significant sedative; secondly, if the child's conscious level does deteriorate, then the clinician's first action should be to assess airway, breathing, and circulation, intervening where appropriate. If these are stable then a dose of naloxone will quickly ascertain whether the diminished conscious level is secondary to morphine or (as is much more likely) represents increasing intracranial pressure. There are significant benefits for the head injured patient in receiving adequate pain relief as the physiological response to pain may increase intracranial pressure.

In the common situation of the patient who has an isolated femoral shaft fracture and a possible head injury, a femoral nerve block may be an effective alternative (see Chapter 24).

Emergency venepuncture and venous cannulation

At present the management of this problem is difficult as anaesthetics take up to an hour to be effective. Alternatives in an emergency include an ice cube inside the finger of a plastic glove placed over the vein to be cannulated or local anaesthetic infiltration (1% buffered lignocaine) using a very fine gauge, e.g. 29 G, needle. Of course, in some instances the urgency of the situation is such that no local anaesthetic can be used.

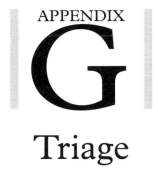

APPENDIX

G
Triage

INTRODUCTION

Nurse triage requires that each child presenting with potentially serious illness or injury is assigned a clinical priority. As such the triage process can be seen to be an extension of the process of recognition of the seriously ill or injured child that has been discussed earlier.

In the United Kingdom (UK), Canada and Australia five part national triage scales have been agreed. The UK scale is shown in the table below. While the names of the triage categories and the target times assigned to each name vary from country to country, the underlying concept does not.

Table G.1. The UK triage scale

Number	Name	Colour	Max time (min)
1	Immediate	Red	0
2	Very urgent	Orange	10
3	Urgent	Yellow	60
4	Standard	Green	120
5	Non-urgent	Blue	240

TRIAGE DECISION MAKING

There are many models of decision making each requiring three basic steps. These are identification of a problem, determination of the alternatives and selection of the most appropriate alternative. The commonest triage method is that developed by the Manchester Triage Group. This method uses the following five steps:

- Identifying the problem
- Gathering and analysing information related to the solution
- Evaluating all the alternatives and selecting one for implementation
- Implementing the selected alternative
- Monitoring the implementation and evaluation of outcomes

Identify the problem

This is done by taking a brief and focused history from the child, their parents and/or any pre-hospital care personnel. This phase is always necessary whatever method is being used.

Gather and analyse information related to the solution

Once the presentation has been identified, discriminators can be sought at each level. Discriminators, as their name implies, are factors that discriminate between patients such that they allow them to be allocated to one of the five clinical priorities. They can be *general* or *specific*. The former apply to all patients irrespective of their presentation, whilst the latter tend to relate to key features of particular conditions. Thus severe pain is a general discriminator, but *cardiac pain* and *pleuritic pain* are specific discriminators. General discriminators would include life threat, pain, haemorrhage, conscious level and temperature.

Life threat
To an APLS provider *life threat* is perhaps the most obvious general discriminator of all. Any cessation or threat to the vital (ABC) functions means that the patient is in the immediate group. Thus the presence of an insecure airway, inspiratory or expiratory stridor, absent or inadequate breathing, or shock are all significant.

Pain
From the child and parents perspective pain is a major factor in determining priority. Pain assessment and management is dealt with elsewhere in this book and not reiterated here. Children with severe pain should be allocated to the very urgent category while those with moderate pain should be allocated to the urgent category. Any child with any lesser degree of pain should be allocated to the standard category.

Haemorrhage
Haemorrhage is a feature of many presentations particularly those following trauma. If haemorrhage is exsanguinating, death will ensue rapidly unless bleeding is stopped. These children must be treated immediately. A haemorrhage that is not rapidly controlled by the application of sustained direct pressure, and which continues to bleed heavily or soak through large dressings quickly, should be treated very urgently.

Conscious level
All unresponsive children must be an immediate priority, and those who respond to voice or pain only are categorised as very urgent. Children with a history of unconsciousness should be allocated to the urgent category.

Temperature

Temperature is used as a general discriminator. It may be difficult to obtain an accurate measurement during the triage process, although modern rapid reading tympanic membrane thermometers should make this aim attainable. A hot child (over 38·5°C) is always seen very urgently, as are children who are cold (less than 32°C).

Evaluate all alternatives and select one for implementation

Clinicians collect a huge amount of information about the children they deal with. The data is compared to internal frameworks that act as guides for assessment. The presentational flow diagrams developed by the Manchester Triage Group provide the organisational framework to order the thought process during triage.

Implement the selected alternative

As previously noted there are only five possible triage categories to select from and these have specific names and definitions. The urgency of the patient's condition determines their clinical priority. Once the priority is allocated the appropriate pathway of care begins.

Monitor the implementation and evaluate outcomes

Triage categories may change as the child deteriorates or gets better. It is important, therefore, that the process of triage (clinical prioritisation) is dynamic rather than static. To achieve this end all clinicians involved in the pathway of care should rapidly assess priority whenever they encounter the child. Furthermore any changes in priority must be noted and the appropriate actions taken.

SECONDARY TRIAGE

It may not be possible to carry out all the assessments necessary at the initial triage encounter – this is particularly so if the workload of the department is high. In such circumstances the necessary assessments should still be carried out, but as secondary procedures by a receiving nurse. The actual initial clinical priority cannot be set until the process is finished. More time consuming assessments (such as blood glucose estimation and peak flow measurement) are often left to the secondary stage.

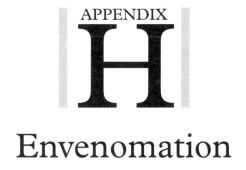

APPENDIX

H

Envenomation

INTRODUCTION

Australia has a wide variety of venomous terrestrial and marine creatures (Table H.1). Of these, the species which cause the most frequent or serious envenomation are some species of snakes, spiders and jellyfish. The number of deaths from snake bite per annum (2–5) is approximately equal to the number of deaths from bee sting anaphylaxis.

Table H.1. Australian venomous creatures, effects of venom and treatment

Creature	Main effects	Main treatment
Snake (many species)	Paralysis (rapid), Haemorrhage	Pressure-immobilisation Antivenom Mechanical ventilation Blood products
Sydney Funnel-web spider	Paralysis (rapid)	Pressure-immobilisation bandage Antivenom
Red-back spider	Pain	Antivenom
Australian paralysis tick	Paralysis (slow)	Remove tick Antivenom
Bees, wasps and ants	Anaphylaxis	Pressure-immobilisation bandage Epinephrine (adrenaline)
Box jellyfish	Paralysis (rapid), Hypotension	Dowsing with vinegar Pressure-immobilisation bandage Antivenom Mechanical ventilation
Blue-ringed octopus	Paralysis (rapid)	Pressure-immobilisation bandage Mechanical ventilation
Stone fish	Pain	Antivenom Analgesia, regional nerve blockade

SNAKE BITE

Australia has over a hundred species of snakes of which about a dozen are among the world's most deadly. The main components of venoms include pre- and post-synaptic neurotoxins which cause the rapid onset of paralysis, and consequent bulbar palsy and respiratory failure. Many venoms also contain prothrombin activators which cause disseminated intravascular coagulation. The coagulopathy is characterised by a consumption of clotting factors including fibrinogen, and often by the secondary generation of fibrin degradation products by endogenous plasmin.

The main consequence of the coagulopathy is spontaneous haemorrhage from mucosal surfaces and from needle sticks. Although the venoms of different species have different effects, the two most common acute threats to life are neuromuscular paralysis with respiratory failure and coagulopathy causing bleeding.

One of the difficulties in the management of snake bite may be to determine whether envenomation has actually occurred irrespective of whether a bite by a snake was observed or not. Snakes may bite and fail to inject venom in approximately 40–50% of occasions. In young children, particularly, snake bite is suspected even though a snake was not observed. In approximately 25% of snake bite presentations envenomation has occurred.

The syndrome of serious envenomation is characterised by a rapid onset of paralysis accompanied by coagulopathy over minutes to several hours. However, an early diagnosis may be made by subtle clinical signs, characteristic symptoms, abnormal laboratory tests of coagulation and a positive test for venom at a bite-site, or in the patient's urine or blood. Some early reliable symptoms of envenomation are headache, abdominal pain and vomiting. Abnormal laboratory tests of coagulation are also very sensitive and reliable – if the bite was by a species with coagulopathic venom.

The onset of weakness of large muscles, including respiratory muscles, is preceded by weakness of the bulbar muscles so that it is imperative to enquire and seek evidence of dysfunction of the external ocular muscles (double vision, ophthalmoplegia), facial muscles (ptosis) and the muscles of speech and swallowing (dysphonia, dysphagia).

The diagnosis may be confirmed with the snake venom detection kit test (CSL Diagnostics). This is a rapid three-step enzyme immunoassay designed for clinical use. It gives a result in approximately 25 minutes and is capable of detecting venom in a concentration of as little as 10 ng/ml. The test can be performed with a swab from the bite site or with the patient's blood or urine. The test indicates which antivenom to use, and does not necessarily identify the species of snake. As with any test there may be false positive or false negative results.

Principles of treatment of snake bite

- To prevent rapid absorption of the venom from the subcutaneous tissue into the circulation by application of a pressure-immobilisation bandage.
- To neutralise the venom by the administration of antivenom.
- To treat the effects of the venom, principally acute respiratory failure and bleeding, and medium term renal failure.

The management of suspected and definite envenomation is summarised in the boxes.

Pressure-immobilisation first-aid

The pressure-immobilisation technique is applicable only to bites on the limbs (where most bites occur). Snake venoms gain access from the subcutaneous tissue to the

Management of suspected snake envenomation

At scene
- Apply pressure-immobolisation bandage
- Transport to hospital

In hospital
- Confirm stock of antivenom
- Check resuscitation equipment
- Remove pressure-immobilisation bandage
- Observe closely
- Perform test of coagulation
- Test urine, blood and bite site for venom

Management of definite snake envenomation

- Resuscitate (airway protection, mechanical ventilation, cardiovascular support)
- Apply pressure-immobilisation bandage or if already applied, do not remove
- Administer antivenom(s), premedicate first
- Test coagulation, treat coagulopathy with antivenom and clotting factors, until resolved
- Remove pressure-immobilisation bandage, reassess

circulation via the lymphatics which can be effectively occluded by the application of a continuous firm crepe bandage. It is initially applied to the fingers or toes (immobilising them), then continued over the bite site and then proximally up the limb. The bandage should be as tight as for a sprained ankle but not as tight as a tourniquet. A splint is then applied to the limb, including the joints on either side of the bite to further immobilise the limb. These measures prevent the use of surrounding muscle groups and hence lymph flow.

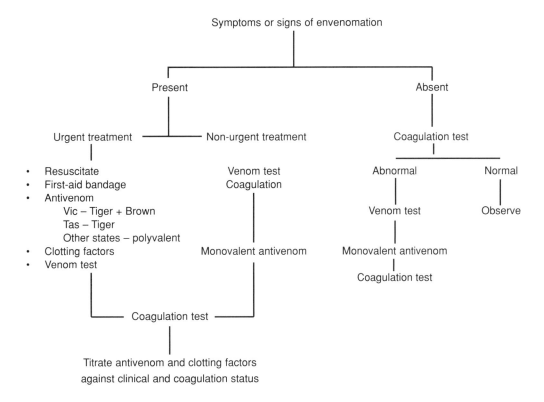

Figure H.1. Management of snake envenomation

Although the technique is a first-aid measure which should be applied at the scene of snake bite to prevent initial absorption of venom, it is also useful in established envenomation in hospital to prevent additional absorption of venom while preparations are being made to administer antivenom. If applied correctly, the bandage can be left in place indefinitely. However, the bandage does not inactivate the venom and should be removed after an asymptomatic patient reaches a hospital which has a stock of antivenom or after an envenomated patient has been given antivenom. Note however, it is dangerous to remove a bandage from an envenomated patient before administration of antivenom because its release allows a substantial additional quantity of venom to gain rapid access to the circulation. The bandage should not be removed solely to allow inspection of the bite site of an envenomated patient as no additional information is to be gained. To allow swabbing of the bite site, a hole may be made in a bandage and the bandage then reinforced.

Antivenom selection

Specific monovalent antivenoms (Commonwealth Serum Laboratories, Melbourne) are available against Tiger, Brown, Taipan, Black, Death Adder and Sea snake envenomation. A mixture of the first five terrestrial antivenoms is available as a polyvalent preparation. Antivenoms are highly purified equine immunoglobulins. Cross reactivity between species is limited, so that it is important to administer the correct antivenom according to the identity of the snake.

If the identity of the snake is not known the type of antivenom to be administered is based on the known snake distribution. In Tasmania, where the snakes are (Black) Tiger snakes and Copperheads, the appropriate antivenom is Tiger snake antivenom. In Victoria where the dangerous species are Tiger, Brown, Black and Copperhead snakes, the appropriate antivenoms are Tiger plus Brown snake antivenom. Elsewhere in Australia, the polyvalent preparation should be chosen.

Premedication before antivenom

Although essential and life saving, antivenoms are foreign proteins and may cause a life-threatening anaphylactoid reaction. However, this may be prevented or ameliorated by premedication with subcutaneous (not intravenously or intramuscularly) epinephrine 5–10 micrograms/kg. Additional protective agents such as a steroid (hydrocortisone) and an antihistamine may be indicated if the patient has a known allergic history.

Dose of antivenom

The dose of antivenom cannot be stated with certainty at the beginning of treatment because the amount of venom injected is unknown. Each ampoule of antivenom contains enough to neutralise the average yield from one snake bite. However, the amount of venom injected at biting is highly variable and bites may be multiple. Children are more susceptible than adults because of the larger venom-to-body-mass ratio. Although the majority of envenomations are treated adequately with 1–2 ampoules, many ampoules are usually required in life-threatening envenomations.

Antivenom should not be withheld if indicated as there is no other satisfactory treatment. Antivenom should be administered if there are clinical signs or symptoms of envenomation after snake bite or if a coagulopathy is present.

Antivenom neutralises venom but it does not, per se, restore coagulation; it allows newly manufactured or released clotting factors to act unimpeded. In the absence of a rapid bedside test for blood venom content, repeated laboratory tests of coagulation (prothrombin time, activated partial thromboplastin time, serum fibrinogen and fibrin degradation products) or bedside tests of bleeding should be performed to determine the need for more antivenom and coagulation factors. The coagulation status is the most sensitive guide to the need for additional antivenom after a bite by a coagulopathic species.

Resuscitation

In the severely envenomated patient, airway protection and mechanical ventilation may be required because of bulbar and respiratory muscle paralysis. Coagulopathy may cause massive haemorrhage from mucosal surfaces and consequent peripheral circulatory failure. Haemorrhage may occur into a vital organ, such as the brain. It is essential to restore the circulatory volume, and to normalise coagulation with antivenom and coagulation factors (fresh frozen plasma) if necessary.

If antivenom therapy is delayed, mechanical ventilation and artificial renal support may be required for many days or weeks.

Avoidable errors in management of snake bite

- Envenomation dismissed because of lack of obvious fang marks
- First-aid bandage released too soon causing rapid collapse
- Early paresis missed by inadequate observation
- Antivenom administered without appropriate premedication
- Wrong antivenom administered because of snake misidentification
- Inadequate quantity of antivenom administered
- Coagulation factors administered without adequate neutralisation of venom
- Coagulopathy allowed to persist untreated
- Renal failure not anticipated
- Antivenom administered to unenvenomated patient

SPIDER BITE

Several thousand species of spiders exist in Australia. Only Funnel-web spiders and Red-back spiders are known to be potentially lethal or cause significant morbidity.

Funnel-web spiders

A robustus (Sydney Funnel-web spider) is a large aggressive spider which has caused the deaths of more than a dozen people inhabiting an area within an approximate 160 km radius of Sydney. The male is more dangerous than the female (in contrast to other species) and are inclined to roam after rainfall, and in doing so may enter houses and seek shelter among clothes or bedding and give a painful bite when disturbed.

Bites do not always result in envenomation but envenomation may be rapidly fatal. The early features of the envenomation syndrome include nausea, vomiting, profuse sweating, salivation and abdominal pain. Life threatening features are usually heralded by the appearance of muscle fasciculation at the bite site which quickly involves distant muscle groups. Hypertension, tacharrhythmias and vasoconstriction occur. The victim may lapse into coma, develop hypoventilation and have difficulty maintaining an airway free of saliva. Finally, respiratory failure and severe hypotension culminate in hypoxaemia of the brain and heart. The syndrome may develop within several hours but it may be more rapid.

Treatment consists of the application of a pressure-immobilisation bandage, intravenous administration of antivenom and support of vital functions which may include artificial airway support and mechanical ventilation. No deaths or serious morbidity has been reported since introduction of the antivenom in the early 1980s.

Red-back spider

This spider is distributed all over Australia and is to be found outdoors in household gardens in suburban and rural areas. The adult female is easily identified. Its body is about 1 cm in size and has a distinct red or orange dorsal stripe over its abdomen. When disturbed it gives a pin-prick like bite. The site becomes inflamed and may be surrounded by local swelling. Over the following minutes to several hours, severe pain, exacerbated by movement, commences locally and may extend up the limb or radiate elsewhere. The pain may be accompanied by profuse sweating, headache, nausea, vomiting, abdominal pain, fever, hypertension, paraesthesias and rashes. In a small percentage of cases when treatment is delayed, progressive muscle paralysis may occur over many hours which would require mechanical ventilation. Muscle weakness and spasm may persist for months after the bite. Death has not occurred since introduction of an antivenom in the 1950s. If the effects of a bite are minor and confined to the bite site, antivenom may be withheld but otherwise, antivenom should be given intramuscularly, preceded by premedication (see Snake Bite) to prevent an anaphylactoid reaction. In contrast to a bite from a snake or Funnelweb spider, a bite from a Red-back spider is not immediately life-threatening. There is no effective first-aid but application of a cold pack or ice may relieve the pain.

JELLYFISH STINGS

Many species may cause significant illness. The most important is the Box jellyfish (*Chironex flecken*).

Box jellyfish

This is the most dangerous venomous creature in the world. It has caused at least 63 deaths in the waters off the north Australian coast. It has a cuboid body up to 30 cm in diameter and numerous tentacles which trail several metres. It is semi-transparent and difficult to see in shallow water. The tentacles are lined with millions of nematocysts which, on contact with skin, discharge a threaded barb which pierces subcutaneous tissue, including small blood vessels. Contact with the tentacles causes severe pain. Envenomation may cause death within several minutes. Death is probably due to both neurotoxic effects causing apnoea and direct cardiotoxicity although the precise mode of action of the venom is still unknown. The skin which sustains the injury may heal with disfiguring scars.

First-aid, which must be administered on the beach, consists of dousing the skin with acetic acid (vinegar) which inactivates undischarged nematocysts. Adherent tentacles can then be removed and a pressure-immobilization bandage applied.

Cardiopulmonary resuscitation may be required on the beach. An ovine antivenom is available but prevention is of paramount importance. Water must not be entered when jellyfish are known to be close inshore. Wet-suits, clothing and "stinger suits" offer protection.

APPENDIX

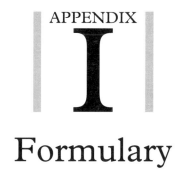

Formulary

The formulary is intended as a reference to be used in conjunction with this book. To this end the drugs mentioned elsewhere are set out alphabetically below, along with their routes of administration, dosage and some notes on their use.

GENERAL GUIDANCE ON THE USE OF THE FORMULARY

The total daily dose of drugs is given. To calculate the actual dose given at each administration, divide the total daily dose by the number of times per day that the drug is to be given.

When dosage is calculated on a basis of per kilogram and a maximum dose is not stated, then the dose given should not exceed that for a 40 kg child.

The exact dose calculated on a basis of per kilogram may be difficult to administer because of the make-up of the formulations available. If this is the case the dose may be rounded up or down to a more manageable figure.

Doses in the formulary are sometimes written as μg or ng. When prescribing such doses these terms should be written in full (micrograms or nanograms respectively) in order to avoid confusion.

More detailed information about individual drugs is available from the manufacturers, from hospital drug information centres, and from the pharmacy departments of children's hospitals.

Abbreviations

The following abbreviations are used:

IO	intraosseous
IM	intramuscular
IV	intravenous
SC	subcutaneous
via ETT	via the tracheal tube

The final responsibility for delivery of the correct dose remains that of the physician prescribing and administering the drug.

Drug	Route	Total daily dose (TDD) 1 month to 12 years	<1 month	Times daily (divide TDD by this figure)	Notes
Acyclovir Injection 250 mg, 500 mg vials	IV infusion	30 mg/kg	30 mg/kg	3	Antiviral Normal or immunocompromised. Administer over 1 hour in 5% dextrose or 0·9% saline. Reduce dose in mild renal impairment
Adenosine Injection 3 mg/ml vials	IV	50 μg/kg to a maximum total dose of 500 μg/kg	50 μg/kg to a maximum total dose of 300 μg/kg	Single dose	Antiarrhythmic Increase to 100 μg/kg then 250 μg/kg
Effect enhanced by dipyridamole, antagonised by theophylline					
Adrenaline: see Epinephrine					
Alprostadil (prostaglandin E$_1$) Injection 0·5 mg/ml ampoules (0·5mg diluted to 500ml = 1μg/ml)	IV infusion	0·05 μg/kg/min **then** 5–20 ng/kg/min (0·3–1·2 μg/kg/h)	0·05 μg/kg/min **then** 5–20 ng/kg/min (0·3–1·2 μg/kg/h)	Continuous Continuous	Prostaglandin Starting dose Maintenance dose Infuse in 5% dextrose or 0·09% saline. Apnoea may occur
Aminophylline Injection 25 mg/ml	IV	5 mg/kg to a maximum dose of 250 mg	Use only with advice	Single dose	Bronchodilator Loading dose over 20 minutes. If plasma level obtained give 1 mg/kg for 2 mg/l desired increase in level
	IV infusion	1 mg/kg/h	Use only with advice	Continuous	Maintenance dose. Dilute to 1 mg/ml in 5% dextrose or 0·9% saline
Monitor plasma levels. Reduce dose in liver disease. Note potential for drug interactions. Plasma levels increased by cimetidine, ciprofloxacin, and erythromycin					

Note: Dose given is total daily dose unless otherwise stated.
If a maximum dose is not stated the dose given should not exceed that for a 40 kg child.

314

Drug	Route	Total daily dose (TDD) 1 month to 12 years	<1 month	Times daily (divide TDD by this figure)	Notes
Amlodarone Injection 50 mg/ml	IV	5 mg/kg	Use only with advice	Single dose	Antiarrhythmic Loading dose over 20–120 minutes at a concentration of up to 2·4 mg/ml in 5% dextrose only. May be given rapidly in VF/pulseless VT
	IV infusion	10 μg/kg/min	Use only with advice	Continuous	
Caution in moderate renal impairment, risk of thyroid dysfunction with accumulation of iodine. Enhances effect of warfarin, increase levels of digoxin (halve maintenance dose) phenytoin, cyclosporin. Increased risk of bradycardia, atrioventricular block and myocardial depression with β-blockers, Ca^{2+} channel blockers. Additive effects with other antiarrhythmics. Toxicity increased with loop diuretics, cimetidine. Plasma level monitoring required					
Amoxycillin	IV	50–100 mg/kg to a maximum dose of 4 g		4	Antibiotic (penicillin) Bolus IV injection or short infusion in 5% dextrose or 0·9% saline over 30 minutes
			Up to 7 days 30 mg/kg	2	
			Over 7 days 30 mg/kg	3	
Reduce in severe renal impairment. Do not mix with aminoglycosides, flush line or separate by 30 minutes					
Ampicillin	IV	50–100 mg/kg to a maximum dose of 4 g		4	Antibiotic (penicillin) Dilute dose to twice volume and bolus over 3–5 minutes
			Up to 7 days 50–75 mg/kg	2	
			Over 7 days 50–75 mg/kg	3	
	IV infusion	400 mg/kg		4	Severe infection Infuse over 30 minutes
			Up to 7 days 100–150 mg/kg	2	
			Over 7 days 150–200 mg/kg	3	
Reduce in severe renal impairment. Do not mix with aminoglycosides, flush line or separate by 30 minutes					

Note: Dose given is total daily dose unless otherwise stated.
If a maximum dose is not stated the dose given should not exceed that for a 40 kg child.

315

Drug	Route	Total daily dose (TDD) 1 month to 12 years	<1 month	Times daily (divide TDD by this figure)	Notes
Atropine sulphate Injection 100 μg/ml Minijet	IV	20 μg/kg (minimum 100 μg; maximum 600 μg)	Do not use in neonates	Single dose	Antimuscarinic *Bradycardia* If increased vagal activity. Administer over 1 minute. IV doses may be given by the intraosseous route; 40 μg/kg may be given via tracheal tube
Benzylpenicillin Injection 600 mg vials	IV infusion	300 mg/kg to a maximum dose of 12 g		6	Antibiotic (penicillin) Dose for severe infection
			Up to 7 days 50 mg/kg	2	Infuse over 30 minutes to reduce irritation and CNS toxicity. Do not mix with aminoglycosides, flush line, or separate by 30 minutes
			Over 7 days 50 mg/kg	3	
		Reduce dose in severe renal impairment, risk of convulsions			
Budesonide	Nebuliser	**Over 3 months** 2 mg	Do not use in neonates	**2**	Croup Can be mixed with salbutamol and ipratropium
Bupivacaine (plain)					Local anaesthetic
	Local infiltration	Up to 2 mg/kg (0·8 ml/kg) to a maximum of 150 mg (60 ml of 0·25%)	Up to 2 mg/kg (0·8 ml/kg)	Single dose not more than every 8 hours	
		Avoid or reduce dose in liver disease			
Calcium chloride Injection 10% (100 mg/ml 6·8 mmol Ca^{2+} in 10 ml) Minijet	IV	20 mg/kg (0·2 ml/kg of 10% injection)	Do not use in neonates	Single dose	*Pulseless electrical activity due to electrolyte imbalance* Slow injection IV doses may be given by the intraosseous route
		Precipitates with sodium and potassium levels. Avoid use with aluminium- and magnesium-containing drugs. Caution with digoxin – levels may be increased. Inadequate dilution may cause impaction of resin			

Note: Dose given is total daily dose unless otherwise stated.
If a maximum dose is not stated the dose given should not exceed that for a 40 kg child.

Drug	Route	Total daily dose (TDD) 1 month to 12 years	<1 month	Times daily (divide TDD by this figure)	Notes
Calcium Gluconate Injection 10% (100 mg/ml or 0·225 mmol Ca^{2+}/ml) ampoules	IV	0·07 mmol/kg (0·3 ml/kg of 10% injection)	0·07 mmol/kg (0·3 ml/kg of 10% injection)	Single dose	Acute calcium supplementation. Slow IV injection
	IV infusion	1 mmol/kg (0·2 ml/kg/h of 10% injection)	0·5 mmol/kg (0·1 ml/kg/h of 10% injection)	Continuous over 24 hours	Maintenance infusion Dilute to at least 0·045 mmol/ml (20 mg/ml) with 5% dextrose or 0·9% saline, maximum infusion rate 0·0255 mmol/ml (10 mg/minute) *Pulseless electrical activity due to electrolyte imbalance*
	IV	0·2 ml/kg 10% injection	0·2 ml/kg 10% injection	Single dose	Administer slowly. IV doses may be given by intraosseous route
Precipitates with sodium bicarbonate. Large doses of Ca^{2+} may cause arrhythmias with cardiac glycosides. Increased risk of hypercalcaemia with thiazide diuretics					
Calcium Resonium powder 1 level 5 ml spoonful = 5 g	Oral or rectal	0·5 g/kg to a maximum of 60 g		3–4	Ion exchange resin for potassium removal. Administer orally with a drink but not fruit squash (high in potassium).
Special rectal suspension			0·5 g/kg	Single dose	Rectal enema prepared by stirring powder into methylcellulose solution
Monitor calcium and potassium levels. Avoid use with aluminium- and magnesium-containing drugs. Caution with digoxin – levels may be increased. Inadequate dilution may cause impaction of resin					
Cefotaxime Injection 500 mg, 1 g, 2 g vials	IV	100 mg/kg to a maximum dose of 2 g		Initial dose	Antibiotic (cephalosporin) Severe infection Given by short infusion
	IV	**then** 200 mg/kg to a maximum dose of 12 g		**then** Subsequent doses 4	Give by short infusion
			Up to 7 days 100 mg/kg	2	Infection
			Over 7 days 150 mg/kg	3	
Reduce dose in severe renal impairment. Bolus over 3–5 minutes or dilute 4–10 times with infusion fluid and administer over 20–60 minutes. Do not mix with aminoglycosides					

Note: Dose given is total daily dose unless otherwise stated.
If a maximum dose is not stated the dose given should not exceed that for a 40 kg child.

Drug	Route	Total daily dose (TDD) 1 month to 12 years	<1 month	Times daily (divide TDD by this figure)	Notes
Ceftazidime Injection 500 mg, 1 g, 2 g vials	IV	150 mg/kg to a maximum dose of 9 g		3	Antibiotic (cephalosporin) Severe infection
Injection 250 mg vials			60–100 mg/kg	2	Infection
Reduce dose in mild renal impairment. Administer over 5–10 minutes as IV bolus or 20 minutes as short infusion. Do not mix with aminoglycosides					
Ceftriaxone Injection 250 mg, 500 mg, 1·0 g vials	IV (IM)	80 mg/kg to a maximum dose of 4 g		1	Antibiotic (cephalosporin) Bolus over 3–5 minutes
		50 mg/kg		1	*Severe infection*
				3	Infuse over 20–30 minutes in 5% dextrose or 0·9% saline
Reduce dose in renal impairment. Do not mix with aminoglycosides					
Chlorpheniramine Injection 10 mg in 1 ml	IV	**1 month–1 year** 250 µg/kg	Do not use neonates	Single dose	Sedative antihistamine Repeat up to four times in 24 hours if necessary. Dilute with 5–10 ml water for injection or 0·9% saline and give over 1 minute. May cause transient drowsiness, giddiness and hypotension especially if administered too rapidly
		1–5 years 2·5–5 mg		Single dose	
		6–12 years 5–10 mg to a maximum of 20 mg		Single dose	
Avoid in liver disease, may produce coma					
Desferrioxamine Injection 500 mg vials	Oral	5–10 g	Use only with advice	Single dose (in 50–100 ml water)	Iron-chelating compound. Leave dose in stomach after lavage. Injection solution may be given orally – unpleasant taste
	IM	1–2 g to a maximum dose of 2 g	Use only with advice	Single dose	To eliminate iron already absorbed. If shocked, hypotensive or seriously ill administer IV. Dose may be repeated every 3–12 hours to a maximum of 6 g/day for adults
	IV infusion	Up to 0·25 mg/kg/min (maximum 80 mg/kg/day)	Use only with advice	Continuous	Decrease rate after 4–6 hours to ensure daily maximum not exceeded. Continue until serum iron less than total iron-binding capacity. Reconstitute 500 mg with 5 ml water for injection and infuse in 5% dextrose of 0·9% saline
Incompatible with heparin. Caution: anaphylaxis and hypotension from rapid IV injection. Use with caution in renal impairment					

Note: Dose given is total daily dose unless otherwise stated.
If a maximum dose is not stated the dose given should not exceed that for a 40 kg child.

Drug	Route	Total daily dose (TDD) 1 month to 12 years	<1 month	Times daily (divide TDD by this figure)	Notes
Dexamethasone Injection dexamethasone phosphate 8 mg in 2 ml (equivalent to 6·7 mg base in 2ml); 4 mg in 1 ml (equivalent to 3·3 mg base in 1 ml)	IV	600 μg/kg	600 μg/kg	4	Corticosteroid – glucocorticoid. Meningitis to reduce meningeal inflammation and incidence of severe hearing loss. Usually given for 4 days. Bolus over 3–5 minutes. Infusion in 5% dextrose or 0·9% saline
		300 μg/kg	300 μg/kg	2	Croup: inhaled budesonide may also be used
All doses are quoted as base		Reduces effects of rifampicin and antiepileptics; antagonises effects of diuretics and antidiabetics. High doses may cause Cushing's syndrome. Withdraw gradually to avoid acute adrenal insufficiency. May suppress growth and increase risk of infection			
Diazepam Diazepam injection 5 mg/ml ampoules Diazepam lipid emulsion for injection 5 mg/ml ampoules	IV	250–400 μg/kg	200 μg/kg	Single dose	Benzodiazepine Slow IV bolus over 3–5 minutes. Repeat after 10 minutes if necessary
Rectal solution 5 mg/2·5 ml, 10 mg/2·5 ml	Rectal	**Up to 1 year** 2·5 mg **1–3 years** 5 mg **4–12 years** 5–10 mg to a maximum dose of 10 mg	2·5 mg	Single dose Single dose Single dose	Repeat dose if necessary after 5 minutes
		Caution: in liver disease, may precipitate coma. Reduce dose in severe renal impairment. Beware respiratory depression in acute use – antagonist flumazenil. Enhanced sedative effects with anaesthetics, opioid analgesics, isoniazid, antihistamines, α-blockers, antihypertensives, baclofen, ulcer healing drugs, omeprazole. Seek advice.			

Note: Dose given is total daily dose unless otherwise stated.
If a maximum dose is not stated the dose given should not exceed that for a 40 kg child.

319

Drug	Route	Total daily dose (TDD) 1 month to 12 years	<1 month	Times daily (divide TDD by this figure)	Notes
Dobutamine Injection 250 mg in 20 ml vials	IV infusion	1–20 μg/kg/min	1–20 μg/kg/min	Continuous	Inotrope Can be increased up to 40 μg/kg/min. Infuse in 5% dextrose or 0·9% saline
		Inactivated by sodium bicarbonate. Caution several drug interactions including hypertensive crisis with monoamine oxidase inhibitors. Seek further advice			
Dopamine	IV	1–5 μg/kg/min	1–5 μg/kg/min	Continuous	Inotrope *Renal dose – renal vasodilatation*
Injection 40 mg/ml ampoules	IV infusion	5–20 μg/kg/min	5–20 μg/kg/min	Continuous	Direct inotropic effect
		Infuse in 5% dextrose or 0·9% saline. Inactivated by sodium bicarbonate. Caution: several drug interactions including hypertensive crisis with monoamine oxidase inhibitors. Seek further advice			
Epinephrine Injection 1:10 000 Minijet ampoules	IV/IO	0·1 ml/kg of 1:10 000 (10 μg/kg) to a maximum dose of 10 ml *of* 1:10 000	0·1 ml/kg of 1:10 000 (10 μg/kg)	First dose	α and β sympathomimetic *Ventricular fibrillation, asystole and pulseless electrical activity* IV dose may be given by intraosseous route flushed with 0·9% saline
			0.1–0.3 ml/kg of 1:10000 (10–30 μg/kg		This is the dose for for resuscitation IV/IO/ET at birth
Injection 1:1000 ampoules	via ETT	0·1 ml/kg of 1:1000 (100 μg/kg)	0·1 ml/kg of 1:1000 (100 μg/kg)	First and subsequent doses	Given via tracheal tube
	IV	0·1 ml/kg of 1:1000 (100 μg/kg)	0·1 ml/kg of 1:1000 (100 μg/kg)	Subsequent doses	If considered appropriate CPR
	IV infusion	0.05 - 2 μg/kg/min	Use only with advice	Continuous	*Inotropic support* Starting dose. Causes marked peripheral vasoconstriction
	IM	0.1 ml/kg of 1:10000 (10 μg/kg)	0.1 ml/kg of 1:10000 (10 μg/kg)	*Single dose*	*Acute anaphylaxis* Dose may be repeated after 5 minutes
	IV infusion	0·05– (2 μg/kg/min)	0·05– (2 μg/kg/min)	Continuous	*Anaphylaxis* if bolus doses not effective in shock
Use injection solution as nebuliser	Nebuliser	2–5 ml of 1:1000	Use only with advice	Single dose	*Emergency treatment of croup* Dilute with 0·9% saline if required, for nebulisation. Repeat every 2–4 hours. Monitor ECG

Note: Dose given is total daily dose unless otherwise stated.
If a maximum dose is not stated the dose given should not exceed that for a 40 kg child.

Drug	Route	Total daily dose (TDD) 1 month to 12 years	<1 month	Times daily (divide TDD by this figure)	Notes
Erythromycin Injection 1g vials (lactobionate)	IV infusion	50–100mg/kg to a maximum of 4 g	50 mg/kg	4	Antibiotic (macrolide) Dilute injection 10 times with 5% dextrose or 0·9% saline, infuse over 15–60 minutes
		Reduce dose in severe renal impairment, use with caution in liver disease. Drug interactions include increased levels of warfarin, carbamazepine, midazolam, digoxin, cyclosporin, theophyllines, disopyramide, alfentanil. Avoid use with terfenadine (metabolism inhibited, arrhythmias possible). Seek advice			
Flecainide Injection 10 mg/ml ampoules	IV	2 mg/kg to a maximum of 150 mg	Do not use in neonates	Single dose	Antiarrhythmic IV bolus over 20 minutes or dilute in 5% dextrose or 0·9% saline and infuse over 30 minutes at a concentration of 0·3 mg/ml. Monitor ECG
		Reduce dose in mild renal impairment. Avoid or reduce dose in liver disease. Drug interactions include increased levels with amiodarone and cimetidine, increased myocardial depression with any antiarrhythmic. Toxicity increased in hypokalaemia, e.g. with diuretics. Monitor plasma levels			
Flucloxacillin Injection 250 mg, 500 mg, vials	IV	50–100 mg/kg to a maximum of 4 g		4	Antibiotic (penicillin) IV can be further diluted to twice the volume in 5% dextrose or 0·9% saline, bolus over 3–5 minutes
			Up to 7 days 50–75 mg/kg	2	
			Over 7 days 75–100 mg/kg	3	
		Do not mix with aminoglycosides, flush line or separate by 30 minutes			
Flumazenil Injection 100 µg/ml ampoules	IV	**Up to 1 year** 50 µg **1–7 years** 100 µg **7–12 years** 150 µg to a maximum dose of 200 µg	Do not use in neonates	Single dose	Benzodiazepine antagonist Initial dose over 15 seconds
		Up to 1 year 25 µg **1–7 years** 50 µg **7–12 years** 75 µg to a maximum dose of 100 µg	Do not use in neonates	Single dose	Repeat dose to be given at 1-minute intervals to maximum dose of 1 mg
		Limited experience in children. Doses quoted for children are derived from adult dose and mean surface area. Contraindicated in prolonged benzodiazepine use in epilepsy			

Note: Dose given is total daily dose unless otherwise stated.
If a maximum dose is not stated the dose given should not exceed that for a 40 kg child.

321

Drug	Route	Total daily dose (TDD) 1 month to 12 years	<1 month	Times daily (divide TDD by this figure)	Notes
Frusemide Injection 10 mg/ml ampoules	IV	1 mg/kg to a maximum dose of 40 mg	1 mg/kg	Single dose	Diuretic (loop) Maximum 4 mg/kg/dose
	IV infusion	2–65 µg/kg/min	2–65 µg/kg/min	Continuous	Infuse in 0·9% saline and not 5% dextrose
Caution: in moderate renal impairment, may need higher doses. Deafness may follow rapid IV injection. May cause hypokalaemia – which may precipitate coma in liver disease. Drug interactions include increased risk of nephrotoxicity with non-steroidal anti-inflammatory drugs and ototoxicity with aminoglycosides, polymyxins, and vancomycin. Antagonises antidiabetic drugs, increases lithium toxicity. Toxicity of cardiovascular drugs and corticosteroids increased in hypokalaemia.					
Gentamicin Injection 10 mg/ml vials	IV (IM)	7·5 mg/kg		3	Antibiotic (aminoglycoside) *Infection*
			Up to 7 days **<2 kg** 3mg/kg **>2 kg** 6mg/kg	Single dose 2	IV bolus over 3–5 minutes or short infusion over 20 minutes in 5% dextrose or 0·9% saline
			Over 7 days **<2 kg** 6 mg/kg **>2 kg** 7·5 mg/kg	2 3	
40 mg/ml vials	IV	9 mg/kg		3	*Cystic fibrosis or pyrexia in neutropenia*
Do not mix with penicillins, cephalosporins, erythromycin. Flush between doses or separate by 30 minutes. Monitor plasma levels. Reduce dose in mild renal impairment. Increased risk of oto- and/or nephrotoxicity with cephalosporins, colistin, polymyxins, amphotericin, cyclosporin, vancomycin, loop diuretics, and in renal impairment. Enhances effects of tubocurarine. Contraindicated in myasthenia gravis					
Hydrocortisone Injection 100 mg (as sodium Succinate = Efcortelan, Solu-Cortef) (as sodium phosphate = Efcortesol)	IV (IM)	4 mg/kg **then** 2–4 mg/kg	2·5 mg/kg **then** 2 mg/kg	Single dose **then** Single dose	Corticosteroid Initial dose Maintenance dose. Repeat every 6 hours. Slow IV over 1–5 minutes. May be mixed with 5% dextrose – or 0·9% saline. IV doses may be given by intraosseous route
Ipratropium bromide Atrovent 20 µg/ activation, Atrovent Forte 40 µg/activation	Nebuliser	**Up to 1 year** 125 µg 1– 5 years 250 µg > 5 years 500 µg	Do not use in neonates	Single dose	Antimuscarinic bronchodilator. Nebuliser solution may be diluted with 0·9% saline and/or mixed immediately before use with other nebuliser solutions except sodium cromoglycate

Note: Dose given is total daily dose unless otherwise stated.
If a maximum dose is not stated the dose given should not exceed that for a 40 kg child.

Drug	Route	Total daily dose (TDD) 1 month to 12 years	<1 month	Times daily (divide TDD by this figure)	Notes
Isoprenaline Injection 20 μg/ml Minijet Injection 200 μg/ml or 1 mg/ml ampoules	IV infusion	0·02–1·0 μg/kg/min	0·02–0·3 μg/kg/min	Continuous	Sympathomimetic IV dose may be given by the intraosseous route. Starting dose, increase if necessary to 1000 ng (1 μg)/kg/min. Infuse in 5% dextrose or 0·9% saline at concentration of 4 μg/ml
Several drug interactions including increased risk of arrhythmias with volatile anaesthetics. Seek further advice					
Labetolol Injection 5 mg/ml ampoules	IV	250–500 μg/kg to a maximum dose of 50 mg	Do not use in neonates	Single dose	β-blockers Loading dose
	IV infusion	30 μg/kg/min	Do not use in neonates	Continuous	Starting maintenance dose Infuse in 5% dextrose or 0·9% saline at a concentration of 1 mg/ml. Must have arterial pressure monitoring. May require atropine to counteract severe bradycardia
Avoid in liver disease, can cause severe hepatocellular injury. Several drug interactions including enhanced hypotensive effect with anaesthetics, other antihypertensives, anxiolytics, hypnotics, and diuretics. Hypotensive effect antagonised by non-steroidal anti-inflammatory drugs, corticosteroids, sympathomimetics. Increased risk of myocardial depression and bradycardia with antiarrhythmics. Risk of heart block with amiodarone, diltiazem. Severe hypotension and heart failure may occur with nifedipine, verapamil. Increased atrioventricular block and bradycardia with digoxin. Seek further advice					

Note: Dose given is total daily dose unless otherwise stated.
If a maximum dose is not stated the dose given should not exceed that for a 40 kg child.

Drug	Route	Total daily dose (TDD) 1 month to 12 years	<1 month	Times daily (divide TDD by this figure)	Notes
Lignocaine					*Ventricular fibrillation or pulseless tachycardia*
Injection 20 mg/ml (2%) Minijet	IV	1 mg/kg to a maximum dose of 100 mg	1 mg/kg	Single dose	If necessary repeat every 5 minutes to maximum 3 mg/kg. IV dose may be given by the intraosseous route; 2 mg/kg may be given via tracheal tube
Injection 5 mg/ml (0·5%), 10 mg/ml (1%), 20 mg/ml (2%) ampoules	IV	0·5–1 mg/kg to a maximum dose of 100 mg	0·5–1 mg/kg to a maximum dose of 100 mg	Single dose	*Antiarrhythmic* Loading dose. Administer over 1 minute
	IV	10–50 infusion	10–50 μg/kg/min	Continuous μg/kg/min	Maintenance dose. Infuse in 5% dextrose or 0·9% saline at a concentration of 2 mg/ml
	Local infiltration	Up to 3 mg/kg	Up to 3 mg/kg	Single dose not more than every 4 hours	*Local anaesthetic*
		Avoid or reduce dose in severe liver disease. Several drug interactions including increased myocardial depression with other antiarrhythmics, β-blockers. Effect antagonised by hypokalaemia, e.g. with loop and thiazide diuretics. Metabolism inhibited by cimetidine. Seek further advice			
Mannitol Injection 10% 20% infusion	IV infusion	0·5–1 g/kg	Do not use in neonates	Single dose over 1 hour	Diuretic (osmotic) May be repeated once or twice after 4–8 hours
Morphine Injection 2·5 mg/ml 10 mg/ml ampoules	IV	**1–3 months** 0·025 mg/kg	0·025 mg/kg	Single dose	Opiate Repeat up to four times in 24 hours
		3–12 months 0·05–0·1 mg/kg		Single dose	Repeat up to four times in 24 hours
		Over 1 year 0·1–0·2 mg/kg		Single dose	Repeat up to six times in 24 hours
		Causes constipation and nausea. Avoid in moderate renal impairment and in liver disease (can precipitate coma). Caution: enhances sedative effects of anxiolytics and hypnotics; antagonises effects of cisapride and metoclopramide. Morphine levels increased by cimetidine. Can cause respiratory depression. Antagonist is naloxone.			

Note: Dose given is total daily dose unless otherwise stated.
If a maximum dose is not stated the dose given should not exceed that for a 40 kg child.

Drug	Route	Total daily dose (TDD) 1 month to 12 years	<1 month	Times daily (divide TDD by this figure)	Notes
Naloxone Injection 20 g/ml 400 g/kg	IV	10 μg/kg	10 μg/kg	First dose	Opiate antagonist Give higher dose if response to first dose is inadequate
		then **<20 kg** 100 μg/kg	**then** 100 μg/kg	**then** Single dose	Repeat doses as necessary to maintain opioid reversal. May be given IM, SC or by intraosseous route if IV not possible
		>20kg 2 mg		Single dose	
	IV infusion	8–30 μg/kg/min	8–30 μg/kg/min	Continuous	Half-life of opioid may be longer than that of naloxonen Considerinfusion in 5% dextrose or 0·9% saline at concentration 4 μg/ml. Adjust rate as required
Paracetamol Suspension 120 mg/5 ml, 250 mg/5 ml Tablets 500 mg Dispersible tablets 500 mg Suppositories 125 mg, 250 mg, 500 mg	Oral or rectal	**1–3 months**	10–15 mg/kg	Single dose	Analgesic and antipyretic Repeat if necessary after 4–6 hours
		10–15 mg/kg		Single dose	
		Over 3 months 15 mg/kg to a maximum dose 0·5–1g		Single dose	
		Avoid large doses in liver disease – dose-related toxicity			
Paraldehyde (injection used rectally)	Rectal	0·4 ml/kg to a maximum dose 5–10 ml	0·3 ml/kg	Single dose	Antiepileptic Dilute with an equal volume of olive oil. May cause rectal irritation
		Use plastic syringe, if administered within 10 minutes			
Phenobarbitone Injection 30 mg/ml, 60 mg/ml ampoules	IV	15 mg/kg	15–20 mg/kg	Single dose	Antiepileptic Administer over 5 minutes. Higher doses have been given to ventilated neonates
		Require drug level monitoring. Avoid administrative via umbilical artery cannulae in neonates due to alkalinity. Use with caution in liver disease – may precipitate coma. Reduce dose in severe renal impairment. Enzyme inducer with many drug interactions including a reduced effect of oral anticoagulants, griseofulvin, calcium channel blockers, corticosteroids, cyclosporin, theophylline, and thyroxine. Toxicity may be enhanced by other anticonvulsants without increase in efficacy. Antagonised by antipsychotics			

Note: Dose given is total daily dose unless otherwise stated.
If a maximum dose is not stated the dose given should not exceed that for a 40 kg child.

Drug	Route	Total daily dose (TDD) 1 month to 12 years	<1 month	Times daily (divide TDD by this figure)	Notes
Phenytoin Phenytoin sodium injection 50 mg/ml ampoules Phenytoin sodium 100 mg = 90 mg phenytoin base	IV	18 mg/kg	18 mg/kg	Single dose	Antiepileptic *Status epilepticus* (only to be given if not currently on phenytoin or if level less than 2·5 mg/l). Loading dose over 20–30 minutes
	IV **then** IV infusion	18 mg/kg **then** 5 mg/kg	18 mg/kg **then** 5 mg/kg	Single dose Single dose	*Antiarrhythmic* Loading dose Maintenance dose. Infuse over 20–30 minutes in 0·9% saline only at maximum concentration 1 mg/ml with ECG monitoring. Monitor plasma level
		Reduce dose in liver disease. Concomitant administration of antiepileptic drugs may increase toxicity without increase in antiepileptic effect. Several drug interactions including increased levels with cimetidine, diltiazem. Enzyme inducer – reduces levels of phenobarbitone, carbamazepine, sodium valproate. Seek further advice			
Potassium chloride Injection 2 mmol/ml (potassium chloride strong 15% w/v)	IV infusion	0·5 mmol/kg	0·5 mmol/kg	Single dose	Potassium supplement Administer in 5% dextrose or 0·9% saline. Shake well to avoid layering. Up to 2 mmol/kg/h have been given in cardiac intensive care
	IV	0·08 mmol/kg/h (2 mmol/kg in 24 h)	0·08 mmol/kg/h (2 mmol/kg in 24 h)	Continuous	Maintenance dose
		Usual maximum concentration 4 mmol/100 ml and rate not more than 0·5 mmol/kg/h. Monitor electrolyte status and ECG. Avoid routine use in moderate renal impairment – high risk of hyperkalaemia. Increased risk of hyperkalaemia with angiotensin-converting enzyme inhibitors, cyclosporin, and potassium-sparing diuretics, e.g. amiloride. Caution: hyperkalaemia may lead to decreased digoxin levels			

Note: Dose given is total daily dose unless otherwise stated.
If a maximum dose is not stated the dose given should not exceed that for a 40 kg child.

Drug	Route	Total daily dose (TDD) 1 month to 12 years	<1 month	Times daily (divide TDD by this figure)	Notes
Prednisolone Tablets 1 mg, 5 mg, 25 mg		1–2 mg/kg	1–2 mg/kg	1–3	Glucocorticosteroid
Tablets (soluble) 5 mg, tablets (enteric-coated) 2·5 mg, 5 mg	Oral	2 mg/kg to a maximum dose of 60 mg	Do not use in neonates	1 or 2	Treat for 3–5 days then stop (no need to taper dose). To be taken in the morning or twice daily, with or after food
Reduces effects of rifampicin, antiepileptics. Effects of diuretics and antidiabetics antagonised					
Propranolol Injection 1mg/ml ampoules					β-Blocker *Cyanotic spells in Fallot's tetralogy*
	IV	100 μg/kg	30 μg/kg	Single dose	Inject slowly under ECG control. Indicated in, repeat as necessary up to 3 or 4 times daily May be used in dysrhythmias, phaeochromocytoma, thyrotoxicosis
	IV	10–50 μg/kg to a maximum dose of 1 mg	10–50 μg/kg	Single dose	*Dysrhythmias* Repeat as necessary up to 3 or 4 times daily
Administer IV slowly with ECG monitoring. Caution in severe renal impairment. May decrease renal blood flow. Reduce oral dose in liver disease. Avoid with verapamil. Seek advice on drug interactions					
Pyridoxine 50 mg in 2 ml	IV	25–100mg			Single test dose in refractory seizures given over 5 minutes

Note: Dose given is total daily dose unless otherwise stated.
If a maximum dose is not stated the dose given should not exceed that for a 40 kg child.

327

Drug	Route	Total daily dose (TDD) 1 month to 12 years	<1 month	Times daily (divide TDD by this figure)	Notes
Salbutamol					Selective β-adrenoceptor stimulant. Bronchodilator Repeat up to 8 times per day, or 12 times per day in hospital with monitoring. Dilute to 3–4 ml with 0·9% saline. May be mixed with ipratropium, beclomethasone, budesonide, or sodium cromoglycate nebuliser solutions
Nebules 2·5 mg in 2·5 ml, 5 mg in 2·5 ml	Nebuliser	**Up to 6 months** Do not use	Do not use in neonates		
		6 months–5 years 2·5 mg		Single dose	
		Over 5 years 5 mg		Single dose	
Inhaler and Autohaler 100 μg per activation	Oral inhalation (aerosol or powder)	**Up to 6 months** Do not use	Do not use in neonates		Maximum acute treatment doses. Infants and children less than 2 years should use large volume spacer with mask, 2–5 years a large volume spacer is recommended, 5–12 years a spacer, dry powder or autohaler
Ventodisk 200 μg 400 μg powder for use in Diskhaler		**6 months–2 years** Up to 2400 μg		6	
		3–4 years Up to 3600 μg		6	
		Over 5 years Up to 7200 μg		6	
Rotacaps 200 μg, 400 μg powder for use in Rotahaler	Oral inhalation (aerosol or powder	**Up to 7 years** 200–400 μg	Do not use in neonates	Single dose	Emergency initial treatment doses A maximum of 400–600 μg can be given in 4 hours
		Over 7 years 200–600 μg		Single dose	A maximum of 800–1200 μg can be given in 4 hours
					100 μg via a large volume spacer can be administered every few seconds until improvement occurs. Use a mask for very young children
Injection 500 μg/ml ampoules	IV	4–6 μg/kg	Use only with advice	Single dose	Status asthmaticus or hyperkalaemia Bolus injection over 5–10 minutes. Repeat if necessary

Note: Dose given is total daily dose unless otherwise stated.
If a maximum dose is not stated the dose given should not exceed that for a 40 kg child.

328

Drug	Route	Total daily dose (TDD) 1 month to 12 years	<1 month	Times daily (divide TDD by this figure)	Notes
Salbutamol (contd) Injection for infusion 1 mg/ml ampoules	IV infusion	1– 5 μg/kg/min	Use only with advice	Continuous	Infusion in 5% dextrose or 0·9% saline at a concentration of 10 μg/ml. Doses have been doubled
Caution: potentially serious hypokalaemia especially in severe asthma. Potentiated by theophylline, diuretics, corticosteroids, hypoxia. Monitor plasma potassium in severe asthma. Efficacy under 18 months of age uncertain					
Sodium bicarbonate					Alkylating agent
Injection 8·4% Minijet	IV	2·5 mmol/kg 2·5 ml/kg 8·4%)	2·5 mmol/kg 2·5 ml/kg of 8·4%)	Single dose	*Acidosis and hyperkalaemia*
1 mmol/ml		1 mmol/kg (1 ml/kg of 8·4%	1 mmol/kg (1 ml/kg of 8·4%	Single dose	*Asystole* Dilute to 4·2% in 0·9% saline or water for injections
Repeat as required. Administer slowly. Monitor blood gases, pH. Inactivates sympathomimetics such as epinephrine (adrenaline), dopamine					
Verapamil Injection 2·5 mg/ml ampoules	IV infusion	**Up to 1 year** Do not use	Do not use in neonates		Calcium channel blocker Antiarrhythmic
		Over 1 year 100–300 μg/kg to a maximum dose of 5 mg		Single dose	Administer over 10 minutes. Monitor ECG
Many drug interactions including increased hypotensive effect of general anaesthetics and risk of atriventricular delay, increased risk of amiodarone-induced bradycardia, atrioventricular block, and myocardial depression. Increases levels of quinidine (extreme hypotension), tricyclics. Enhances effect of digoxin (atrioventricular block and bradycardia), carbamazepine, cyclosporin, lithium, non-depolarising muscle relaxants, theophylline. Decreased levels with rifampicin, reduced effect with phenytoin. Enhanced hypotension effect with antipsychotics, severe hypotension, and heart failure with β-blockers. Seek further advice					

Note: Dose given is total daily dose unless otherwise stated.
If a maximum dose is not stated the dose given should not exceed that for a 40 kg child.

329

INDEX